PATHOPHYSIOLOGY — A PLAIN ENGLISH APPROACH

Mechanisms and Treatment of Disease

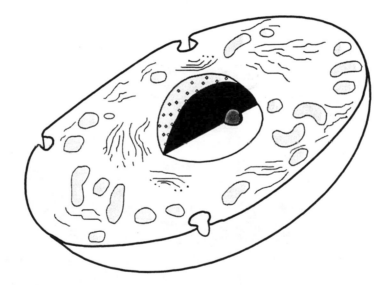

Mikel A. Rothenberg, MD
[C] 2001

INTRODUCTORY MATERIAL

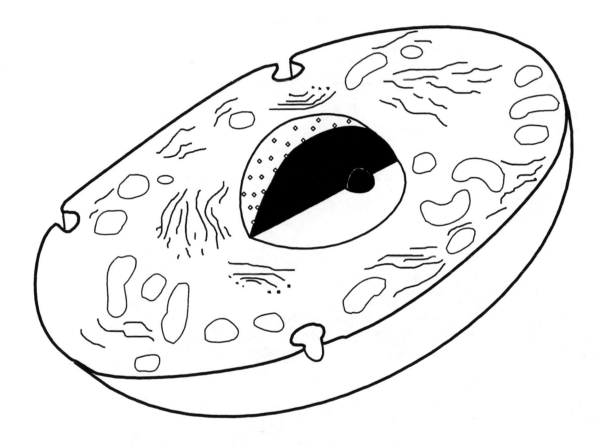

Published by:

PESI HEALTHCARE, LLC
PO Box 1000
200 Spring Street
Eau Claire, Wisconsin 54702

Printed in the United States

**For information on this and other PESI HealthCare manuals
and audiocassettes, please call**

800-843-7763

or visit our website:
www.pesihealthcare.com

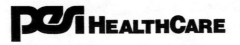

BRIEF TABLE OF CONTENTS

Mechanisms and Treatment of Disease
PATHOPHYSIOLOGY
A Plain English Approach

Table of Contents

By Mikel A. Rothenberg, MD

Crossword Puzzle Review – The Answers

Index

FORWARD

To appreciate the mechanisms of disease, it's essential to understand how things work normally. It then becomes straightforward to appreciate how normal structure and function are altered, resulting in illness. Laboratory medicine, biochemistry, pharmacology, and pathophysiology are integrally related to each other. As such, I've incorporated liberal portions of each into the discussions.

It's my expectation that the concepts here will be *perfectly clear* to you. If not, I haven't done my job. As an aid, I've relied on lots of metaphors, figures, and downright silly mnemonics — I really want you to understand this material completely. As a result, you'll own it forever. And, you'll be able to put it into clinical practice immediately!

I'm assuming that many readers will have tried to wade through physiology and pathophysiology in a "previous life" — sometimes with difficulty. If this is your first experience, great — don't worry about the past. I promise to teach you right the first time, providing information in a way that you *will* understand, remember, and be able to use in your day to day practice.

This book is not intended to be all-inclusive — I have selected the topics based on diseases we often see in a wide range of practices. I've included lots of figures and tables summarizing the common clinical presentations, physical and test findings, and standard treatments. I've done this to try to provide a "one-stop shopping experience" for the information you *really need to know* about the selected topics.

Learning is supposed to be fun — have a great time!

Mikel

Mikel A. Rothenberg, MD
North Olmsted, OH

FUN IN LEARNING — THE CROSSWORD PUZZLE REVIEW

At the end of each chapter, I have made a crossword puzzle for you to use as a review tool. Admittedly, the print size of the "hints" is somewhat small (a software limitation), but feel free to copy and enlarge this for your own personal use. The answers are near the back of the book. Numerous studies show that puzzles help in learning and concept retention.[1] I hope you find these useful.

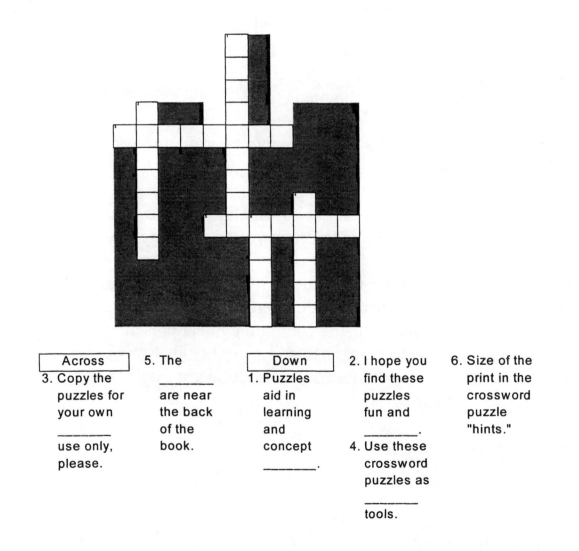

Across		Down		
3. Copy the puzzles for your own _____ use only, please.	5. The _____ are near the back of the book.	1. Puzzles aid in learning and concept _____.	2. I hope you find these puzzles fun and _____. 4. Use these crossword puzzles as _____ tools.	6. Size of the print in the crossword puzzle "hints."

---

[1]Bailey, C.M., et al., *Educational puzzles for understanding gastrointestinal physiology.* Am J Physiol 276 (Adv Physiol Educ 21): S1-S18, 1999.

THANK YOU, THANK YOU . . .

An undertaking of this magnitude is impossible without help. Thank you, Diane, Marc, and Kara (my family), for tolerating my obsessive-compulsive behavior — I love you more than words can ever express.

I owe much gratitude to Kathleen Dubin, JD for her excellent editorial job on this manuscript. It is rare that a single person has such intelligence, attention to detail, and wonderful personality wrapped up in "one package."

Gracious thanks to Dale Dubin, MD for his continuing friendship and support. Without Dr. Dubin's teaching me the beauty of simplistic elegance, I would never have learned how to convey complex concepts in "Plain English."

Last and never least, thanks to my Higher Power for creating a world so complex, yet elegantly easy to understand.

UNDERSTANDING IS OWNING — LEARN IT FOREVER!

I learned the philosophy of "understanding is owning" more than thirty years ago. Since then, I've tried to apply this advice in all of my teaching. It seems pretty clear to me — if you understand something in the first place, you remember it. Yet, if you memorize, the concept is gone right after the test (sometimes, even sooner!).

As I gain experience, it becomes increasingly evident that most of what we (which includes *all* health care professionals, since we all work together equally for the patient's benefit) do in medicine is based on simple, yet elegant, rules. Those of us who refuse to accept the beauty of simplicity are really missing the boat — and our patients may be the unknowing victims.

Our analytical mind ("left brain") can be our best friend or our worst enemy, depending on how we use it. Typically, it rears its head early in the medical thinking process, interfering with free-form thinking ("brainstorming") and giving us "tunnel vision." Put differently, the left brain seems to exist, at times, for the sole purpose of taking something that's perfectly simple and making it confusing! Like it or not, my friends, left brains come with being human. And, the more education we get, the more likely our left brain will "overthink" something into oblivion.

WARNING: The left brain seems to exist, at times, to overthink something that is *perfectly clear* into something *totally incomprehensible*.

Fortunately, the other half of the "human package" is intuition or "gut feelings" ("right brain"). The day we're born, each of us is smarter than *any* "test" we ever obtain on a patient. Add your interest, training, and experience to this innate ability and the potential is incredible. It's this "right brain" approach that works best in the initial evaluation of a patient — consider *all* the possibilities. Then, incorporate analytical thinking ("left brain") to refine your thoughts into a differential diagnosis.

Graphically, the thinking process is called "triangulation" or the "diagnostic triangle." The crux of this approach is the difference between a *finding* and a *diagnosis*. Findings are relatively fixed — in other words, a WBC of 12,500, or a systolic murmur, or ST-segment elevation, or an infiltrate on the chest x-ray is there and not about to change instantly, regardless of the cause. On the other hand, there are multiple explanations for these various findings. We then incorporate other information and formulate a likely list of diagnostic probabilities, commonly called the "differential diagnosis."

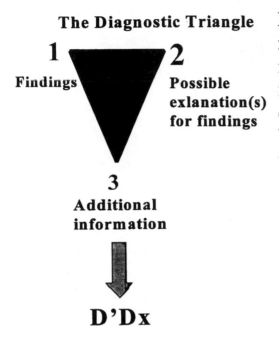

The Diagnostic Triangle

1 Findings

2 Possible exlanation(s) for findings

3 Additional information

D'Dx

Let's take, for example, a right middle lobe infiltrate on a chest film. The *finding* of an infiltrate is fixed (at least on that particular film, taken at one particular time). The list of possible causes would take up an entire book by itself, so we'll be brief — infection, tumor, trauma, inflammation (and lots of others I didn't list!). Let's assume the film belongs to a 23-year old male with a productive cough, WBC of 14,000, physical signs of consolidation over the right middle lobe, and a T-shirt that says "I need an antibiotic, now!" The *most likely* explanation for the *entire* picture is an infectious process, probably pneumonia (e.g., diplococcus or mycoplasma). We arrive at this profound conclusion only after brainstorming ("right brain") possibilities and then refining them ("left brain"), based on what we know clinically. By doing this, rather than memorizing diagnoses, we leave our minds open to the possibility that something other than what seems to be immediately obvious might be going on.

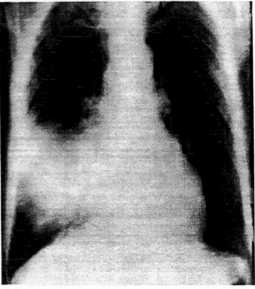

I encourage you to approach the study of pathophysiology with an open mind — remember to take advantage of those "simple, but elegant" truths. Use them to make yourself even better than you already are at what you do.

PRINCIPLE: Be open-minded; use your *right brain* first to consider many possibilities. Then, refine them into an educationally sound, medically correct, and legally defensible list of "probabilities" using the *left-brain*.

A WORD TO EDUCATORS . . .

If you're reading this, congratulations — I know you're part of a group I really want to reach. The health care professions (all of them) need more educators like you.

When we leave high school, we depart a world of teachers who are trained to teach. In all more advanced pursuits, including undergraduate and graduate school, technical training, and professional schools, we all play a game of chance as to whether our "professor" will be knowledgeable in the techniques of adult education or not. All of us have experienced the "prof" who was an expert in his or her field, but who couldn't explain even the most basic concept to a student.

This book, as well as everything else I write and teach, is not intended to be the "bottom line" reference to all known scientific detail on the subject. It is meant to teach a "system" of thinking that incorporates both right and left brain, and takes advantage of all adult learning domains — visual, auditory, and kinesthetic. Figures, mnemonics, and metaphors are used liberally.

I've chosen topics that are common in a wide variety of primary care practices to apply these techniques. In this way, your students will learn the thinking process as well as clinical information that will be *immediately applicable* in real-life situations. I've included summary tables and figures of clinical presentations, physical and lab findings, and common treatments as well.

For the topics covered, my goal is to provide "one-stop shopping," so the reader is not forced to consult other references for basic information. I do not apologize for deliberately skipping some topics — rather, I thank you in advance for recognizing my main purpose in writing this book. In Chapter 8, I have summarized the major educational principles emphasized throughout the text, as well as given you my "hints" on how to use this material for evaluation purposes.

Medical thinking should not be difficult — especially since the laws of physics and nature that underlie our professions *are* elegantly simple. Thank you for seeing the innate beauty of simplicity and letting it work for you and your students. Once they are familiar with the underlying concepts outlined in this text, it's relatively easy to look up other topics of interest. And, it's intellectually exciting to see how these, too, fit the generic models I've discussed here. Enjoy and pass the word: "Understand is owning!"

PRINCIPLE: **An apple fell from the tree, hitting Sir Isaac Newton, because of *gravity*. Like all laws of Nature, we're not about to change this fact any time soon.**

CORROLARY: **The main reason we don't understand concepts is that we try to rewrite the Laws of Nature.**

GLOSSARY OF ABBREVIATIONS AND ACRONYMS

Note: Chemical symbols are not listed

AA — amino acid
AAT — alpha-1 antrypsin
ABCs — airway, breathing, circulation
ABGs — arterial blood gases
Abs — antibodies
ABs — antibiotics
ACE — angiotensin converting enzyme
Acetyl-CoA — acetyl-coenzyme A
ACTH — adrenocorticotropic hormone
ADH — antidiuretic hormone
ADP — adenosine diphosphate
Ags — antigens
AI — adrenal insufficiency
ALT — alanine amino transferase
AM — adrenomedullin
AMA — against medical advice
AMI — acute myocardial infarction
AMPLE — allergies, medications, past history, last meal, events
APE — acute pulmonary edema
AQP — aquaporins
ARBs — angiotensin receptor blockers
ARDS — adult respiratory distress syndrome
ARF — acute renal failure
ASA — aspirin
AST — aspartate aminotransferase
AT-I — angiotensin I
AT-II — angiotensin II
AT-III — angiotensin III
ATP — adenosine triphosphate
AVPU — level of consciousness scale
BAL — bronchoalveolar lavage
BD — benzodiazepines
BDP — beclomethasone dipropionate
BG — blood glucose (blood sugar)
BiPAP — biphasic positive airway pressure
BOHB — beta-hydroxy butyrate

BPM — beats/breaths per minute
BRG — bilirubin diglucuronide
BS — blood sugar
BU — unconjugated bilirubin
BUN — blood urea nitrogen
CAD — coronary artery disease
cAMP — cyclic adenosine monophosphate
CARS — compensatory anti-inflammatory response syndrome
CB1 — cannabinoid receptor in the central nervous system
CB2 — cannabinoid receptor in the peripheral tissues
CBF — cerebral blood flow
CD14 — monocyte surface glycoprotein
cGMP — cyclic guanosine monophosphate
CHF — congestive heart failure
CK — creatine kinase
CNS — central nervous system
CO — carbon monoxide
COPD — chronic obstructive lung disease
COX — cyclo-oxygenase
CPAP — continuous positive airway pressure
CPK — creatine phosphokinase
CPK-MB — cardiac specific creatine phosphokinase
CPR — cardiopulmonary resuscitation
Cr — creatinine
CRF — corticotropin releasing factor
CRHs — counterregulatory hormones
CRP — C-reactive protein
CTL — cytotoxic T lymphocyte
CVA — cardiovascular accident (stroke)
CXR — chest x-ray
D10W — ten percent dextrose in water
D5W — five percent dextrose in water
DA — dopamine

DAG — diacylglycerol
DBT — dobutamine
DIC — disseminated intravascular coagulation
DKA — diabetic ketoacidosis
DNA — deoxyribonucleic acid
DW50 — 50 percent dextrose in water
E — epinephrine
ECF — extracellular fluid
EDRF — endothelial derived relaxing factor
EF — ejection fraction
EKG — electrocardiogram
EMS — emergency medical system
Epi — epinephrine
ERV — expiratory reserve volume
ESR — erythrocyte sedimentation rate
F — furosemide
FAD — flavin adenine dinucleotide
FADH$_2$ — reduced form of flavin adenine dinucleotide
FBS — fasting blood sugar
FDA — United States Food and Drug Administration
FEV$_1$ — forced expiratory volume in one second
FFAs — free fatty acids
FIO$_2$ — percentage of inspired oxygen concentration
FRC — functional reserve capacity
G6PD — glucose 6-phosphate dehydrogenase
GABA — gamma aminobutyric acid
GCS — Glasgow Coma Scale
GDP — guanosine diphosphate
GFR — glomerular filtration rate
GI — gastrointestinal
GMCSF — granulocyte macrophage-colony-stimulating factor
GOT — glutamate oxaloacetate transaminase
GPT — glutamate pyruvate transaminase
GTP — guanosine triphosphate
Hb — hemoglobin
HbA$_{1-c}$ — glycosylated hemoglobin
HBP — high blood pressure (hypertension)

Hct — hematocrit
HDLs — high density lipoproteins
HES — hydroxyethyl starch
Hg — hemoglobin
HHNC — hyperosmolar hyperglycemic nonketotic coma
HS — hypertonic saline
HSD — hypertonic saline + 6% dextran-70
HSP — heat shock proteins
IC — inspiratory capacity
ICAM — intracellular adhesion molecule
ICF — intracellular fluid
IgE — immunoglobulin E
IL — interleukin
IM — intramuscular
INR — international normalized ratio
IRV — inspiratory reserve volume
KBLs — Kerley B lines
LDLs — low density lipoproteins
LFTs — liver function tests
LOC — level of consciousness
LPM — liters per minute
LPR — late phase reaction
LPS — lipopolysaccharide bacterial endotoxin
LPS-BP — LPS-binding protein
LTB4 — leukotriene B4
LV — left ventricle; left ventricular
LVEDP — left ventricle end diastolic pressure
MAC — membrane attack complex
MAP — mean arterial pressure
MAST — pneumatic anti-shock garment
MDF — myocardial depressant factor
MI — myocardial infarction
MIF — migration inhibitory factor
MODS — multiple organ dysfunction syndrome
MOSF — multiple organ system failure
MPOS — myeloperoxidase system
mRNA — messenger RNA
MS — morphine sulfate
MSH — melanocyte stimulating hormone
MXs — methylxanthines
NAD$^+$ — nicotinamide adenine dinucleotide

NADH — reduced form of nicotinamide adenine dinucleotide

NADP⁺ — nicotinamide dinucleotide phosphate

NADPH — reduced form of nicotinamide dinucleotide phosphate

NE — norepinephrine

NG — nasogastric

NK — natural killer

NO — nitric oxide

NRS — normal regulatory system

NSAIDs — nonsteroidal anti-inflammatory drugs

NTG — nitroglycerin

PAF — platelet activating factor

PAWP — pulmonary artery wedge pressure

PDE5 — phosphodiesterase type 5

PEF — peak expiratory flow

PET — positron emission tomography

PF — plasma ultrafiltration

PFTs — pulmonary function tests

P$_i$ — high energy phosphate

PMNs — polymorphonuclear cells

PMX — Polymyxin B immobilized fiber

PNS — peripheral nervous system

PRN — as needed

PT — prothrombin time

PTT — partial thromboplastin time

PTX — pentoxifylline

RAAS — renin-angiotensin-aldosterone-system

RBCs — red blood cells

RES — reticuloendothelial system

RIND — reversible ischemic neurologic defect

RNA — ribonucleic acid

RR — respiratory rate

rRNA — ribosomal RNA

RUQ — right upper quadrant

RV — residual volume

SIRS — systemic inflammatory response syndrome

SLI — sublingual injection

SLUMPED — acronym for causes of metabolic acidosis

SQ — subcutaneous

SVR — systemic vascular resistance

T&R — treat and release

T3 — tri-iodothyronine (thyroid hormone)

T4 — thyroxine

TGs — triglycerides

TIA — transient ischemic attack

TLC — total lung capacity

TM — thrombomodulin

TNF — tumor necrosis factor

tPA — tissue plasminogen activator

TRH — thyroid releasing hormone

tRNA — transfer RNA

UA — urinalysis

UBs — urobilinogens

UGIB — upper gastrointestinal bleeding

VC — vital capacity

VCAM-1 — vascular cell adhesion molecule 1

VF — ventricular fibrillation

VLDLs — very low density lipoproteins

V$_t$ — tidal volume

WBCs — white blood cells

CHAPTER 1
BACK TO BASICS

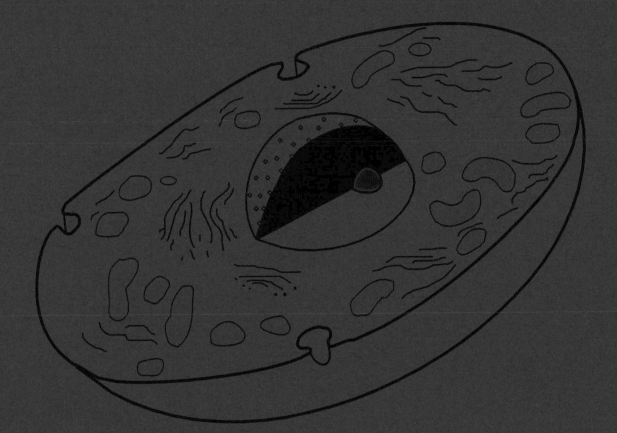

CHAPTER 1 — BACK TO BASICS

Contents

Objectives
Introduction

PART I — "SCIENTIFIC BASICS"
Homeostasis and Normal Regulatory Systems
Bad Stuff Happens — the Pathophysiological Model
Basic Molecular Genetics — a Quick Review
How Cells Communicate
Metabolism 101 — Basics of Biochemistry
Cell Injury and Death — Basic Pathology
Chemical Mediators of Inflammation

PART II — "CLINICAL BASICS"
The ABCs
General Approach to a Sick Patient
Take an AMPLE History
Patient Assessment — the "Thinking Cook" Approach
The "Heart-Lung-Brain" Triad
The Four Fixes
Principles of Laboratory Tests
Principles of X-rays

Summary
Crossword Puzzle Review
References

Objectives (Part I and Part II)

After reading this chapter, you'll be able to:

Describe and give examples of normal regulatory systems.

Draw and describe a model to summarize features common to the pathophysiology of many serious medical conditions.

- Delineate and explain the three major means of intercellular communication.

Outline, in general, the body's metabolism of ingested sugars, proteins, and fats.

Define and explain a G-protein mediated reaction.

Defend the concept: "The majority of the body's vital processes are G-protein mediated."

Summarize the molecular steps that take place when a protein is synthesized by the cell.

Describe how white blood cells (leukocytes) kill bacteria.

Define the role of oxidation-reduction reactions, free radicals, and antioxidants in both normal physiology and in disease states.

Define and describe the role of apoptosis in both normal physiology and in disease states.

Define cytokines — describe their normal role in the inflammatory process.

Define and explain what is meant by an "AMPLE" history.

Give two examples where failure to take an adequate medication history may result in misdiagnosis, bad patient outcome, or both.

Describe and apply in your clinical practice major patient assessment principles.

Delineate the basic principles of patient care.

Draw and summarize the significance of the "Heart-Lung-Brain" triad.

List and explain the significance of "The Four Fixes."

List and explain two rules that conceptualize and summarize the principles of laboratory tests.

- List and explain two rules that conceptualize and summarize the principles of x-ray tests.

Introduction

Rothenberg's Rule of Advanced Life Support states: "For every advanced skill we learn, we *forget* two basic ones." Like it or not, our natural tendency as we acquire more and more fancy techniques, tests, and equipment is to rely on these instead of what really matters — the basics. This chapter presents information that forms the *foundation* of everything we do in health care. When things get tough, chances are you'll do better by going back to these basics rather than relying on the latest tricks.

I've always subscribed to what I call the "Law of the Apple." Remember Sir Isaac Newton? The apple fell off the tree, hitting him on the head, because of _____?? Gravity, right?

> *REMEMBER:* **Don't try to rewrite the laws of physics. Use them to benefit you and your patients!**

This is an unchangeable law of physics and we all know it. Many of the major principles of medicine are similar — fixed laws of nature. We have two choices: use these unchangeable laws to benefit our patients, or try to rewrite the laws of physics. I suggest we go with the former approach; let these laws work for you and your patients.

One of the major goals of this text is to illustrate recurrent "themes" or "principles" that apply to a wide variety of conditions. These are highlighted throughout. Remember, there are far more *similarities* among the body's cells and systems than *differences*.[1] For example:

- Most cells combine oxygen with the breakdown products of carbohydrate, fat, or protein to release energy for normal functioning.

- Most cells have the ability to reproduce.

> *COROLLARY:* **By concentrating on *similarities* rather than *differences*, you only need to learn the underlying "principles" once. The rest involves *applying* the principle *with understanding* to various diseases.**

- Often, when tissue is destroyed, the remaining cells regenerate new ones until the appropriate number is restored.

- All cells are bathed in extracellular fluid (ECF), the contents of which are precisely controlled. The ECF includes all fluid that is not within the cell (e.g., in the interstitial tissue and circulatory system).

What goes on in the basic science laboratory now often has direct applicability in the clinical setting. No longer are clinicians and researchers on different planets. It's important to have a working understanding of scientific principles to be able to give our patients the best clinical care.

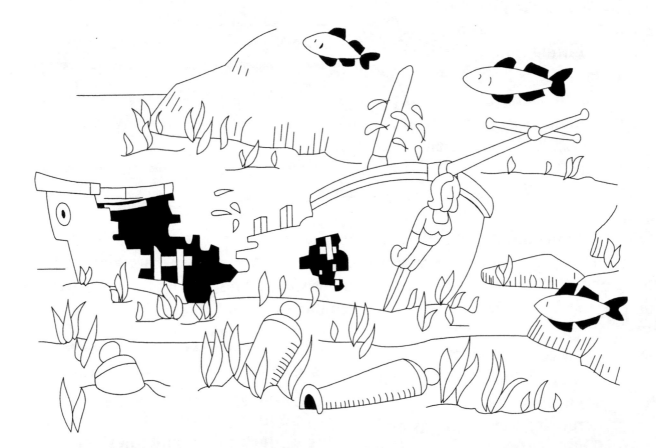

Appearances are sometimes deceptive — the underwater environment is a well-organized ecosystem. In this, it resembles human physiology, where numerous normal regulatory systems maintain homeostasis.

PART I — "SCIENTIFIC BASICS"

Homeostasis and Normal Regulatory Systems
Bad Stuff Happens — the Pathophysiological Model
Basic Molecular Genetics — a Quick Review
How Cells Communicate
Metabolism 101 — Basics of Biochemistry
Cell Injury and Death — Basic Pathology
Chemical Mediators of Inflammation

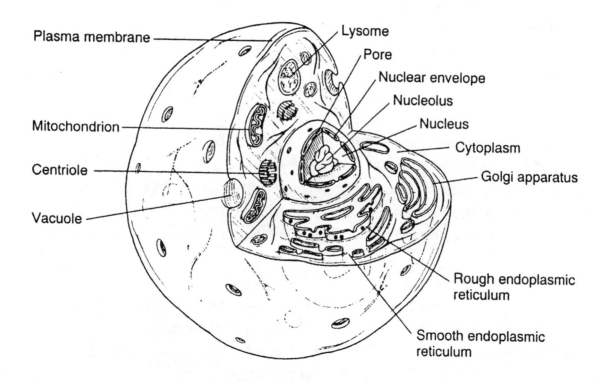

MAJOR CELL COMPONENTS (ORGANELLES)

Homeostasis and Normal Regulatory Systems

> ## OBJECTIVE: Describe and give examples of normal regulatory systems.

Homeostasis is a steady state in the internal environment of the body, maintained by various feedback and control mechanisms. Though all body systems play a role, the nervous and endocrine systems reign supreme in maintenance of homeostasis. Each cell contributes to, as well as benefits from, normal on-going processes. Physiologists have termed this reciprocal interaction

> **PRINCIPLE:** Homeostasis is maintained by interactions of numerous "normal regulatory systems" of the body.

automaticity. This balance continues unless one or more of the systems loses the ability to maintain its "share" of the function. At this point, all body cells suffer. Moderate dysfunction leads to illness, while severe dysfunction leads to death.

I've coined the term **normal regulatory system (NRS)** for the myriad of checks and balances that we have in our bodies. Each of our bodily processes has a "yin" and a "yang." For every system that does one thing, there is one or more that does the opposite. The purpose, of course, is to keep things in balance, maintaining homeostasis. When alterations disrupt the NRS balance, disease occurs.

The best metaphorical example of a NRS I know is a ceiling fire sprinkler, as in a hotel room. Think about it — what is its "job description?" Of course, to put out fires. So, you'd agree that if there is a fire, it's a darn good thing that the sprinkler head senses it and turns on the water, correct? Well, this is a normal regulatory system doing what it is supposed to do in response to an *appropriate* stimulus. What if there were a fire and no water came out of the sprinkler? Not such a healthy situation, eh? So, if a NRS fails to respond in response to an appropriate stimulus, trouble is likely.

Now, what if some joker held a lit match up to the sprinkler (please don't try this — trust me, it works!)? The device would sense fire and a rainstorm would ensue. This time, however, there really wasn't a fire. The sprinkler just *thought* there was. Its job description, then, is very limited: sense fire, make rain! This NRS responds to fire — in one case, the stimulus is appropriate (a fire in the room); in the other, it is inappropriate (joker with lit match). The sprinkler can't tell the difference between the real thing and a match; the stimulus is the same, yet the results differ vastly. **[FIGURE 1-1]**

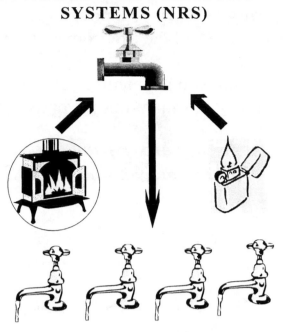

NORMAL REGULATORY SYSTEMS (NRS)

Figure 1-1: Fire sprinklers are an excellent example of a normal regulatory system.

So we can summarize:

1. When an appropriate stimulus triggers a normal regulatory system, things are good.

2. When an appropriate stimulus fails to trigger a normal regulatory system, things are bad.

PRINCIPLE: **Most disease arises from loss of a normal regulatory system (NRS) or normal activation of a NRS under abnormal circumstances, or both.**

3. When an inappropriate stimulus (e.g., a lit match) triggers a normal regulatory system, things are still bad.

In two of the three scenarios above, the normal regulatory system was doing *exactly* what it was supposed to do; it just didn't know the difference between a room fire and the fire from a lit match.

Make sure you are comfortable with the concept of a normal regulatory system — this underlies the basis of all disease:

Most disease arises from failure of a normal regulatory system (NRS) or normal activation of a NRS under abnormal circumstances, or both.

Bad Stuff Happens — the Pathophysiological Model

OBJECTIVE: Draw and describe a model to summarize features common to the pathophysiology of many serious medical conditions.

The beauty of medical science is its intrinsic simplicity — elegant, yet simple. As a result, there is a somewhat humorous *and* highly accurate generic model for the pathophysiology of just about any condition. *Something* happens ("the event"), resulting in the release or production of "abnormal stuff." This is a generic term for any of a number of different biochemical mediators that we'll talk about later. Alternatively, some diseases result from loss of "normal stuff."

"BAD STUFF HAPPENS" — THE PATHOPHYSIOLOGICAL MODEL:

"THE EVENT"

LOSS OF "GOOD STUFF" **PRODUCTION OF "BAD STUFF"**

"BAD STUFF"

"WORSE STUFF"

"DEAD STUFF"

As you might guess, the loss of normal "stuff" or the production of "abnormal stuff" has to do with normal regulatory systems (NRSs). If a NRS works, there is no disease. If it doesn't produce normal "stuff" or if it produces normal "stuff" at the wrong time (making the latter "abnormal stuff"), disease results. Production of "abnormal stuff" or loss of "normal stuff" causes "bad stuff" to happen. Untreated, "worse stuff" then "dead stuff" results.

Let's apply this to our fire sprinkler system. Silly as it seems (and I think it's right up there on the laughter scale!), this model is incredibly valid, as well as useful. We only have to substitute the type of "stuff" involved and the effects of its presence or absence. I urge you to try to fit the pathophysiology of any disease you study into this model — it really works!

How does the principle of "stuff" apply to patient care? There are several perfectly simple and logical conclusions that we may draw from the "laws of stuff":

1. If lack of "stuff" contributes to the problem, give 'em back the necessary "stuff" to improve things!

2. If "stuff" leads to problems, give "anti-stuff" to stop the formation of "stuff," block its action, or both.

3. Some "stuff" outlasts "anti-stuff." If the "stuff" outlasts the treatment, there's still a problem.

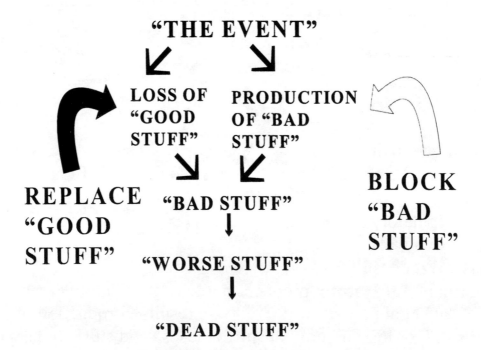

Basic Molecular Genetics — a Quick Review

> ***OBJECTIVE:*** **Define and explain transcription, translation, and protein synthesis in molecular genetics terms.**

How does molecular genetics fit into pathophysiology?
"Like a charm," many would say. The more we learn about the genetic code, the closer we come to treating diseases thought untreatable only a few years ago. Gene therapy has become reality, though in its infancy. Already, patients with refractory angina and congestive heart failure have benefited. The entire field of molecular genetics is linked integrally with the mechanisms of disease.

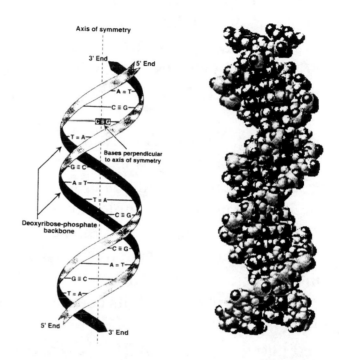

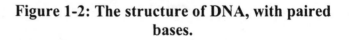

Figure 1-2: The structure of DNA, with paired bases.

Genes control protein synthesis. Each **gene** is a double-stranded helical molecule of deoxyribonucleic acid (**DNA**) that controls formation of ribonucleic acid (**RNA**) in the nucleus. RNA moves to the cytoplasm and attaches to ribosomes where it controls the formation of a specific protein. There are over 100,000 genes in our chromosomal DNA that code for various proteins. In addition, mitochondria possess their own separate collection of DNA (called a **genome**).

What is the genetic code? The **genetic code** consists of triplets of three successive bases on a DNA strand, each coding for a specific protein. Each triplet is called a **codon**. There are four possible bases on a strand of DNA: two **purines** (**adenine** and **guanine**) and two **pyrimidines** (**thymine** and **cytosine**). The purine base adenine of one strand always bonds with the pyrimidine base thymine of the other strand of DNA. Similarly, guanine always binds with cytosine. [**FIGURE 1-2**]

TRANSCRIPTION OF mRNA

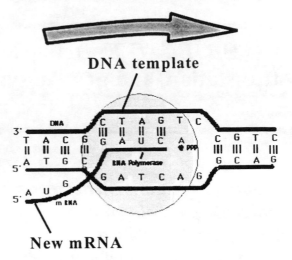

DNA template

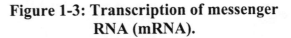

New mRNA

Figure 1-3: Transcription of messenger RNA (mRNA).

How is RNA made? RNA is made in the cell nucleus, using DNA as a template. This is the process of **transcription**. The two strands of DNA separate; one side acts as a template causing the formation of complementary code triplets (codons) in the RNA. The RNA codons control the amino acid sequence that will eventually be synthesized. An enzyme called **RNA polymerase** moves along the template, forming a single strand of RNA based on the code on the DNA. As in DNA, each purine is replaced with its complementary pyrimidine. In RNA, the base **uracil** is substituted in place of thymine. The RNA strand is then released into the cytoplasm. [**FIGURE 1-3**]

What are the types of RNA? There are three different types of RNA:

1. **Messenger RNA** (mRNA) — carries the genetic code to the cytoplasm to control the formation of proteins.
2. **Ribosomal RNA** (rRNA) — forms the ribosomes, where the proteins are actually assembled.
3. **Transfer RNA** (tRNA) — transports amino acids to the ribosomes to be used in the assembly of proteins.

How does mRNA lead to synthesis of a particular protein? Once transcribed, the strand of mRNA exits the cell nucleus and enters the cytoplasm. From here, it moves to the **ribosome**. Much like a magnetic tape reader, the ribosome "reads" the code, along its length, on the mRNA and binds together the appropriate amino acids. The amino acids are brought to the ribosome by tRNA. Once all of the coded amino acid sequences are bound together by peptide bonds, the final protein is released from the ribosome. The process of synthesizing a protein by the ribosome's "reading" the genetic code on mRNA is called "**translation**." Often, though not always, proteins undergo further modification (post-translational modification) by enzymes in the cytoplasm of the cell. **[FIGURE 1-4]**

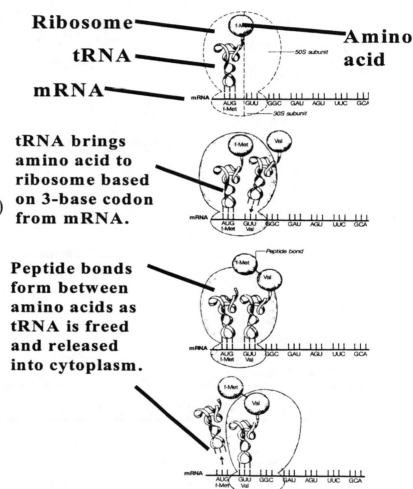

Ribosome — **Amino acid**

tRNA —

mRNA —

tRNA brings amino acid to ribosome based on 3-base codon from mRNA.

Peptide bonds form between amino acids as tRNA is freed and released into cytoplasm.

Figure 1-4: Translation of mRNA into proteins takes place at the ribosomes. Transfer RNA (tRNA) brings in amino acids that are joined by peptide linkages to form proteins.

How Cells Communicate

OBJECTIVE: Delineate and explain the three major means of intercellular communication.

The intracellular and extracellular environments are different.
Communication between cells occurs in the face of radically different intracellular fluid (ICF) and extracellular fluid (ECF) chemical mileus ("environments"). The basic differences are: **[FIGURE 1-5]**

Figure 1-5: Major differences in the composition of ECF and ICF

SUBSTANCE	INTRACELLULAR	EXTRACELLULAR
Sodium (mmol/liter)	10	142
Potassium (mmol/liter)	140	4
Chloride (mmol/liter)	4	108
Bicarbonate (mmol/liter)	10	24
Phosphates (mmol/liter)	75	4
Protein (mg/dl)	16	2

- ECF has a high concentration of sodium and a low concentration of potassium. The opposite is true for ICF.

- ECF contains a high chloride concentration compared with ICF.

- The concentrations of potassium, phosphates, and proteins in the ICF are greater than those in ECF.

How does transport through the cell membrane occur? The two most common means are diffusion and active transport.

- **Diffusion** is the random movement of molecules either through spaces in the membrane or in combination with a carrier protein (**facilitated diffusion**). No "special" energy source is required.

- **Active transport** involves movement of substances across a membrane in combination with a carrier protein *against* a concentration gradient. A source of energy is required.

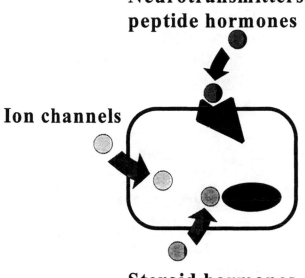

Neurotransmitters, peptide hormones

Ion channels

Steroid hormones

Figure 1-6: There are three major mechanisms for intercellular communication.

Cells communicate by three methods. There are three different means by which cells communicate with each other. Two of these involve specific receptors (cell membrane receptors or intracellular cytoplasmic receptors), while the third involves protein-lined channels. **[FIGURE 1-6]**

Molecules move through protein channels in the cell membrane. These channels are selectively permeable for the transport of one or more specific molecules. Characteristics of an individual channel are determined by its diameter, shape, and electrical charge. Specific channels exist for the movement of electrolytes (ions), such as sodium, potassium, and calcium, both between cells and from the ICF to the ECF. Channels through which ions move are called **ion channels**.

Channels open or close in response to stimuli, which are usually either changes in voltage or chemicals. This control process is called **gating**:

- Voltage gating — changes in electrical potential across the cell membrane lead to a change in the molecular conformation of the gate proteins, either allowing or preventing passage of a substance.

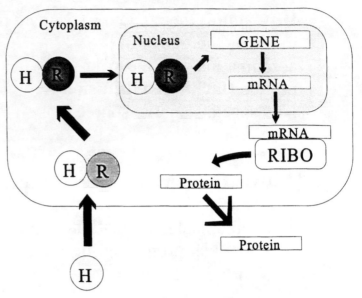

- Chemical gating — the binding of another molecule with the gate protein leads to a configurational change, which either "opens" or "closes" the gate.

Figure 1-7: Ligands (such as hormones) bind intracellular receptors, initiating a set of events that eventually leads to synthesis of one specific protein. [(H) = hormone, (R) = intracellular receptor]

Intracellular receptors. These receptors are located within the cell cytoplasm. The "stimulant" substance (e.g., neurotransmitter or steroid) crosses the cell membrane and binds to the intracellular receptor (shortly, we'll rename "stimulants" ligands). A series of molecular events then takes place, eventually leading to synthesis of one final protein product: [**FIGURE 1-7**]

1. The "stimulant" and receptor form a complex.

2. The complex undergoes a conformational change such that a three base segment of DNA (codon) is exposed. The complex then moves into the nucleus.

3. This single codon, known as the **recognition codon**, binds to a single complementary codon on the chromosomal DNA.

4.   Binding of the recognition codon triggers the process of messenger RNA (mRNA) transcription.

5.   A specific mRNA for the intended final protein product is produced and sent to the cytoplasm.

6.   In the cytoplasm, the mRNA binds with the ribosome. Here, the mRNA is translated into protein, based on the nucleic acid base sequence.

The most common "stimulants" to bind to intracellular receptors are the steroid hormones (e.g., aldosterone). Note that once the receptor is bound, a set of reactions must take place *before* any final result occurs. That's why steroids don't work instantaneously — at least an hour is required for the necessary protein synthesis to take place.

Cell surface receptors — the "lock and key" model. Many cellular interactions involve a substance ("stimulant"), such as a neurotransmitter, that binds to the part of the receptor located in the cell membrane. The receptor is an integral part of the membrane, and it has both an exterior and an interior portion. **[FIGURE 1-8]** Interactions of "stimulants" with these receptors have been described by the "lock and key" model of stimulus-receptor (enzyme-substrate) interaction. Basically, this model is still correct, but the words have changed. Physiologists have expanded our knowledge to the *molecular level*!

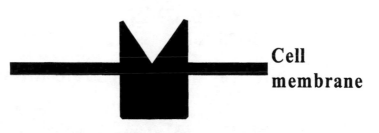

External portion of receptor

Cell membrane

Internal portion of receptor

Figure 1-8: Membrane receptors have both external and internal components.

The following is the classic "lock and key" model of transmitter-receptor interaction: A "stimulant" (the "key") binds to its receptor (the "lock"). The combination of "lock and key" catalyzes a chemical reaction. Once the reaction takes place, the "lock and key" separate and return to the "work pool" unchanged.

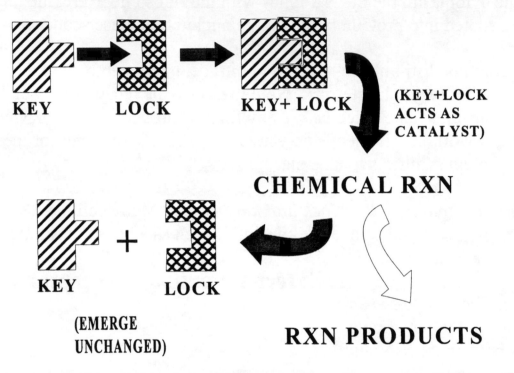

KEY   LOCK   KEY+ LOCK   (KEY+LOCK
                                              ACTS AS
                                              CATALYST)

CHEMICAL RXN

KEY   +   LOCK

(EMERGE   **RXN PRODUCTS**
UNCHANGED)

"Lock and Key" Model of Transmitter-Receptor Interaction

> ## OBJECTIVE: Define and explain a G-protein mediated reaction.

> ## OBJECTIVE: Defend the concept: "The majority of the body's vital processes are G-protein mediated."

"Keys" ("stimulants") are now called ligands; "locks" are receptors.
Ligands are molecules that temporarily bind to other molecules (e.g., receptors), the combination of which triggers a biological reaction. Once the reaction starts, the pair separates and the original molecular components emerge unchanged. This differs from the *bonding* of two substances, which results in the formation of a new compound, completely and permanently changed from its individual components.
[FIGURE 1-9]

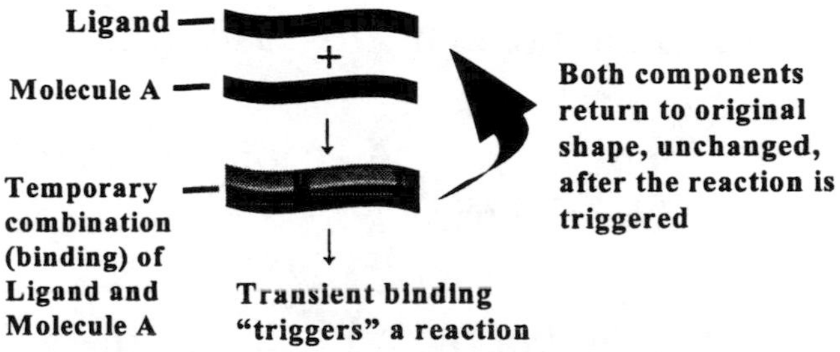

Figure 1-9: Ligands emerge unchanged when the end reaction is complete.

Two new pieces of the puzzle.
Newer work has shown that the ligand-receptor complex, by itself, doesn't really catalyze the end reaction. Two additional elements are required: energy (supplied by a **G-protein**) and a **second messenger**.

G-proteins. G-proteins are regulatory proteins that bind to various phosphorus-containing molecules, such as guanosine diphosphate (GDP) or guanosine triphosphate (GTP). Once a ligand has bound the external portion of a receptor, the phosphate-bound G-protein in the cytoplasm combines with the intracellular portion of the receptor.

I-19

In their inactive form, G-proteins are bound to GDP. When they bind a ligand-receptor complex, the GDP is replaced by a molecule of GTP, activating the G-protein. The "triplex" of ligand, receptor, and G-protein provides a high-energy phosphate, P_i, that energizes another molecule, the "second messenger," to complete the end reaction. [**FIGURE 1-10**] Essentially, G-proteins at the inner cell membrane surface couple outer surface membrane receptors to their second messengers.

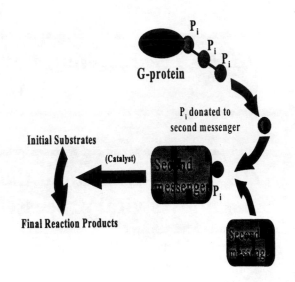

Figure 1-10: G-proteins supply high energy phosphates to second messengers which then catalyze the final reaction.

G-protein mediated reactions are very common, accounting for nearly 90% of the major biochemical reactions in our bodies (e.g., virtually all catecholamine-mediated reactions). Protein lined ion channels are often gated by G-protein mechanisms, as well.

Second messengers. A second messenger is a compound that becomes activated by the triplex of ligand-receptor and G-protein. It is this second messenger that that catalyzes the end reaction, *not* the initial receptor-ligand complex.

What are the common second messengers? Compounds commonly involved as second messengers include:

- Cyclic AMP (cAMP) — Stimulation of adenyl cyclase results in the formation of cAMP. cAMP activates

REMEMBER: G-proteins at the inner cell membrane surface couple surface membrane receptors to their second messengers.

REMEMBER: The most common second messengers are cyclic AMP (cAMP) and intracellular calcium.

protein kinase A, which leads to phosphorylations that either activate or inactivate various target enzymes. Think of phosphate groups as a "switch." The presence or absence of this group, depending upon the enzyme, either activates or deactivates it. This is why **kinases** (which add phosphate groups) and **phosphorylases** (which remove phosphate groups) are of vital importance in the study of pathophysiology.

- Calcium — Ligand-receptor interactions activate calcium channels, permitting calcium ions to enter the cell, as well as to be mobilized from intercellular stores. Calcium ions bind with the protein **calmodulin**. The calmodulin-calcium complex alters the activity of calcium-dependent enzymes and reactions. [***NOTE:*** in contractile tissue (e.g., cardiac muscle), calcium from the sarcoplasmic reticulum binds **troponin** to facilitate muscle contraction. In other tissues, the endoplasmic reticulum serves as a major calcium source.]

- Plasma membrane phospholipids — Ligand-receptor interactions activate the membrane-bound enzyme phospholipase C, which causes phospholipids in the cell to split into the second messengers diacylglycerol and inositol triphosphate. Inositol triphosphate mobilizes calcium, activating protein kinase C, which either activates or inactivates enzymes. Diacylglycerol enhances the action of protein kinase C, and is also hydrolyzed to arachidonic acid, the precursor to prostaglandins. Prostaglandins also influence hormonal responses.

PROCESSES INVOLVING SECOND MESSENGERS:

- **Growth factors — cell growth, neoplasia**
- **Hormones — metabolism, secretion, absorption**
- **Blood processes — inflammation, hemostasis**
- **Catecholamines — cardiovascular, metabolic, fluid and electrolytes**

- Cyclic GMP (cGMP) — via G-proteins, cGMP mediates the effects of atrial natriuretic peptide.

This is the "new DNA".
Remember how we felt when first learning about DNA and the double-helix? Less than twenty years later, my kids were learning the same thing in elementary school! We've come a long way —

REMEMBER: A *kinase* is an enzyme that adds a high energy phosphate ($\sim P_i$) to a molecule. A *phosphorylase* hydrolyzes (removes via the addition of water) $\sim P_i$ from a molecule.

and the same thing will happen with G-proteins and second messengers. We're going to hear a lot about them in the coming years.

So, let's review it one more time. Stated somewhat differently (remember, it's really all just a "fancy version" of the old "lock and key" enzyme activation model):

1.   Ligands bind a receptor.

2.   G-proteins bind the ligand-receptor complex.

3.   The G-protein donates a $\sim P_i$ to a second messenger.

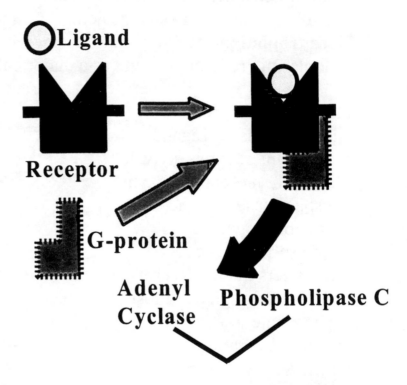

Second Messenger Formation (cAMP, increased intracellular calcium)

Figure 1-11: Summary of G-protein interactions, leading to activation of either cyclic AMP or intracellular calcium as second messengers.

4.   The second messenger then triggers the end reaction, usually by catalyzing a set of chemical reactions.

5.   The ligand and receptor emerge unchanged.

The "gory" details. Since G-protein mediated reactions are so common and so important, I thought I'd share the biochemical details for those of you who are interested. Many G-protein mediated reactions result in the production of cyclic AMP (cAMP), increased intracellular levels of calcium, or both. cAMP and calcium are the most common second messengers. **[FIGURE 1-11]**

G-proteins consist of three subunits (α, β, and γ) bound to either GDP or GTP. When the subunits are bound to GDP, the G-protein is *inactive*. To become activated, GTP displaces GDP from the G-protein subunits. The activated G-protein, α, β, and γ subunits bound to GTP, binds to the inner portion of the membrane receptor.

The α-subunit of the G-protein, along with GTP, breaks away from the rest of the triplex. The α-subunit-GTP complex activates either adenyl cyclase, leading to the production of cAMP, or

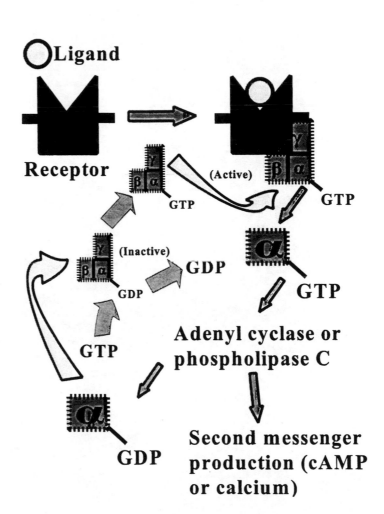

Figure 1-12: Details of G-protein interactions resulting in donation of ~P_i to a second messenger. The energized second messenger completes the chemical reaction.

I-23

phospholipase C, resulting in phosphorylation (and subsequent activation) of other proteins and increased intracellular calcium concentrations.

Once the reaction is completed, the α-subunit is inactivated, since it is now only bound to GDP (a high energy phosphorus was donated to activate the reaction). For the G-protein to become activated again, the GDP must be displaced by GTP. **[FIGURE 1-12]**

Metabolism 101 — Basics of Biochemistry

> ## *OBJECTIVE:* Outline, in general, the body's metabolism of ingested sugars, proteins, and fats.

Though it took me a few years to realize it, biochemistry really underlies all of the medical sciences. It takes the structures, mechanisms, and chemical processes vital to life and describes them in molecular terms — the "molecular logic of life." To understand the role of various hormones and enzymes in both health and disease, we need to review some basic biochemistry. Don't fear — I'll keep it on my level ("Plain English"). If you're interested in more detail, look in your favorite Biochemistry text.

Our sources of energy are carbohydrates (mostly as glucose), fats, and proteins. Ultimately, glucose serves as the main cell "food," whether taken in orally, parenterally, or made from conversion of stored fats and proteins. A major cause of and contributor to disease is failure of the body to make sufficient energy.

Carbohydrate Metabolism

Digestion of carbohydrates begins in the mouth and stomach. The salivary enzyme ptyalin (salivary amylase or α-amylase) hydrolyzes starch into maltose. Recall that a "hydrolysis" reaction really just means adding some

$$H-R-R-R-OH \; + \; H_2O \; \rightleftharpoons \; H-R-OH \; + \; H-R-R-OH$$

Hydrolysis = splitting with water

Figure 1-13: Hydrolysis is the splitting of a molecule by addition of water. "R" refers to any carbon-containing organic molecule ("radical").

water and breaking the bigger molecule into smaller ones. **[FIGURE 1-13]**

I-25

The process continues in the stomach for about an hour, until the activity of α-amylase is blocked by stomach acid.

After gastric chyme empties into the duodenum, pancreatic α-amylase takes over; this enzyme is several times more powerful than salivary amylase. Prior to leaving the duodenum, nearly all starches are converted into maltose or other small glucose polymers. These are then hydrolyzed into monosaccharides by intestinal epithelial enzymes. Glucose represents more than 80% of the final products of carbohydrate digestion:

- Lactose ⇨ galactose + glucose
- Sucrose ⇨ fructose + glucose
- Maltose ⇨ glucose

Facilitated diffusion and phosphorylation. So, the final products of carbohydrate digestion in the gut are glucose, fructose, and galactose. These small sugars attach to carrier molecules and pass through the intestinal mucosal cell membranes via *facilitated diffusion*, an energy-requiring process. Insulin is not required. Glucose and galactose leave the mucosal cells by facilitated diffusion and by simple diffusion to enter the portal circulation. The mechanism by which fructose enters the circulation is unknown. From the portal circulation, the sugar molecules are transported to various cells throughout the body.

Storage as glycogen. Once absorbed into the cell, glucose may be used immediately for fuel or stored as glycogen. Though all cells are capable of storing sugar as glycogen, the liver and muscle tissues have the greatest glycogen stores:

- **Glycogenesis** is the process of glycogen formation.

- **Glycogenolysis** is the process of glycogen breakdown to re-form glucose. It is not simply the reverse of glycogenesis. A specific enzyme is required; it normally resides in an inactive form within the cell.

Metabolism of one molecule of glucose yields up to 32 molecules of ATP.
Three processes are involved in the metabolism of glucose:

1.   **Glycolysis** splits glucose into two molecules of pyruvic acid. There are ten reactions in the process, each catalyzed by a specific enzyme. Glucose is the sole source of metabolic energy in erythrocytes, renal medulla, brain, and sperm. Glycolysis is a relatively inefficient energy-producing process, and only generates two moles of ATP for each mole of glucose used (remember — a "mole" is 6.02×10^{23} molecules of a substance). Pyruvic acid is then converted to acetyl-coenzyme A (acetyl-CoA), with no additional gain of ATP. Acetyl-CoA, however, then enters the mitochondrial citric acid cycle (Krebb's cycle), producing additional energy. [**FIGURE 1-14**]

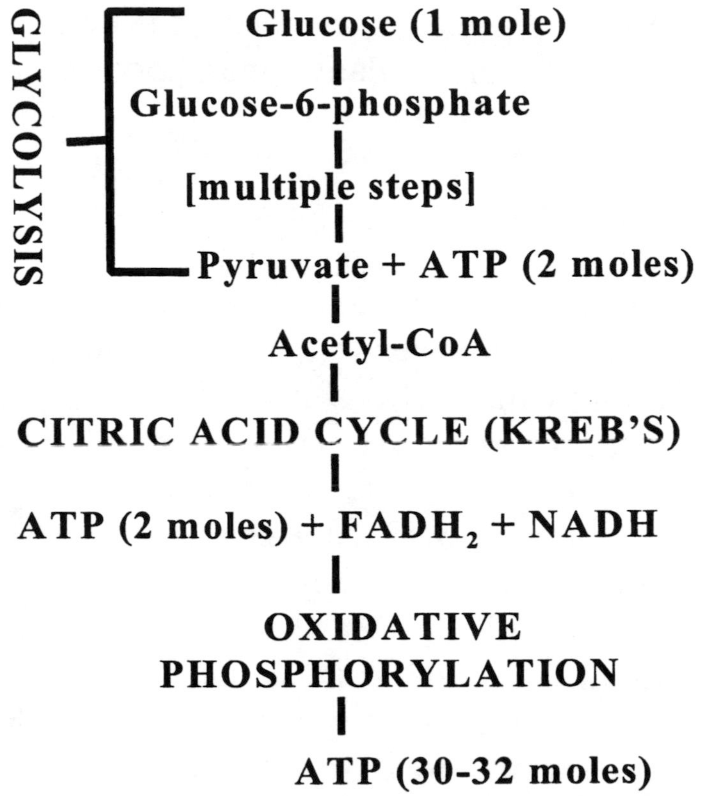

GLYCOLYSIS

Glucose (1 mole)
|
Glucose-6-phosphate
|
[multiple steps]
|
Pyruvate + ATP (2 moles)
|
Acetyl-CoA
|
CITRIC ACID CYCLE (KREB'S)
|
ATP (2 moles) + FADH$_2$ + NADH
|
OXIDATIVE PHOSPHORYLATION
|
ATP (30-32 moles)

Figure 1-14: Glycolysis converts glucose into pyruvate, which is converted to Acetyl Co-A to enter the citric acid cycle. Products of this cycle undergo oxidative phosphorylation to produce large amounts of ATP.

2. During the **citric acid cycle** (also known as the Krebb's cycle), acetyl-CoA is converted to carbon dioxide and hydrogen. For each molecule of glucose metabolized, two molecules of ATP are formed. Most of the ATP generated from glucose, however, occurs during oxidative phosphorylation. **[FIGURE 1-15]**

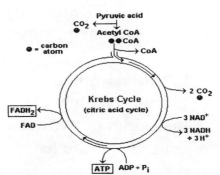

Figure 1-15: The citric acid (Kreb's) cycle produces NADH and FADH$_2$ which then undergo oxidative phosphorylation, producing ATP.

3. **Oxidative phosphorylation** involves conversion of hydrogen atoms (made during the citric acid cycle) into hydrogen ions and electrons. Oxygen (O_2) is reduced to water (H_2O) with electrons donated by NADH and FADH$_2$. The electrons from hydrogen enter a series of reactions, known as the **electron transport chain**. They are shuttled between highly specialized proteins known as **cytochromes**. The process is catalyzed by the enzyme **cytochrome oxidase**. Eventually, the electrons combine with dissolved oxygen, forming hydroxyl ions. Two hydroxyl ions combine to yield water! (Neat, huh?) The movement of hydrogen ions between cytochromes establishes an electrochemical gradient that produces energy. This energy is used to catalyze the conversion of ADP to ATP by the enzyme **ATP synthetase**. **[FIGURE 1-16; FIGURE 1-17]**

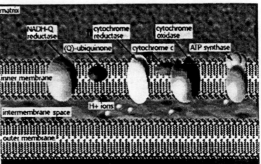

Figure 1-16: The electron transport chain involves the movement of H$^+$ ions between cytochromes, with release of energy at each step along the way.

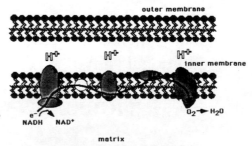

Figure 1-17: Oxidative phosphorylation utilizes energy from the electron transport chain to convert ADP to ATP. Water is produced as a final product.

Tell me, please, how do we get a total of 32 molecules of ATP? The net energy yield is either 30 or 32 molecules of ATP from each glucose molecule. More ATP molecules are made in the liver, kidney, and heart muscle (2.5 molecules per pair of electrons) than in skeletal muscle and brain (1.5 molecules per pair of electrons). This occurs because slightly different pathways are utilized in certain steps during oxidative phosphorylation. A summary of the energy yield from the complete oxidation of glucose is beyond the intended scope of this text, but is well-summarized in standard biochemistry texts.

Interestingly, the net efficiency of the above processes is only 66%. The remainder of the energy generated becomes heat, helping maintain body temperature.

Lipid Metabolism

The first step in digestion of fat is emulsification. Emulsification is the process of breaking fat globules into smaller pieces via the combined actions of bile salts and lecithin. This process leads to a marked increase in the surface area of ingested fats. Lipases, such as pancreatic lipase (the most important), then attack fat surfaces. This action digests nearly all triglycerides into free fatty acids and monoglycerides.

MIXED MICELLE

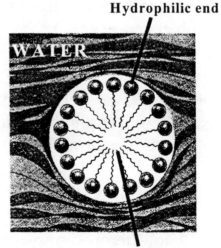

Hydrophilic end

Hydrophobic end

Since the breakdown of triglycerides is highly reversible, bile salts combine rapidly with monoglycerides and free fatty acids, forming **mixed micelles**. These are clusters of **amphiphatic** lipids, meaning that one end of the molecule contains a **hydrophobic** (non-water soluble) group and the other, a **hydrophilic** (water soluble) one. Micelles carry the fat breakdown products (monoglycerides, free fatty acids) to the intestinal brush border for absorption. As a result, reaction equilibrium is shifted in favor of further breakdown of triglycerides to monoglycerides and free fatty acids. **[FIGURE 1-18]**

How is fat transported from the GI tract to the blood?
Essentially all fats are absorbed from the intestine into lymphatics in the form of **chylomicrons**, small "packages" of triglycerides. They travel via the lymphatic channels to the venous circulation. Chylomicrons are removed from the plasma in adipose tissue and in the

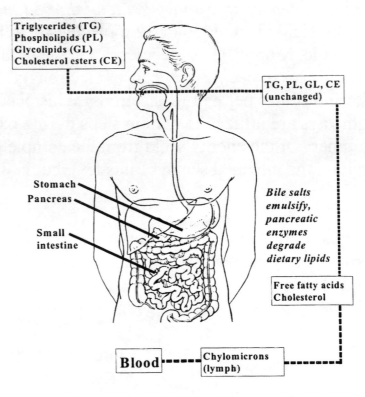

Figure 1-18: Initial digestion and absorption of ingested fats. Chylomicrons move via lymphatic channels into the blood.

liver. Once removed from the plasma, the enzyme lipoprotein lipase hydrolyzes triglycerides into fatty acids and glycerol. The fatty acids diffuse into the liver and adipose cells and are then resynthesized into triglycerides.

How does fat get to other tissues?
Free fatty acids are transported in the plasma bound to albumin. In addition, the liver forms lipoproteins, which transport lipids throughout the body:

- **Very low density lipoproteins** (VLDLs) contain high concentrations of triglycerides and moderate concentrations of phospholipids and cholesterol. Triglycerides are made in the liver, mostly from carbohydrates, and are transported to the tissues via VLDLs.

- **Low density lipoproteins** (LDLs) contain relatively few triglycerides but a very high concentration of cholesterol. LDLs are the cholesterol and phospholipid residues left after VLDLs have delivered most of their triglycerides to adipose tissue.

- **High density lipoproteins** (HDLs) contain roughly a 50-50 mixture of proteins and lipids. HDLs transport cholesterol from the periheral tissues to the liver and play an important role in prevention of atherosclerosis.

How are triglycerides used as fuel? They are first hydrolyzed into fatty acids and glycerol, which are transported to active tissues and oxidized to release energy. Most cells, with the exception of brain tissue, can use fatty acids interchangeably with glucose for energy. Oxidation of fatty acids takes place only in the mitochondria. They must first cross the mitochondrial membrane in a carrier-mediated process, using carnitine. [**FIGURE 1-19**] Once inside the mitochondrion:

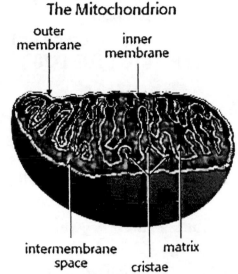

The Mitochondrion

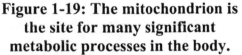

Figure 1-19: The mitochondrion is the site for many significant metabolic processes in the body.

1. Fatty acids are degraded by beta oxidation to two-carbon segments, forming acetyl-coenzyme A (acetyl-CoA). In the process, NADH and $FADH_2$ (energy-containing reduced [hydrogen-containing] coenzymes) are produced. Each coenzyme donates a pair of electrons to the electron transport chain. Via oxidative phosphorylation, ATP is formed from ADP and inorganic phosphate.

2. Acetyl-CoA formed from oxidation of fatty acids enters the citric acid cycle (Krebb's cycle) and is metabolized to hydrogen (as NADH and $FADH_2$).

3. Hydrogen from NADH and $FADH_2$ is subsequently oxidized by mitochondrial enzymes (oxidative phosphorylation, electron transport chain) to form ATP. [**FIGURE 1-20**]

What happens to the glycerol component? Glycerol released during the breakdown of triglycerides is phosphorylated and eventually converted to glyceraldehyde 3-phosphate, which is oxidized via glycolysis.

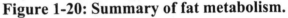

Free Fatty Acid
|
[multiple steps]
|
$FADH_2$ + NADH
+
Acetyl-CoA
|
CITRIC ACID
CYCLE (KREB'S)
|
ATP + $FADH_2$ + NADH
|
OXIDATIVE
PHOSPHORYLATION
|
ATP

Figure 1-20: Summary of fat metabolism.

Does the liver use all of the acetyl-CoA it makes? Despite the fact that fatty acid breakdown to acetyl-CoA occurs in the liver, it only uses a fraction of the acetyl-CoA produced for its own metabolism. The rest is converted to acetoacetic acid; much of this is then converted to β-hydroxybutyric acid and a small amount of acetone. Acetoacetic acid and β-hydroxybutyric acid diffuse out of the liver into the blood, where they are carried to other tissues. There, acetyl-CoA molecules are reformed, then enter the citric acid cycle and are oxidized for energy.

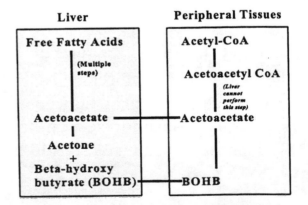

Figure 1-20A: The production and metabolism of ketone bodies (acetoacetate, acetone, beta-hydroxybutyrate). These are a part of normal body processes. Excess accumulation, however, may be dangerous, because they dissociate in serum, leading to acidosis.

Acetone, acetoacetic acid, and β-hydroxybutyric acid are collectively known as **ketone bodies**. They are a normal part of metabolism, providing a handy alternative fuel source for cells, especially during fasting. These are important in normal physiology: **[FIGURE 1-20A]**

1.   Ketone bodies are soluble in aqueous solution and don't need to be carried by albumin or incorporated into lipoproteins, as do other lipids.

2.   Ketone bodies are produced in the liver when the amount of acetyl-CoA present exceeds the liver's oxidative capacity.

3.   Ketone bodies are metabolized by extrahepatic tissues (e.g., skeletal and cardiac muscle, renal cortex) in proportion to their blood concentration.

4.   The brain is able to use ketone bodies as a fuel source, especially during prolonged periods of fasting.

Aren't ketone bodies produced in diabetic ketoacidosis (DKA)? Correct — and they are also produced in any state of starvation and during ingestion of a ketogenic diet (low carbohydrate, high protein, variable fat content). When the rate of formation is greater than the rate of their use, ketone levels rise in the blood and in the urine (ketonuria). Ketone bodies dissociate in the blood, resulting in free hydrogen atoms:

$$KH \rightarrow K^- + H^+ \qquad (\text{"K" stands for ketone body})$$

A significant elevation of ketone bodies in the blood may result in acidosis. The net effect on serum pH and bicarbonate levels of ketosis secondary to starvation, fasting, or dieting is negligible. However, during DKA, sufficient concentrations of ketone bodies *are* present to result in acidosis.

Can carbohydrates and proteins be converted to triglycerides? Triglycerides may be synthesized from carbohydrates and proteins. Fat synthesis from carbohydrate, is important because most body cells have limited capacities to store carbohydrate as glycogen. The average person has nearly two hundred times as much energy stored in the form of fat as in the form of carbohydrates! Remember, each gram of fat contains approximately 2.25 times the number of calories of usable energy as each gram of glycogen. Many amino acids can be converted into acetyl-CoA, which is then converted into triglycerides. On the other hand, fatty acids are *not* converted to glucose in mammals.

Didn't we forget about cholesterol? No, just saved it for last. . . Cholesterol is present in all diets and is absorbed via the intestinal lymphatics. A large quantity is also made by the liver. Cholesterol is an essential component of all cell membranes. The liver converts cholesterol that is not used to form membrane components to cholic acid. This cholesterol, in conjunction with other substances, forms bile salts, which promote digestion and absorption of fats. Finally, a small amount is used by the endocrine system:

- Adrenals — to manufacture adrenal cortical hormones.
- Ovaries — to make progesterone and estrogen.
- Testes — to make testosterone.

Protein Metabolism

Digestion of proteins begins in the stomach. Pepsin in the stomach digests the majority of collagen ingested. Most other proteins are digested in the duodenum by pancreatic enzymes: **[FIGURE 1-21]**

- Trypsin and chymotrypsin split larger proteins into small polypeptides.

- Carboxypolypeptidase cleaves amino acids from the carboxyl ends of polypeptides.

- Proelastase is converted to elastase, which digests elastin fibers (such as in meat).

Amino acids represent more than 99% of protein digestive products. The final step in protein digestion occurs at the intestinal lining cell level:

- Peptidases at the brush border break larger polypeptides into small ones.

- Peptidases within the cells digest virtually all the remaining dipeptides and tripeptides into amino acids before they enter the blood.

We're a lot of protein, baby. Nearly 75% of the solids in our body are proteins, the principle constituents of which are amino acids. These are connected by **peptide linkages** (peptide

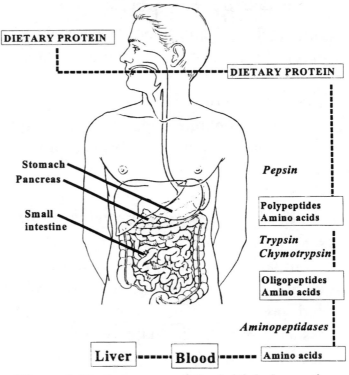

Figure 1-21: Summary of the initial absorption and digestion of proteins.

Generic Amino Acid (AA)

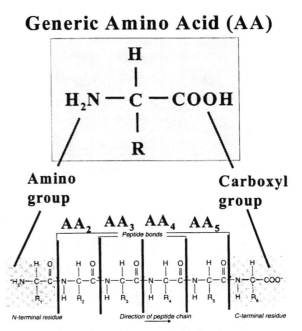

Figure 1-22: Proteins consist of amino acids linked together by peptide bonds.

bonds). **[FIGURE 1-22]** These are covalent (shared electrons) amide bonds between the α-carboxyl of one amino acid and the α-amino group of another. The carbon of the carboxyl and the nitrogen of the amino group share an electron pair. Separate peptide chains may be bound or linked together to form complex polypeptides.

Amino acids are stored as proteins within the cells. Within seconds of passing intracellularly (via a carrier mechanism), most amino acids are formed into proteins. When needed, proteins can be hydrolyzed to release necessary amino acids. This reversible process is common, with three exceptions:

1.   Chromosomal proteins.
2.   Structural proteins (collagen).
3.   Contractile proteins (muscle).

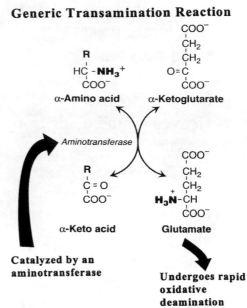

Figure 1-23: A "generic" transamination reaction. The result is glutamate, which then undergoes oxidative deamination.

These proteins are rarely hydrolyzed to release amino acids. Otherwise, whenever the plasma levels of amino acids fall, storage proteins are degraded and the released amino acids transported across the cell membrane into the blood.

Proteins are also used for energy. No big surprise here. Once cellular protein stores are full, additional amino acids in the body fluids are metabolized for energy or converted to fat or glycogen. Metabolism of proteins takes place in the liver:

●   **Transamination** is the first step in the catabolism of most amino acids. It involves the transfer of their α-amino group to another compound, α-ketoglutarate. By accepting the amino group, α-ketoglutarate becomes glutamate. The amino groups of most amino acids are ultimately funneled to glutamate production, since glutamate is the only amino acid able to undergo rapid oxidative deamination. [**FIGURE 1-23**]

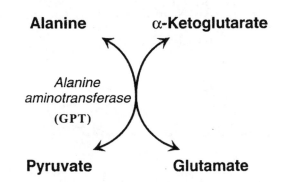

Figure 1-24: The ALT (SGPT) reaction.

- **Oxidative deamination** results in the production of free ammonia. The reaction takes place primarily in the liver and kidneys. The end products are α-ketoacids (used in energy production) and ammonia. Ammonia generated during the deamination process is removed from the blood by hepatic conversion to urea (via the urea cycle).

Even in the absence of food intake, there is an obligatory breakdown of 20-30 grams of body proteins each day. Thus, to prevent a net loss of protein from the body, one must ingest at least 20 to 30 grams of protein daily.

What does transamination have to do with clinical practice?
Transamination reactions are catalyzed by specific enzymes called **aminotransferases**. Each aminotransferase is specific for a small number (usually one) of amino group donors. The two most important reactions are catalyzed by **alanine aminotransferase** (ALT) and **aspartate aminotransferase** (AST).

ALT is also known as **glutamate pyruvate transaminase** (GPT), and is present in many tissues. It catalyzes the transfer of alanine's amino group to α-ketoglutarate, resulting in the formation of pyruvate and glutamate. [**FIGURE 1-24**]

AST is also known as **glutamate oxaloacetate transaminase** (GOT). It transfers amino groups from glutamate to oxaloacetate. The transfer initiates aspartate formation, which is used as a source of nitrogen in the urea cycle. The biochemical details are interesting, but somewhat complex because the amino group is not directly transferred from glutamate to oxaloacetate. Rather, **pyridoxal phosphate** (a derivative of vitamin B_6) plays an essential intermediate role as a coenzyme.

If you're interested, here are the details: **[FIGURE 1-25]**

1. Glutamate is deaminated to form α-ketoglutarate (reaction [1] in Figure 1-25).

2. The removed amino group binds to the coenzyme pyridoxal phosphate, forming pyridoxamine phosphate (reaction [1] in Figure 1-25).

3. Pyridoxamine phosphate then transfers the amino group to oxaloacetate, forming aspartate (reaction [2] in Figure 1-25) and reforming pyridoxal phosphate.

4. Aspartate enters into the urea cycle, as shown in **FIGURE 1-26**.

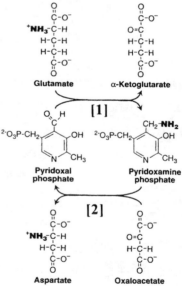

Figure 1-25: The AST (SGOT) reaction involves a complex interaction with vitamin B_6 derivatives.

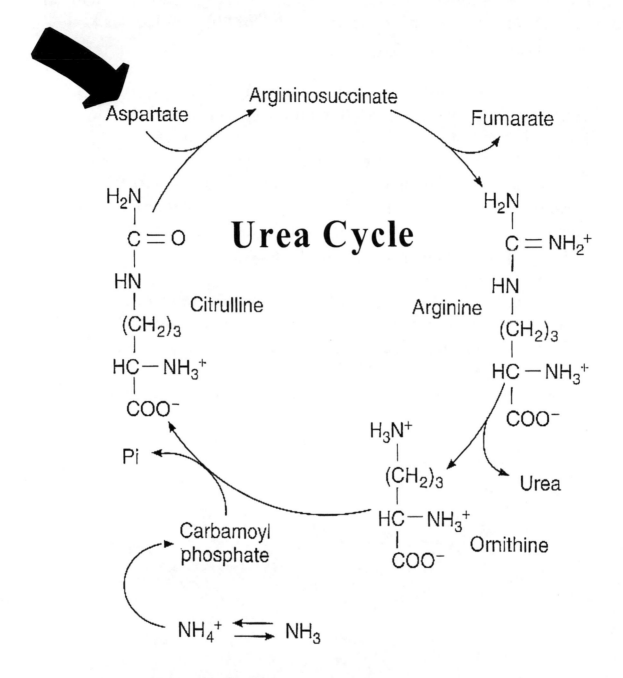

Figure 1-26: The urea cycle

Catabolism in a nutshell — Catabolic reactions serve to capture chemical energy in the form of ATP from the breakdown of "fuel molecules." Catabolism involves three stages:

1.   Hydrolysis of complex molecules into components — proteins to amino acids, polysaccharides to monosaccharides, triglycerides to free fatty acids and glycerol.

2.   Conversion of components to simple intermediates — further breakdown of monosaccharides, free fatty acids, and amino acids to acetyl CoA and a few other simple molecules. Some energy is captured at this stage, but relatively little as compared to the third stage.

3.   Oxidation of acetyl CoA: the citric acid cycle (Kreb's cycle) is the final common pathway in the breakdown of "fuel molecules." Acetyl CoA is oxidized to to CO_2 molecules. Four pair of electrons are transferred to NAD^+ and FAD to produce NADH and $FADH_2$. Large amounts of ATP are generated as these two compounds undergo oxidative phosphorylation.

The **Figure** below summarizes the initial catabolic (breaking down) processes in normal human metabolism:

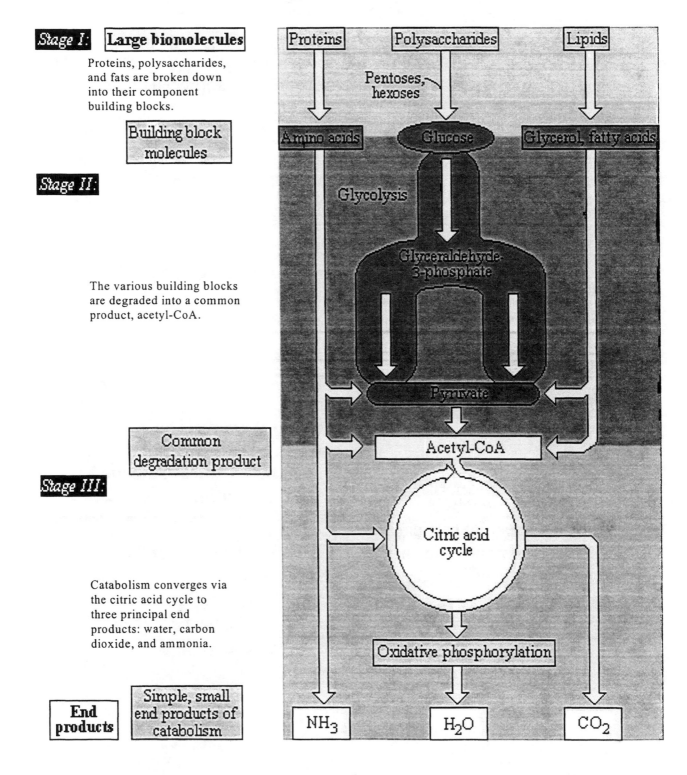

Cell Injury And Death — Basic Pathology

Molecular mechanisms of cell injury and death. In the past, there was very little direct correlation between "basic science" research and actual clinical practice. Those days are gone. A significant majority of what we do clinically is directly related to and based upon "basic science" research. The two are no longer separate — we *must* understand and appreciate both.

Four intracellular systems are particularly vulnerable to injury. These are:

1. Aerobic respiration — mitochondrial oxidative phosphorylation and the production of adenosine triphosphate (ATP).

2. Integrity of cell membranes — the ionic and osmotic homeostasis of the cell depends upon proper function of the cell membrane. Regardless of the cause, virtually all cell injury results in damage to cell membranes.

3. Protein synthesis.

4. Genetic apparatus of the cell.

REMEMBER: **Alterations in function become apparent early. Structural changes occur later, and are usually noted only after critical biochemical damage has *already* occurred.**

All body systems are intertwined — dysfunction in one inevitably affects others. Functional alterations become readily apparent early in a disease process; morphologic changes are only noted some time after critical biochemical damage has *already* occurred. Put another way, disruptions in one normal regulatory system lead to problems in others. Remember, homeostasis depends on a critical "yin-yang" type of balance. When this balance is upset, the "scales" shift in an unfavorable direction.

Types of biochemical damage. There are five; none is mutually exclusive of the others. They include:

1. **Decreased ATP synthesis and ATP depletion** — these are common consequences of both ischemic and toxic injury.

2. **Oxygen-derived free radicals** — free radicals are a species of highly reactive molecules produced as a byproduct of chemical reactions. They are very unstable and may damage many types of cells. Any imbalance between the body's normal free radical-scavenging system and free-radical formation leads to **oxidative stress**. Free radicals are extremely important in human physiology.

3. **Loss of calcium homeostasis** — normally, intracellular calcium concentrations are very low. An energy-dependent system maintains this gradient. Cell injury leads to increased intracellular calcium, which activates phospholipases (degrade membrane phospholipids), proteases (break down membrane and structural proteins), ATPases (break down ATP), and endonucleases (fragment chromatin). Both ischemia and toxins can affect normal calcium homeostasis.

4. **Changes in membrane permeability** — membranes can be damaged by toxins, physical or chemical agents, and intrinsic cell products (e.g., complement).

5. **Irreversible mitochondrial damage** — various types of injury result in formation of an abnormal high conductance channel — the **mitochondrial permeability transition** (MPT) **channel** — in the inner mitochondrial membrane. This nonselective pore formation may be reversible early on following an injury, but soon becomes permanent. This leads to leakage of cytochrome C and activation of cellular apoptotic ("programmed cell death") pathways.

OBJECTIVE: Define the role of oxidation-reduction reactions, free radicals, and antioxidants in both normal physiology and in disease states.

Free radical. **Free radicals** are highly-reactive chemical intermediates that are short one electron in their outer orbital shell. Though uncharged, the presence of an odd, unpaired electron results in chemical instability. Free radicals form as a result of enzyme-catalyzed reactions in the body. They play a major role in both normal physiology and in disease. Free radicals are represented as molecular formulas with a "dot" in the upper right corner: $O_2^{\cdot}$. There are three chemical steps in free radical reactions:

1. **Initiation** — the formation of radicals at the beginning of a reaction.
2. **Propagation** — continuation of the reaction in a series of steps in which a radical reacts with a molecule to yield another radical as one of the products. The propagation steps can continue to form a **chain reaction**.
3. **Termination** — combination of two radicals to form a stable compound. In nature, this may occur spontaneously or as a result of enzyme actions.

Free radicals play a major role in many normal life processes, including aging and bacterial killing by white blood cells (WBCs).

How do WBCs kill bacteria? Once WBCs (predominantly neutrophils) reach the "scene" of a bacterial invasion, they ingest (by phagocytosis) and kill the invaders. There are two mechanisms by which WBCs perform their duties: **[FIGURE 1-26]**

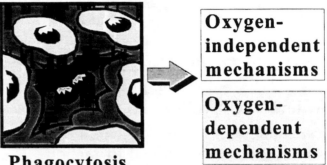

Phagocytosis

- **Non-oxygen dependent mechanisms** — release of enzymes from lysosomes and phagolysosomes (lysosomes within phagocytic vesicles).

Oxygen-independent mechanisms

Oxygen-dependent mechanisms

- **Oxygen dependent mechanisms** — formation of oxygen-derived free radicals.

Figure 1-26: Mechanisms of bacterial killing by leukocytes.

These systems include the **myeloperoxidase system** (MPOS) and other means to generate free radicals in the presence of oxygen. The MPOS is the more potent of WBC bactericidal mechanisms.

How does the MPOS operate? Following phagocytosis, the enzyme **NADPH oxidase** (located in the WBC membrane) converts molecular oxygen from surrounding tissues into the **superoxide free radical (O_2^-)**. This is a rapid reaction and consumes large quantities of oxygen — this stage is appropriately called the **respiratory burst**. Next, superoxide dismutase converts superoxide into hydrogen peroxide (H_2O_2). In the presence of chloride ions (Cl^-), the lysosomal enzyme **myeloperoxidase** (MPO) catalyzes H_2O_2 to one **hypochlorite free radical** ($HOCl^-$) and one **hydroxy free**

> ***DID YOU KNOW?*** **Hypochlorous acid is responsible for the greenish color of pus?**

radical(OH⁻). Both destroy bacterial membranes and internal bacterial contents. (By the way, HOCl⁻ is also known as **hypochlorous acid**, the main component of household bleach.) Once they have accomplished their "mission," excess hypochlorite and hydroxy free radicals are neutralized by the enzymes catalase and glutathione peroxidase to form water and chloride ions. [**FIGURE 1-27**]

What happens if a person's MPO level is low? As you might imagine, low levels of myeloperoxidase (MPO) impair the major "killing step" of leukocytes — free radical formation. The compromised individual is susceptible to severe and persistent bacterial infections. The most common cause is a genetic condition, known as **chronic granulomatosis**.

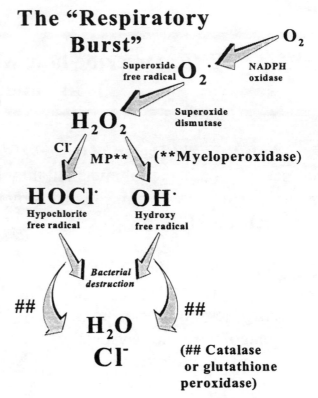

Figure 1-27: The myeloperoxidase system is the most potent white cell bacterial "killing mechanism."

Can free radicals be harmful? You bet — they are very nondiscriminating and will "eat up" anything in their path. Imagine the release of free radicals at an inappropriate time. If not eliminated promptly, cell membrane damage is likely to occur. In fact, this is the mechanism by which several common diseases take their toll on the body: hypoglycemia, stroke, myocardial infarction, congestive heart failure. So, under normal conditions, free radicals may be life-saving (killing bacteria); other times, they are potentially fatal. A classic example of a normal regulatory system,

> *REMEMBER:* Free radical formation during many diseases is a "classic" example of a normal regulatory system's responding "normally" to an inappropriate stimulus.

activated under "inappropriate" circumstances! Since free radical reactions involve oxidation-reduction, antioxidant agents (e.g., vitamin C, certain fish oils) have been used therapeutically in an attempt to decrease damage.

What happens in persons with glucose 6-phosphate dehydrogenase (G6PD) deficiency? G6PD catalyzes the conversion of glucose 6-phosphate to 6-phosphogluconolactone in the hexose monophosphate pathway (a means to make ribose compounds, and NADPH). (The big names aren't really as important as the concept.) When G6PD catalyzes this reaction, the high energy phosphate compound NADPH is formed. And, the presence of NADPH is essential for glutathione peroxidase to convert peroxide free radicals to water. So, if G6PD is deficient, lesser amounts of NADPH are formed, increasing the number of free radicals in cells.

G6PD deficiency also impairs the ability of the RBCs to form NADPH, resulting in hemolysis. When red blood cells in patients with G6PD deficiency are exposed to antimalarial drugs (primaquine) or sulfa antibiotics, the red cells generate free radicals that cannot be broken down normally. The result — hemolysis of red blood cells, jaundice, and sometimes, renal failure. The same thing happens when these patients eat fava beans, leading to the descriptive term "favism."

> # *OBJECTIVE:* Define and describe the role of apoptosis in both normal physiology and in disease states.

Apoptosis. **Apoptosis** is normal, genetically-programed cell death. It exhibits characteristic nuclear changes (chromatin condensation and DNA fragmentation). Typically, cells die in well-defined clusters rather than in a random fashion. The molecular mechanism of cell death is

DID YOU KNOW? **Evidence of inflammation is completely lacking in cells that have undergone apoptotic death?**

activation of genes that code for proteins known as **chymases** or **caspases**. Think of these as cellular "cyanide," since their production essentially leads to cell suicide. Unlike death from other causes, proteins and DNA undergo controlled degradation that allows them to be taken up and reused by neighboring cells. Apoptosis thus allows the body to eliminate a cell, yet "recycle" many of its components. Pathologically, there is a characteristic *lack* of inflammation in areas that have undergone apoptotic death. This is strikingly different, for example, from cells that have undergone necrosis from hypoxia or cellular toxins — an inflammatory response is typical.

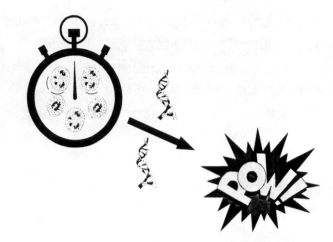

APOPTOSIS = genetically-programmed cell death

Apoptosis is unique in that it is genetically programmed into the cell as a part of normal development, organogenesis, immune function, and tissue growth. Apoptosis plays a normal role in aging, early development, menses, lactating breast tissue, thymus involution, and RBC turnover every 120 days. It can also be activated prematurely by pathological factors, such as cell injury.

Premature stimulation of apoptosis results in early cell death, such as in congestive heart failure. Another example of pathologic apoptosis is the death of hepatocytes (liver cells) in patients with viral hepatitis. The dying cells form chromatin lumps of chromatin, typical in apoptosis, known in hepatitis as Councilman bodies. Factors that inhibit the normal course of apoptosis result in unwanted cellular proliferation. Examples include cancer and rheumatoid arthritis (uncontrolled synovial tissue proliferation).

Recent data[2] have demonstrated the existence of **sentrin**, an anti-apoptotic protein. Patients with rheumatoid arthritis (RA) have up-regulation (*increased* sensitivity) of sentrin receptors. The result — decreased normal apoptosis of synovial tissue. This is now thought to explain the proliferation of synovial tissue in RA versus in other common arthridites (e.g., osteoarthritis). Synovial proliferation is not a feature of osteoarthritis.

Another recent study showed that administration of the drug indomethacin (Indocin®) led to induction of apoptosis in colon cancer cells. Though very exciting, the role of this agent, if any, in the routine therapy of colon cancer remains to be elucidated.[3] These findings are compatible with the finding that a normal pro-apoptotic gene, p53, is altered in over 50 percent of patients with cancer.

Ischemic and hypoxic injury. Ischemia and hypoxia are responsible for most cell injury seen in clinical practice. There are three types: reversible injury, irreversible injury, and reperfusion injury.

1.   **Reversible injury** may reverse, up to a certain point, if proper treatment is made available (including oxygen).

2.   **Irreversible injury** occurs once cells have passed a "point of no return," after which no treatment will help.

3.   **Reperfusion injury** results when blood flow is restored to cells that have been previously ischemic, leading to exacerbation of injury. This is a particularly important in the pathogenesis of myocardial infarction and stroke.

Chemical Mediators of Inflammation

OBJECTIVE: Define cytokines — describe their normal role in the inflammatory process.

Chemical mediators are substances that carry out various normal (and, at times, abnormal) tasks in the body. They are derived either from the plasma or from cells. Most perform their functions by binding to specific receptors on target cells. Some mediators stimulate the release of other mediators, leading to a vicious cycle. Others are relatively short-lived. Chemical mediators are another excellent example of the body's natural system of checks and balances — most mediators have both beneficial *and* potentially harmful effects.

There are lots of "big words" in the material that follows — it's the nature of the scientific beast. Those that are of the most practical importance, in my humble opinion, are placed in a larger font.

Vasoactive amines. Histamine and serotonin are some of the first mediators released in acute inflammation. They cause vasodilation and increased vascular permeability. Numerous stimuli lead to their release from mast cells, basophils, and platelets.

Plasma proteases. Three inter-related systems of plasma mediators formulate the plasma protease system — complement, kinins, and the clotting factors.

- Complement. The complement cascade is a series of events that occur resulting in formation of the **membrane attack complex** (MAC), which lyses bacterial cell membranes. Complement is activated either by antigen-antibody complexes, endotoxins, polysaccharides, or globulins.

- Kinin system. **Kinins** are vasoactive peptides generated from kinogens by specific proteases called kallikreins. The ultimate result is the formation of bradykinin. The cascade is activated when clotting factor XII is activated to factor XIIa and converts plasma prekallikrein into kallikrein. **Bradykinin** is a potent stimulator of increased vascular permeability, vasodilation, and bronchoconstriction.

- Clotting system. During activation of the clotting pathway, fibrinopeptides are formed that induce vascular permeability and are chemotactic (attractive) for leukocytes. In addition to clotting properties, thrombin also has anti-inflammatory properties, causing increased leukocyte adhesion to endothelium. Once factor XIIa is formed, it activates the fibrinolytic system, producing plasmin. Plasmin is involved in the cleavage of complement components, as well as in the formation of fibrin split products, which increase vascular permeability. Plasmin also activates factor XII, amplifying the response.

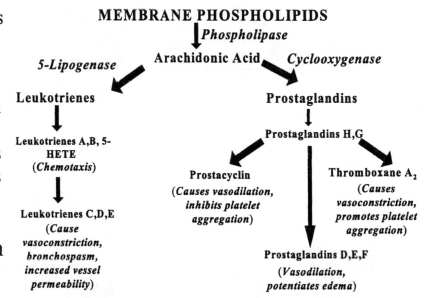

MEMBRANE PHOSPHOLIPIDS

↓ *Phospholipase*

Arachidonic Acid

5-Lipogenase   *Cyclooxygenase*

Leukotrienes   **Prostaglandins**

Leukotrienes A,B, 5-HETE (*Chemotaxis*)

Prostaglandins H,G

Leukotrienes C,D,E (*Cause vasoconstriction, bronchospasm, increased vessel permeability*)

Prostacyclin (*Causes vasodilation, inhibits platelet aggregation*)

Thromboxane A$_2$ (*Causes vasoconstriction, promotes platelet aggregation*)

Prostaglandins D,E,F (*Vasodilation, potentiates edema*)

Figure 1-28: The arachidonic acid pathway

Arachidonic acid metabolites — a generic response of cells to inflammatory stimuli is the formation of lipid mediators. These are referred to as **eicosanoids** and are synthesized from arachidonic acid by two sets of enzymes: **[FIGURE 1-28]**

- Cyclo-oxygenases generate **prostaglandins** and **thromboxanes**.
- Lipoxygenases produce **leukotrienes** and **liposins**.

Each of the following compounds has a slightly different role in the inflammatory cascade:

- Prostaglandin I_2 (prostacyclin) and prostaglandin E_2 cause vasodilation.

- Thromboxane A_2 causes vasoconstriction as do leukotrienes C_4, D_4, E_4. These leukotrienes also increase vascular permeability.

- Leukotriene B_4 has a powerful chemotactic effect.

- Liposins are thought to regulate leukotrienes.

[*NOTE: membrane phospholipids are the major source of arachidonic acid (via phospholipase A2), however, some is also produced via the metabolism of diacylglycerol (DAG) by lipase (not shown in **Figure 1-28**)*].

Platelet-activating factor. Platelet-activating factor (PAF) is produced by mast cells and leukocytes following a variety of stimuli, including Ig-E mediated allergic reactions. It causes platelet aggregation, as well as bronchoconstriction, vasodilation, increased vascular permeability, increased leukocyte adhesion, and leukocyte chemotaxis.

REMEMBER: **All mediators have normal functions, especially in the inflammatory response. Excess levels or "inappropriate" release results in disease.**

Cytokines. Cytokines are proteins produced by activated lymphocytes and macrophages that modulate the function of other cells. There are five classes:

1. Cytokines that regulate lymphocyte function — IL-2 (interleukin-2) and IL-4 promote lymphocyte growth, while IL-10 and transforming growth factor-β have inhibitory effects.

2. Cytokines involved with natural immunity — This group includes tumor necrosis factor alpha (TNF-α), interleukin-1β (IL-1β), interleukin-6 (IL-6), and the interferons.

3. Cytokines that activate inflammatory cells — This group includes various interferons, TNF-α, IL-5, IL-10, and IL-12.

4. Chemokines — cytokines that have chemotactic activity (attractants) for leukocytes. Chemokines perform their activities by binding to G-protein-linked receptors.

5. Cytokines that stimulate hematopoiesis. These cytokines influence growth and differentiation of leukocytes: examples include IL-3, granulocyte-macrophage colony stimulating factor (GM-CSF), macrophage colony stimulating factor (M-CSF), granulocyte-CSF (G-CSF), and stem cell factor.

Nitric oxide. Also known as endothelium-derived relaxing factor, nitric oxide (NO) vasodilates, inhibits platelet aggregation and adhesion, and may act as a free radical. It is important both in inflammation and in the host response to infection.

Neuropeptides. These compounds play a major role in the initiation of an inflammatory response. **Substance P** transmits pain signals, regulates blood pressure and vascular permeability, and stimulates secretion by immune and endocrine cells.

Please note again that *all* of the above cytokines have a *normal* function as part of the body's normal regulatory systems. However, when released under "inappropriate" circumstances, they worsen the situation. **[TABLE 1-1]**

MEDIATOR	SOURCE	VASCULAR LEAKAGE	CHEMOTAXIS
Histamine, serotonin	Mast cells, platelets	✔	✖
Bradykinin	Plasma	✔	✖
C3a	Plasma	✔	✖
C5a	Macrophages	✔	✔
Prostaglandins	Mast cells, membrane phospholipids	Potentiates other mediators	✖
Leukotriene B	WBC	✖	✔
Leukotrienes C,D,E	WBC, mast cells	✔	✖
Oxygen metabolites	WBC	✔	✖
Platelet activating factor	WBC, mast cells	✔	✔
Interleukin-1, tumor necrosis factor	Macrophages	✖	✔
Chemokines	WBC	✖	✔
Nitric oxide	Macrophages, endothelium	✔	✔

Table 1-1 — Chemical Mediators

[✔] = has an effect; [✖] = no effect

PART II — "CLINICAL BASICS"

The ABCs
General Approach to a Sick Patient
Take an AMPLE History
Patient Assessment — the "Thinking Cook" Approach
The "Heart-Lung-Brain" Triad
The Four Fixes
Principles of Laboratory Tests
Principles of X-rays

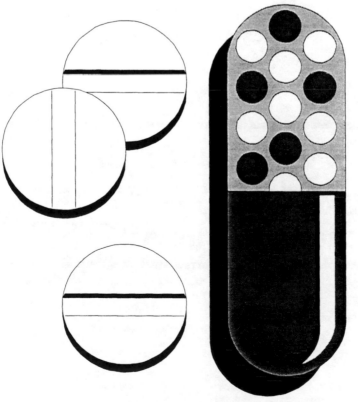

The ABCs

As complex as the human body is, the reasons people live and die (at least from a medical point of view) are simple — air enters the lungs when we breathe, oxygen circulates to the tissues, and waste products are eliminated. When any of these processes fail, regardless of the reason, we're in big trouble — agreed? As I've said earlier, the more fancy drugs and skills we acquire, the more likely we are to develop "tunnel vision" and lose track of the fact that most people get better or worse because of Airway, Breathing, and Circulation (the ABCs), *not* the latest drug in the Journal of Advanced Pharmacologic Esoterics (please don't try to find this one on MedLine — it's a Rothenberg creation!!).

Please don't get me wrong — I love research and the scientific method. My only objection is when it blinds us to reality; the basics are still the most important thing. Over my nearly 30 years of practice, I've found that when the going gets rough, the best thing to do is to assume that the real problem lies with the ABCs and look there. And, I intend to show you that many of our "newer" treatments for disease are based on re-establishing the integrity of airway, breathing, and circulation — as they should be. Please don't forget the basics — they will save you and your patient every time!

PRINCIPLE: All physiology/pathophysiology starts and ends with the ABCs!

General Approach to a Sick Patient

OBJECTIVE: Delineate the basic principles of patient care.

Whether acute (e.g., emergency department) or chronic (e.g., clinic setting), the generic approach to patient care should be the same:

1. *Am I safe?* Though most of us think of the "scene survey" as an out of hospital technique, we're wrong. All clinicians must establish and ensure their personal safety. For whatever reason, if we are too sick or injured to do our job, nobody benefits! Some situations are obvious, such as a violent patient. Those aren't the ones that get us into trouble — it's the subtle ones. Take, for example, the person with a "little cough." That patient's tuberculosis forced twelve staff members in one emergency department to take isoniazid (INH) for a year. And, there's one friend of mine who still can't walk right after being kicked in the back by a hypoglycemic patient who was abruptly woken up by a dextrose (DW50) bolus.

    Those of us who work in a trauma center expect to be exposed to all types of flying secretions. And, several studies point out that the more "blood and crud" is present, the less widespread is the use of "universal precautions," "body substance isolation precautions," or whatever the latest catch-all term happens to be. The bottom line — it's OK and *very important* to take care of ourselves first![4]

General Approach to a Sick Patient:

- **Am I safe?**
- **Life-threatening -problems?**
- **Do I need help?**
- **What's going on?**
- **What am I going to do?**

---

2. ***Is there something that I'd better fix NOW or the patient dies?***
    Regardless of the setting, once we've ensured our own safety, our job is
    to identify rapidly any potentially life-threatening problems and fix
    them. The ABCs always comes first.

3. ***Do I need help now?*** It's far easier to call out the troops and then
    apologetically send them back after a false alarm than to call too late.
    This step of "who do I call first when I need help?" applies equally well
    to all health care settings. In the field, calling an advanced life support
    unit or helicopter is obvious. In the clinic, it might mean calling an
    ambulance. In the hospital, "help" means things ranging from calling a
    "code" to obtaining a consult. Depends on who and where you are.

4. ***What's going on?*** One you've taken care of protecting yourself,
    keeping the patient alive, and getting help on the way, the next step is
    to figure out what's wrong. This does not necessarily mean that you
    must make a "final diagnosis." In the clinic, field, or emergency
    department setting, the most important thing to ascertain (after dealing
    with immediate life threats) is "how sick is the patient?" I've admitted
    many patients to the hospital from both the clinic and the emergency
    department with "provisional diagnoses," some of which turned out to
    be wrong. And, the patient *still* needed to be in the hospital!

5. ***What am I going to do about it?*** The decisions here depend on your
    location and legal scope of practice, as well as the patient (*real* sick
    versus not very sick). Applying an understanding of basic (yet elegant)
    pathophysiology, combined with always remembering the importance
    of ABCs, will guide you best here. This last step in our approach to
    patient care forms the "meat" of the rest of this book.

Take an AMPLE History

OBJECTIVE: Define and explain what is meant by an "AMPLE" history.

I'm not a big fan of acronyms (or of memorizing), because it's easy to forget what the letters stand for! There are a couple, though, that we all need to know. The most important is "ABC" (Airway, Breathing, and Circulation),

---

PRINCIPLE: You're only as good as the information you have to work with.

---

followed by "AMPLE." It's important to acquire rapidly all the relevant information possible, and the way to do this is to take an "**AMPLE**" history:

- **A** = **A**llergies
- **M** = **M**edications
- **P** = **P**ast History
- **L** = **L**ast Meal
- **E** = **E**vents (what happened?)

OBJECTIVE: Give two examples where failure to take an adequate medication history may result in misdiagnosis, bad patient outcome, or both.

A word about the "**M.**" It's easy, especially if you're busy, to simply ask, "Do you take any medications?" If the patient answers no, we're on to the next question. Let me suggest that this question is one of the most important historical items we ever ask. As such, it *must* be more detailed:

1. *Do you take any medications with or without a prescription, including over-the-counter drugs, birth control pills, pills for impotence, or herbal preparations?* Some people don't think of birth control pills as medications unless we specifically remind them. Some of the impotence preparations for erectile dysfunction have a potential interaction with nitrates, since both lead to the production of nitric oxide, a vasodilator. Conceivably, the combination could result in life-threatening hypotension.

DID YOU KNOW? Excessive use of over-the-counter ephedra alkaloid products has led to more than a dozen reported deaths, often due to heart failure?

The majority of currently available herbals do not come under the control of the FDA. Because of this, many people (including health care professionals) forget that these still contain *drugs*. Whether "officially" regulated or not, herbals have pharmacologic activity.[5] (See **Table 1-2**, immediately below).

DID YOU KNOW? St. John's Wort induces an enzyme responsible for the metabolism of more than 73 medications, including oral contraceptives, antiepileptics, calcium channel blockers, and some antibiotics? This leads to increased rates of drug clearance and may affect a patient's response.

Table 1-2: COMMON HERBAL MEDICINES

HERB	USE	SIDE EFFECTS	DRUG INTERACTIONS
Aloe vera	Burns, skin injuries, cosmetics (external use)	None known	None known
Cascara sagrada	Stimulant laxative	Intestinal cramping	Loss of potassium with chronic use may cause digitalis toxicity and cardiac arrhythmias
Capsium (Cayenne, hot pepper)	Pain relief in shingles, arthritis	Hypersensitivity	May interfere with MAO inhibitors; may increase liver metabolism of various drugs
Chamomile	Antispasmodic for indigestion, flatulence, GI tract inflammation	None known	None known
Cranberry	Prevention of urinary tract infection	None known	None known
Dandelion	Natural diuretic (leaves)	None known	None known
Dong quai	"Female tonic" to treat muscle cramps and pain during menstrual period	Contraindicated during pregnancy and lactation	Increases activity of blood thinning drugs (anti-coagulants, anti-platelet drugs)
Echinacea	Wound treatment; strengthening of immune system; treatment of colds and flu	Contraindicated in progressive systemic diseases (TB, MS)	May interfere with immuno-suppressive therapy

Evening primose	Menstrual irregularities; arthritis pain	Mild headache, abdominal pain; not recommended for patients diagnosed with schizophrenia	Increased risk of temporal lobe epilepsy in schizophrenic patients being treated with phenothiazines (e.g., Thorazine)
Feverfew	Pain relief; menstrual cramps; migraine headache	Occasional mouth ulceration or gastric disturbance	None known
Garlic	Cardiovascular conditions; high cholesterol or triglycerides; prevention of colds and flu	Rare GI symptoms	May increase the activity of warfarin (Coumadin) anti-coagulants
Ginger	Nausea, motion sickness, vomiting	Heartburn; may aggravate gallstone disease	Large doses may interfere with cardiac, antidiabetic, or anticoagulant therapy
Ginkgo	Conditions associated with aging (memory loss, poor-circulation); tinnitus (ringing in the ears); vertigo	Contraindicated in pregnancy and lactation	None known
Ginseng	Increase resistance to all types of stress; increase energy and endurance	None known; avoid in acute illness, hypertension	Stimulants, coffee, antipsychotic drugs, MAO inhibitors
Goldenseal	Wound healing; colds and flu	Contraindicated during pregnancy and lactation; also in high blood pressure	May oppose the anticoagulant action of heparin
Hawthorn	Heart conditions (angina)	None known	None known

Kava kava root	Nervous anxiety, stress, restlessness; insomnia	Contraindicated in endogenous depression, pregnancy and lactation	May potentiate alcohol, barbiturates, and various psychopharmacological agents
Licorice	Inflammation; adrenal gland stimulation	Headache, lethargy, sodium and water retention, excessive loss of potassium, high blood pressure	Loss of potassium may increase sensitivity to digitalis glycosides
Milk thistle	Improvement of liver function	Mild laxative effect	None known
Passion flower	Mild sedative for insomnia	None known	None known
Peppermint	Antispasmodic action on stomach and intestinal tract	None known	None known
Psyllium	Major source of fiber; used as bulk laxative	Intestinal cramping	None known
Saw palmetto	Benign prostatic hypertrophy (BPH); increases urine flow and reduces frequency of nightime urination	Headaches, diarrhea	None known
Senna	Laxative	Long-term dependence may develop	None known
St. John's wort	Mild to moderate depression	Photosensitization; contraindicated during pregnancy	May potentiate MAO inhibitors; should not be used at the same time as prescription antidepressants
Valerian	Sedative, sleep aid; said to be nonhabit forming	None known	None known

[Adopted from Dictionary of Medical Terms, 4th Edition; Mikel A. Rothenberg, MD; Barron's Medical Guides 2000, with permission]

2. *Do you ever use drugs or drink alcohol?* I know that the chances of getting "the truth, and nothing but the truth" are sometimes slim, but we still need to ask. Then, there's always the patient who tells me "I just drink beer, I never drink alcohol." Go figure. . .

3. *Have you changed or stopped any medications within the last two weeks?* This is probably the most important part of the question and the most frequently omitted. There are several medications that result in potentially life-threatening situations when they are abruptly stopped. These include clonidine, β-blockers, and alpha-methyldopa. Used to be that the patient was the one to "cold turkey" the drug because it caused more ill effects (tiredness, impotence) than the condition it was prescribed for (hypertension). Now, the health care provider (*read my lips — us!*) is the likely culprit.

With the proliferation of new drugs and associated television advertising, we often receive lots of free samples. The patient is given the new drug and told to stop the old one abruptly. We forget that the new drug may take two or more days (two to three pharmacological half-lives) to reach an adequate serum level. Meanwhile, the old drug is metabolized and eliminated from the body. The net result is that there is a period of time during which the patient is not covered by any drug, "old" or "new."

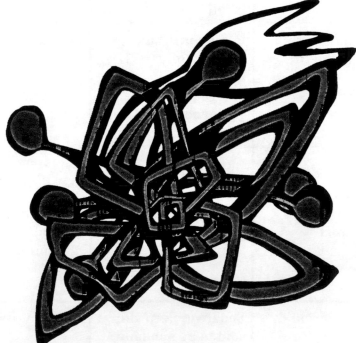

Drug interactions are a common source of patient problems.

Patient Assessment — the "Thinking Cook" Approach

> **OBJECTIVE:** Describe and apply in your clinical practice major patient assessment principles.

This section is not intended to replace standard texts on physical examination. Rather, I want to give you some principles that will allow you to remember *details* by understanding the "*whys*." These principles work as well in an emergency department as they do in

> **PRINCIPLE:** There's nothing wrong with a "cookbook approach," as long as there's a thinking cook!

a primary care office, and anywhere else you choose. Many consider the traditional approach to assessment a "cookbook." As long as a "thinking cook" is using the "cookbook," I've got no problem. And, I assume that if you've read this far into this book, you are *definitely* a "thinking cook."

Vital signs and the primary survey. After ensuring our own safety, assess the patient's vital signs. In emergency medicine, the approach is termed the **primary survey** or **initial assessment**. The logic, regardless of your "playing field," is the same: rapidly assess the adequacy of **Airway, Breathing**, and **Circulation**. As we'll see later,

> **REMEMBER:** The primary survey rapidly evaluates integrity of Airway, Breathing, and Circulation (the ABCs).

the primary survey forms the *basis* of the causes and treatment of diseases. Depending on the situation, you may or may not stop to obtain a full set of vital signs at this point. First:

- **A** — The **A**irway is at least partially open if the patient is able to vocalize.

- **B** — Rapidly auscultate both sides of the chest to ascertain that **B**reathing (breath sounds) is adequate and symmetrical.

- **C** — Estimate adequacy of **C**irculation by evaluating peripheral pulses and capillary refill. As a rough estimate, you can estimate systolic BP by the presence or absence of palpable peripheral pulses (radial = 80 mm Hg; femoral = 70 mm Hg; carotid = 60 mm Hg). Capillary refill, in an adult, should normally be less than two seconds, and is unreliable in a cold environment.

  Capillary refill has been the subject of debate in recent years. Remember that it is *one* subjective aid in your *entire* evaluation of the patient, not the bottom line. Now, the controversial data: in patients who had significant hypovolemia (defined as > 450 cc of blood loss acutely), only 64% had delayed capillary refill. The investigators suggested that capillary refill is not useful for detecting mild-to-moderate hypovolemia in adults. They also noted that orthostatic vital signs were more sensitive and specific.[6] Unfortunately, other data have questioned the value of orthostatic vital signs in similar groups of patients (mild to moderate hypovolemia).[7]

- **D** — Disability; many experts add this letter to the acronym as a way of reminding us also to evaluate rapidly a patient's mental status. We'll talk about the Glasgow Coma scale next. In the initial approach to a patient, the "AVPU" scale is quicker. Our "mini-neurological exam" at this point consists of pupillary evaluation (size, equality, and reactivity), as well as a patient's AVPU level of consciousness (**A** = alert; **V** = responds to vocal stimuli; **P** = responds to painful stimuli; **U** = unresponsive).

Most of us are used to the **Glasgow Coma Scale** (GCS). Remember, this is only a guide, and was originally developed to monitor head-injured adults. In brief, the patient receives points for the best motor, verbal, and eye opening response (motor = 6; verbal = 5; eye opening =4). Thus, the best possible score is "15." Statistically, a score below "9" in an adult independently portends a bad outcome. Other scales are more helpful in small children. By the way — we like to use the term "alert and oriented times three" (person, place, time) — imagine how silly it looks if you write that a two-month child is "A&O X3!" This is laughable. I prefer to state that a baby follows me with the eyes, or that a toddler "gives me five with enthusiasm." Seems a lot clearer when inquiring minds really want to know. . .☺

A few comments on "vital signs" are essential at this point:

1.   Though most of us are taught that the normal adult respiratory rate is less than 20 BPM, data suggest that at least in emergency department patients, the average rate is 21 BPM. And, this is in patients with *no* respiratory complaints. So, the "normal" respiratory rate may actually be higher (or at least, the range somewhat wider) than suggested in most of the medical literature.[8]

2.   Pulse oximetry is often relied upon as the "fifth vital sign." Though a fair amount of supportive data exist, I saw perfectly competent health care providers act "stupid"

> **PRINCIPLE**: If the patient looks *sick* and the test looks good, the patient is still *sick*!

when these devices first became widespread. The reason — as long as the oxygen saturation was over 90%, we started to assume that all was well in "patientland." NOT!! If the patient looks sick and the test looks good — guess what? The patient is likely sick. Don't let a machine overrule your instincts.

3. Temperature — a favorite technique, especially in primary care, is the ear thermometer (tympanic membrane temperature). Again, you can find data on both sides of the fence, which I won't delve into here. Just remember that the TM temperature is an *estimate* that works in many, but not all, people. It's also a great scream (especially in little kids) and time saver. On the other hand, if there is a case (e.g., hypothermia, sepsis) where you *really care what the temperature is*, rectal temperature remains the "gold standard."

4. Breath sounds — I've witnessed more arguments over what to "call" various breath sounds than just about any other subject in health care. The bottom line is simple: studies have repeatedly shown that we really don't know the difference between "rhonchi" and "rales." (At least, I don't know what you really mean, and vice versa.) Before you report me to the local Medical Board, look at the data just below.

    The International Lung Sounds Association is a group dedicated to the understanding of intrathoracic acoustics. They have performed several studies — all with the same result. Investigators took groups of health care providers (different disciplines) and played tape recordings of breath sounds. The listeners used a checklist to record if they thought the breath sounds were wheezes, rhonchi, or rales. Turned out, no one agreed. Most important was the fact that they retested the same group with the *same* recordings two weeks later. This time, investigators determined whether you agreed with *yourself* two weeks ago. Guess what? We didn't agree with each other *or* with ourselves![9] Numerous other studies have confirmed these results — our communication of what we hear is far less than ideal.[10] And, the problem seems to extend to the scientific literature. One study of lung sound terms in the scientific literature concluded that: "It is evident that current usage varies widely, even in the terminology of the basic categories of sounds."[11]

That's why I'd rather use descriptive terminology (e.g., "wet sounding," "crackles") than ill-defined, but sometimes popular terms (e.g., rhonchi, rales). By the way, most studies agreed on the sound of wheezing, so I think we're relatively safe there.

Hints to make things smoother for everyone. When we learn physical diagnosis, we're generally so busy learning to use new equipment and memorizing findings that we lose track of the basics (so, what's new??). There are two simple and elegant rules that will help:

1. *We are symmetrical* — With few exceptions, much of what happens on one side of the body should also occur on the other. Think about it — breath sounds, neurological findings, pupillary responses — the *absence of symmetry* is a big "red flag" that something might be wrong. Use it to your and to the patient's advantage.

2. *If you know the normal, the abnormal is usually obvious* — I use this principle all the time. We all know that the normal heart sounds something like "lub-dub," right? Well, if we hear "lub-da-dub" or "lub-splash-dub" or some other heartsong

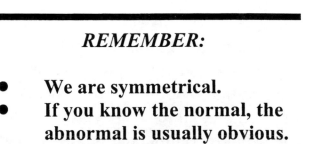

REMEMBER:

- **We are symmetrical.**
- **If you know the normal, the abnormal is usually obvious.**

(besides "lub-dub"), we should immediately recognize that something's different. The exact cause and pathological significance is of less immediate concern than recognizing that "something's wrong with this picture." And, we can apply this to breath sounds, fundoscopic examination. . . in fact, to just about any part of patient evaluation. Your assignment — think about how many different areas of patient assessment (including lab and x-ray studies) you can apply this principle to. In so doing, you will also improve your patient care skills exponentially!

The "Heart-Lung-Brain" Triad

> **OBJECTIVE:** Draw and summarize the significance of the "Heart-Lung-Brain" triad.

Pathophysiology involves an understanding of inter-relationships between various organ systems. Nowhere is this more true than in the interplay between heart, lungs, and brain. I have termed this the "Heart-Lung-Brain Triad" [**FIGURE 1-29**] and the bottom line is clear: *when something goes wrong with one system, the others are inevitably affected.*

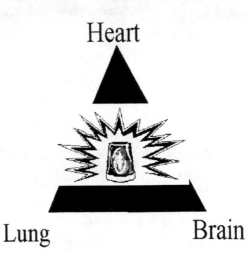

Figure 1-29: The heart-lung-brain triangle.

I originally taught this concept in relationship to neurological events, before I realized that it applies to *all* types of patient problems. Patients with stroke, for example, all tend to hypoventilate, regardless of their clinical appearance. The usual recommendation, then, is to apply nasal oxygen (2-3 LPM) for at least the first 24 hours.

Persons with subarachnoid hemorrhage often have EKG changes, such as symmetrically inverted T-waves. Many of us were taught that this represents simply "CNS changes" of no particular importance. In some cases, though, these "classic" (sarcasm implied) CNS changes have been shown, in fact, to represent concomitant myocardial ischemia, due to the massive release of catecholamines as a result of the irritant effect of subarachnoid blood. . . and there are many more. Rather than memorize specific instances, it's safest to assume that these inter-relationships are present in a wide variety of patient problems. That way, you won't miss anything.

The Four Fixes

OBJECTIVE: List and explain the significance of "The Four Fixes."

First, the disclaimer — many of us are used to protocols, clinical guidelines, and other "cookbook" types of directions. And, it's real easy to get into trouble if we don't think. As I mentioned earlier, I have absolutely no problem with "cookbook medicine," as long as there is a "thinking cook." So, when I present a generic approach, I know that each of you will use your common sense and professional judgement in applying it to a real patient. Of course, we all have to deal with scope of practice and other legal issues, though they will not be discussed in detail here. Thanks, now I feel better.

My disclaimer considered, wouldn't it be nice if we came up with a short list of "easy to diagnose things that make people sick in lots of ways?" You bet — and here it is:

- Hypoxia.
- Hypoglycemia.
- Hypovolemia.
- Hyposhockemia.

The above list, though far from all-inclusive, is associated intimately with the ABCs, and presents four conditions that may cause a wide variety of clinical syndromes. It's easy to "diagnose" all of these, and even empirically treat the first three with very little risk to the patient. There are many clinical presentations of hypoglycemia (e.g., coma, seizures, altered level of consciousness, tachycardia), hypoxia, hypovolemia, and hyposhockemia

I-71

(dysrhythmias). I suggest that you always consider that any or all of these could cause or contribute to a patient's condition. Just as you should always go back to the ABCs, use these "Four Fixes" to find and correct common causes of a wide variety of patient problems.

Finally, notice how the "Four Fixes" relate to the ABCs. Hypoxia is obvious (airway, breathing), as should be hypovolemia and hyposhockemia (circulation, but with a liberal dose of airway and breathing thrown in, due to the need to keep tissues oxygenated). Hypoglycemia can manifest in a variety of ways, including respiratory depression. Always think: oxygen, sugar, fluids, electricity. Remember, common things are common! Use it to your patient's advantage.

The Four Fixes:

ALWAYS THINK: OXYGEN, SUGAR, FLUIDS, ELECTRICITY!

- **Hypoxia.**
- **Hypoglycemia.**
- **Hypovolemia.**
- **Hyposhockemia.**

Principles of Laboratory Tests

OBJECTIVE: List and explain two rules that conceptualize and summarize the principles of laboratory tests.

To understand laboratory tests, it's essential to have a grasp on the underlying physiology. I've incorporated relevant "tests" into many of the discussions in the upcoming chapters for exactly this reason. Right now, I want to give you an easy, but very helpful overview that applies to most lab tests we use.

The most important rule for *any test* is: "A normal test doesn't mean a normal patient." Remember, you were smarter than any test from the day you were born — and you only get better with increasing training and experience. When in doubt, rely on your intuition, brains, and experience! If the test looks *good* and the patient looks *bad* — guess what? — The patient is *BAD*! Don't let a "test" change what your "medical intuition" tells you.

PRINCIPLE: A normal test *doesn't* mean a normal patient!

Without getting too picky, it's safe to assume that most lab results, especially "blood tests," fall into two possible categories — normal or abnormal. We can break "abnormal" down further into "too high" or "too low" for most tests. Thus, the possibilities for a test result are: normal, too high, or too low — agreed? As a general rule, normal is better than abnormal (too high, too low), though please remember that a normal test does not necessarily mean a normal patient.

Many lab results are reported as concentrations (e.g., meq/L). As such, we can apply a simple principle — the most common thing that affects our bodies, as reflected in abnormal lab results, is *fluid balance*. Think about it — dehydration or overhydration causes either hemoconcentration or hemodilution, which will be reflected in a myriad of lab tests. These range from urine specific gravity to hemoglobin/hematocrit to serum sodium. And, many endocrine diseases result in abnormal levels of hormones that either directly or indirectly affect water balance (e.g., hyperaldosteronism, Cushing's disease).

The next principle is directly related — *drugs* are the other "generic" explanation for the majority of laboratory abnormalities. Many drugs (e.g., diuretics, angiotensin converting enzyme inhibitors) have potential effects on fluid balance. There are three common categories of drugs that often affect lab values:

1. **Oxygen.** Surprised? You shouldn't be, since oxygen is a drug as well as a basic essential of life. However, when the O_2 levels are altered, they don't affect just the pO_2; chronic hypoxia also leads to other changes, such as increased hematocrit.

2. **Nonsteroidal anti-inflammatory drugs** (NSAIDs). As a group, these drugs are well-tolerated in most patients. The low incidence of side effects is counterbalanced by the fact that so many people take these drugs, with and without a prescription. Thus, we're *real* likely to see some type of side effect from them, whether it be gastritis, GI (gastrointestinal) bleeding, or a lab abnormality.

> ***REMEMBER:***
>
> - *Fluids* and *drugs* are **responsible for many laboratory abnormalities.**
> - **If the patient is on *any* medication, consider it a *possible cause* of the problem until proven otherwise!**

3. **Antibiotics (ABs).** As with the NSAIDS, the majority of "culprits" here are very safe and *very* commonly used. The net result is the same; we're bound, in the average primary care setting, to see problems. Sulfa drugs, cephalosporins, and fluoroquinolones lead the list in frequency of use, and thus, frequency of causing lab abnormalities. **[FIGURE 1-30]**

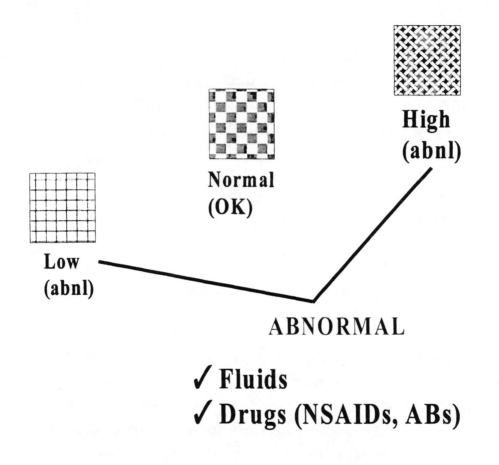

High (abnl)

Normal (OK)

Low (abnl)

ABNORMAL

✓ **Fluids**
✓ **Drugs (NSAIDs, ABs)**

Figure 1-30: Fluids and drugs are the most common cause of laboratory abnormalities.

Principles of X-rays

X-rays are another example of elegant simplicity. I'll give you the basics right now. If you're interested in more detail, please see my text, "Understanding X-Rays — A Plain English Approach" (Professional Education Systems Healthcare Division, Eau Claire, WI).

The easiest way to understand x-rays is to accept the fact that there is a *significant* difference between "clinical anatomy" and "x-ray anatomy." The anatomy that most clinicians learn is based upon colors, textures, and shapes as viewed in three dimensions. Things look the way they do because of their composition (muscle, bone, blood, etc.) and shape. When we open up the chest cavity, we see various organs and structures in full color and three dimensions.

If we take an x-ray of the *identical* area, however, it looks different. We have a two-dimensional view of a three-dimensional patient, and our "colors" are limited to black and white, with shades of gray in between (gray-scale). What we see on an x-ray is based on ***radiological (x-ray) density*** and shape. X-ray density is not the same as physical density. X-ray density is the ability of a structure or substance to *absorb* x-rays. The more radiodense (radiopaque) a structure, the more x-rays it absorbs, and vice-versa for radiolucent materials. Thus, by absorbing more x-rays, radiodense materials

PRINCIPLE: Radiographic density is different from physical density. XR density refers to the ability of a substance to *absorb* (block) x-rays.

effectively block or attenuate passage of the beam (by absorbing x-rays to a variable degree, depending upon their radiodensity), resulting in *fewer* x-rays hitting the film plate. Radiolucent materials let more x-rays through (because they absorb *less*), allowing *more* x-rays to hit the film.

The difference between x-ray and physical density is extremely important. A block of lead (physically dense *and* x-ray dense) has the same x-ray density as a cup of liquid x-ray contrast material (physically not very dense [liquid], but as x-ray dense as lead). Thus, an x-ray of either, side by side, should look the same.

The reason any x-ray looks the way it does is related directly to the number of x-rays that strikes a given portion of the film. In my x-ray course and book, I call this the "More of me, less of me" rule. "Me" refers to the x-ray beam:

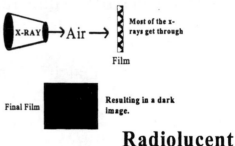

- The *more of me* (x-rays) that hits the film, the *darker* that area turns once the film is processed ("developed").

- The *less of me* (x-rays) that hits the film, the *lighter* that areas turns following processing. **[FIGURE 1-31]**

Radiolucent
"More of me. . ."

"More of me, less of me" is the reason *any* x-ray looks the way it does, whether it's of a body part, a car, or a toaster. If we know what the normal "x-ray color" of an object is, we can then determine what might be wrong when a film or area on a film is "too dark" or "too light." ("Colors" refer to black, white, and shades of gray in between.)

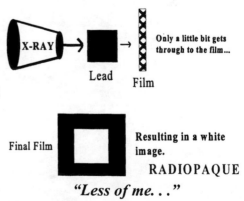

RADIOPAQUE
"Less of me. . ."

Figure 1-31: "More of me, less of me" tells it all regarding understanding of x-rays. [Reproduced, with permission, from "Understanding X-Rays: A Plain English Approach, Mikel A. Rothenberg, MD, 1999; PESI]

"Too dark" or "too light," in x-ray terms ("more of me, less of me"), means either *too much* or *too little* radiation hit the film, as compared to normal, right? Generically, the reasons for this are limited to one of two:

1. Too much or too little radiation is "shot through" *normal* tissue — an overpenetrated or underpenetrated film ("technical factors") — resulting in too many or too few x-rays hitting the film.

2. The correct amount of radiation is "shot through" *abnormal* tissue that either lets too much through or absorbs more than normal. The result is too many or too few x-rays reaching the film.

The net effect, regardless of which of the above causes is responsible, is that either too much or too little radiation hits the film, resulting in an area that is either too light or too dark.

Since it's a given that x-ray anatomy and clinical anatomy are different, our job is to simultaneously "translate" between the "two languages." When we talk about disease processes, we describe what goes on pathophysiologically and anatomically. By translating "clinical anatomy" into x-ray anatomy, understanding the x-ray is straight-forward (though not always "easy").

Take, for example, an area on a film that is lighter than usual. That means *too little* radiation hit the film (i.e., less than normal). Based on the rules above, the choices are either that the film is underpenetrated or that the tissue itself is more radiodense than usual — OK so far? Well, an underpenetrated film should result in the *entire film's* being too light, rather than one isolated area. Unless the entire film is too dark or too light, technical considerations are unlikely to be responsible. With isolated "too dark" or "too light" areas, it's most likely a normal exposure with an abnormal tissue (either more radiodense or radiolucent than usual). In our example, we surmise since just a localized area is too light, that whatever structure or structures this area corresponds to anatomically has absorbed more x-rays than usual (ie., become more radiodense), allowing fewer than normal to hit the film. The result — an area that is "too light" as compared to normal. **[FIGURE 1-32]**

Depending on the film, the above change ("too light") could represent many disease states. On a chest x-ray, "too light" over the lung fields often means an infiltrate, due to accumuled abnormal matter (e.g., pus, blood, lymph, serum) within the lung parenchyma that absorbs more x-ray than normal lung tissue. As a result, less hits that area of the film and it turns "lighter" than usual.

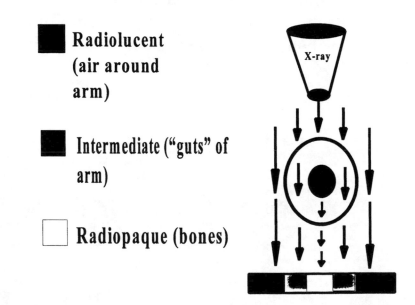

Figure 1-32: Lighter areas indicate that *fewer* x-rays have hit the film, while darker areas mean *more* x-rays have hit. [Reproduced, with permission, from "Understanding X-Rays: A Plain English Approach, Mikel A. Rothenberg, MD, 1999; PESI]

Summary

The beauty of medical thinking lies in its intrinsic simplicity. The "whys" of disease and patient care are elegant, yet basic. The "basics" are truly the foundation of everything we do in health care. Despite a proliferation of information in the new millenium, we cannot lose sight of the rules of the game. Patients live and die because of Airway, Breathing, and Circulation. Our mission is to relate our understanding of pathophysiology and treatment back to this cardinal principle, regardless of how complex the issue in question appears to be. Accept that the basics are, indeed, the most important pathophysiological concept (deal with it!) and everyone benefits. "Understanding is owning!"

PRINCIPLE: **When it "hits the fan," go back to basics!**

PRINCIPLE: **You're only as good as the information you have to work with.**

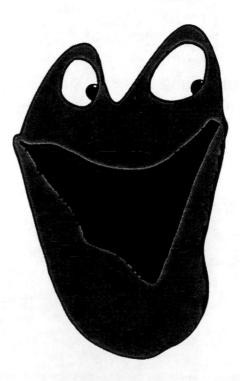

Understanding is owning. . .

I-80

Crossword Puzzle Review

Path Chap 1 -- The Basics

Across

1. The amino groups of most amino acids are ultimately funneled to _____.
5. Movement of substances across a membrane in combination with a carrier protein against an energy gradient.
9. Genetically-programmed cell death.
10. Chronic granulomatosis results from congenital deficiency of sufficient _____.
11. Always take an _____ history.
15. _____ are eventually broken down to acetyl CoA from fat digestion, which enters into the citric acid cycle.
17. Ketones _____ in the blood, resulting in free hydrogen ions.
18. During the _____ _____ _____ (3 words), acetyl CoA is converted to water and carbon dioxide, and ATP is produced.
20. Compound that becomes activated by the triplex of ligand-receptor and G-protein (two words).
21. Carries the genetic code to the cytoplasm to control the formation of proteins (abbrev).
24. Catalyzes conversion of ADP to ATP during oxidative phosphorylation.
25. The myriad of "checks and balances" in the body (abbrev).
26. Process where glycogen is broken down into glucose.
30. Remove phosphate groups from molecules.
32. Add phosphate groups to molecules.
34. Each cell contributes to and benefits from normal on-going processes.
38. There are more _____ among the body's systems than differences.
39. Main toxic product of the urea cycle.
40. Attached to activated G-proteins.
41. Electrons are shuttled between compounds known as _____ as they pass through the electron transport chain.
42. Potent stimulator of increased vascular permeability, vasodilation, and bronchoconstriction.
43. _____ is a steady state in the internal environment.
44. Proteins produced by activated lymphocytes and macrophages that modulate the function of other cells.
45. Carry sodium, potassium, chloride, and calcium ions between cells.
46. _____ splits glucose into two molecules of pyruvic acid (pyruvate).
46. Glycerol released from the metabolism of triglycerides is eventually metabolized via _____.

Down

2. Pyruvate is converted to _____.
3. All physiology and pathophysiology begins and ends with the _____.
5. Use cell membrane receptors, G-proteins, and second messengers.
6. Transports amino acids to the ribosomes to be used in the assembly of proteins (abbrev).
7. During starvation, ingestion of a ketogenic diet, or DKA, levels of ketone bodies _____ in the blood.
8. Each _____ is a double-stranded helical molecule of deoxyribonucleic acid (DNA) that controls formation of ribonucleic acid (RNA).
12. _____ is the first step in the catabolism of most amino acids.
13. During oxidative phosphorylation, _____ from hydrogen enter a series of reactions, known as the electron transport chain.
14. The first step in digestion of fat.
16. Typically use intracellular receptors, leading to de novo synthesis of new proteins.
17. Random movement of molecules through spaces in the membrane.
19. Process of making RNA from DNA.
22. _____ are highly-reactive chemical intermediates that are short one electron in their outer orbital shell.
23. Excess acetyl CoA from fat breakdown is converted to _____ _____ (2 words).
27. Characteristically lacking in cells that have undergone apoptosis.
28. General term for products made from arachadonic acid.
29. Attached to inactivated G-proteins.
31. The _____ consists of triplets of three successive bases on a DNA strand, each coding for a specific protein.
33. The "respiratory burst" results in the formation of hypochlorous acid, more commonly known as _____.
35. The main digestive product of proteins.
36. Carbohydrates do not require _____ to be absorbed through the intestinal mucosa.
37. Intracellular calcium and _____ are the two most common second messengers.
40. Stimuli that open or close ion channels.

References

1. Modell, HI. *How to help students understand physiology? Emphasize general models.* Adv Physiol Educ 2000; 23: 101-7.

2. Gay, SF, et al. *Sentrin highly expressed in synovial tissues in patients with rheumatoid arthritis.* Arthritis Rheum 2000; 43:599-607.

2. Hull, MA, et al. *NSAIDs exert their effects on colorectal cancer cells via diverse mechanisms.* Eur J Cancer 2000; 36:664-64.

4. Kim, LE, et al. *Compliance with universal precautions among emergency department personnel: implications for prevention programs.* Am J Infect Control 1999 Oct; 27(5):453-5.

5. See: Clin Pharmacol Ther 2000; 67:451-57, for article on St. John's Wort and metabolism of several commonly prescribed drugs.

6. Schriger, DL and Baraff, LJ. *Capillary refill — Is it a useful predictor of hypovolemic states?* Ann Emerg Med June 1991; 20:601-05.

7. Olziol-McLain, J, et al. *Orthostatic vital signs in Emergency Department patients.* Ann Emerg Med June 1991; 20:606-10.

8. Hooker, EL, et al. *Respiratory rates in Emergency Department patients,* J Emerg Med 1989; 7:129-132.

9. Mikami, R, et al. *Symposium on Lung Sounds. Synopsis of proceedings.* Chest 1987 Aug; 92(2):342-5.

10. See, for example: Wilkins, RL and Dexter, JR. *Comparing RCPs to physicians for the description of lung sounds: are we accurate and can we communicate?* Respir Care 1990 Oct; 35(10):969-76.

11. Bunin, NJ, et al. *Lung sound terminology in case reports.* Chest 1979 Dec; 76(6):690-2.

CHAPTER 2
ENDOCRINE AND METABOLIC PROBLEMS

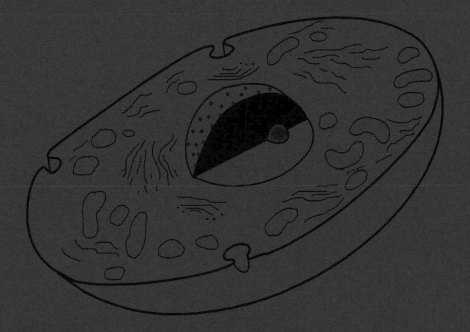

CHAPTER 2 — ENDOCRINE AND METABOLIC PROBLEMS

Contents

Objectives

After reading this chapter, you'll be able to:

Explain the major hormonal factors that regulate the blood glucose level, including insulin and counter-regulatory hormones.

Summarize the major actions of insulin on the metabolism of carbohydrates, proteins, and fats.

List and explain the mechanisms by which glucagon and epinephrine affect the blood glucose level.

Summarize the role of counter-regulatory hormones in the body's "early warning system" for hypoglycemia.

Summarize at least one therapeutic strategy that may be tried to improve awareness of early hypoglycemia.

Describe the Somogyi Phenomenon ("dawn phenomenon") — why it occurs; when it should be suspected; potential treatments.

Explain the pathophysiological basis for many of the neurological effects of prolonged hypoglycemia.

Describe at least two common situations where unsuspected hypoglycemia may be responsible for a patient's condition.

Describe the mechanism by which angiotensin converting enzyme (ACE) inhibitors increase a person's risk of hypoglycemia.

Explain the physiological basis for administering glucagon in suspected hypoglycemia.

List at least three clinical situations where a hypoglycemic patient should be observed for a period of several hours, rather than T&R'd (treated and released); what is the common pathophysiological parameter linking each of these clinical situations?

Illustrate the pathophysiology of diabetic ketoacidosis based on the "when insulin does, when insulin doesn't" concept.

Defend the concept that fluids are often the first and best therapy for DKA.

- Defend the concept that most patients in DKA are total-body potassium-depleted, regardless of their serum level.

Summarize the primary roles of sodium, potassium, chloride, and bicarbonate in the body.

Demonstrate how to use the measured serum bicarbonate level to determine the presence of metabolic acidosis or metabolic alkalosis.

- Summarize the kinetics of potassium in the presence of metabolic acidosis.

Define the acronym "SLUMPED" and defend its clinical utility.

Defend the statement: "The anion gap, as performed in most clinical laboratories, is of no benefit and may be dangerously misleading."

Enumerate the body's typical physiologic response to cold exposure; what are the implications of this response for the health care provider, regarding volume therapy?

What are the implications of the above responses for rescue and movement of hypothermic patients, especially from cold water situations?

- Illustrate and explain the "kinetics of bilirubin," and the origin and significance of urobilinogen.

Defend the statement: "the dip UA is the single best initial screening test for the jaundiced patient."

Formulate a plan to use the dip UA and no more than two "blood tests" to categorize the most likely cause(s) of jaundice in a given patient.

Introduction

The full gamut of endocrine and metabolic problems ranges far beyond the intended scope of this text. At the same time, the generic approach to pathophysiology is *universal*. In this chapter, we'll look at common problems from an "understanding is owning" point of view, so we can really know why the best treatments involve careful attention to the ABCs.

Glucose Homeostasis

OBJECTIVE: Explain the major hormonal factors that regulate the blood glucose level, including insulin and counter-regulatory hormones.

Since glucose is the major source of energy for all human cells, it is important to understand the normal regulatory systems (NRSs) that affect glucose homeostasis. What's the body's goal? Of course — to keep the cells "well fed" and to maintain a normal blood sugar (BS) level. Though many hormones and other factors are involved, the major "yin-yang" balance of glucose homeostasis involves insulin on one side of the equation, and the counter-regulatory hormones (CRHs) glucagon and epinephrine on the other. **[FIGURE 2-1]**

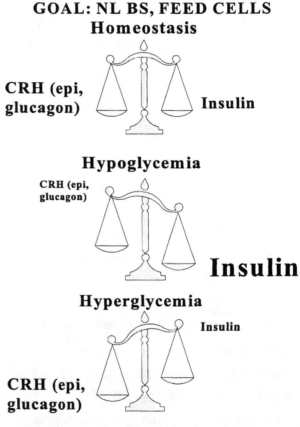

GOAL: NL BS, FEED CELLS
Homeostasis

CRH (epi, glucagon)   Insulin

Hypoglycemia

CRH (epi, glucagon)

Insulin

Hyperglycemia

Insulin

CRH (epi, glucagon)

Figure 2-1 — Glucose balance in the body is determined by insulin and the counter-regulatory hormones, glucagon and epinephrine.

Insulin's main job is to facilitate the transport of glucose into the cells (intracellular transport or "feeding the cells") and its storage as glycogen. It also affects a myriad of other metabolic processes, including the anabolism of fatty acids to triglycerides and amino acids to proteins. Insulin tends to *lower* the BS level. On the other hand, CRHs, primarily glucagon and epinephrine, have the opposite effects. Their tendency is to *raise* the blood sugar level. Hypothalamic stimulation by hypoglycemia also results in the release of ACTH (leading to cortisol production in the adrenal gland) and growth hormone. Both increase the blood sugar, but these responses have little effect in acute hypoglycemic states.

The beaver pond analogy — physiologists have equated the body's tightly regulated control of blood glucose concentration to the control of the water level in a beaver pond:

> "A beaver must maintain a constant water level in the pond for the proper functioning of the lodge, just as blood glucose concentrations must be maintained for brain function. The beaver controls the water level by changing the outflow over the dam and the inflow from stream beds. Water flow over the dam is analogous to glucose leaving the blood for tissues, which is controlled by insulin. Inflow of water from streams is analogous to glucose absorption from the GI tract and glucose release from the liver, the latter being controlled by glucagon and other counterregulatory hormones."[1]

REMEMBER: Insulin has anabolic effects (building large molecules up), while CRHs have catabolic effects (breaking large molecules down).

Why is glucose stored as glycogen and not just as a glucose monomer?
Glycogen is a single large polymer consisting of many glucose monomers linked together. It contributes very little to the intracellular osmolarity. On the other hand, individual glucose monomers contribute far more because of the greater total number of molecules. This would set up an osmotic gradient that might rupture the cell. So, the preferred storage form of glucose is as glycogen.

Isn't insulin an anabolic hormone? Absolutely — think of insulin as an anabolic hormone (building bigger molecules). On the other hand, the counter-regulatory hormones are catabolic — they tend to break molecules down (such as glycogen to glucose). This simple difference is cardinal to your understanding in diseases of blood sugar regulation (e.g., hypoglycemia, diabetic ketoacidosis).

BIOCHEMICAL PRINCIPLE: **Many major chemical reactions in the body involve either the *addition* of phosphate or its *removal* from a molecule, often an enzyme. Depending upon the particular substance, this results in either *activation* or *inactivation*.**

Does insulin act via receptors and G-proteins? Yes and no. There *are* insulin receptors on the cell surface. However, insulin does not mediate its effects through second messengers, as do most protein hormones. Rather, it acts via *autophosphorylation* of its own receptor. Let's translate this to English. The receptor consists of two portions — one lies outside the membrane, while the other penetrates the membrane and protrudes into the cytoplasm. Insulin binds the outside portion of the receptor. This triggers the enzyme tyrosine kinase in the receptor's internal portions. As a result, tyrosine residues on the internal portion of the receptor are phosphorylated. The result is continued phosphorylation of other intracellular proteins and enzymes, leading to multiple cellular responses. **[FIGURE 2-2]**

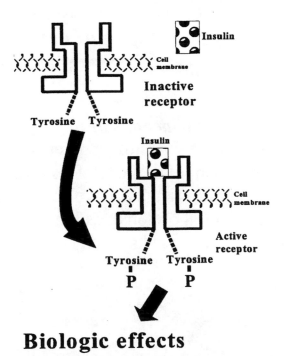

Note that *glucose transport* into the cells is effected via a different mechanism. Since glucose cannot diffuse directly into the cell, it enters via one of two transport mechanisms:

Figure 2-2 — The insulin receptor has two parts. The binding of insulin to the exterior portion causes autophosphorylation of the inner part. This activates the entire receptor, leading to the biologic actions of insulin. (P = phosphate)

1. **Facilitated transport** is the most common mechanism. Here, glucose transport is mediated by one of several glucose transporters (**glucose transport vesicles**) in the cell membrane. Five have been described so far. Each has a tissue-specific pattern of expression. The GLUT-4 transporter, for example, is prevalent in adipose tissue and skeletal muscle. Its activity there is increased by insulin. Facilitated transport of glucose follows a concentration gradient, moving glucose from areas of higher to areas of lower concentrations. Galactose utilizes a similar carrier. The mechanism for fructose, however, is unknown.

2. **Cotransport** is an energy-requiring process that transports glucose against a concentration gradient. It is carrier-mediated and couples the movement of glucose to the transportation of sodium into the cell at the same time.

OBJECTIVE: **Summarize the major actions of insulin on metabolism of carbohydrates, proteins, and fats.**

What are the actions of insulin? Overall, insulin serves to facilitate the use of available foodstuffs and energy. It affects carbohydrate, fat, and protein metabolism. For those of you who are really interested in the "nitty gritty" biochemical detail, I have summarized it in the **TABLE** below. I consider this material optional, as long as you understand that the major role of insulin is to "feed the cells sugar" and prevent the breakdown of fat and muscle.

	Effects of Insulin on Carbohydrate Metabolism
TISSUE	ACTIONS
Muscle	Promotes uptake and metabolism of glucose: • Stimulates intramuscular movement of glucose by increasing the number of *glucose transporter vesicles* in the cell membrane. • Glucose transported into muscle undergoes glycolysis and is stored as glycogen.
Liver	Promotes glucose uptake and storage; inhibits glucose production by: • Increasing the flux of glucose into cells — insulin induces the enzyme glucokinase, which phosphorylates glucose to glucose-6-phosphate, facilitating intracellular movement of the latter. • Activating glycogen synthetase — increases the formation of glycogen. • Increasing the activity of phosphofructokinase and pyruvate kinase, key enzymes in the process of glycolysis. • Decreasing the hepatic output of glucose in several ways: 1. Impairs glycogenolysis by inhibition of glycogen phosphorylase. 2. Decreases exit of glucose by inhibiting glucose-6-phosphatase. 3. Inhibits gluconeogenesis by decreasing amino acid uptake into the liver, and by decreasing activity of two key gluconeogenic enzymes, pyruvate carboxylase and fructose-1,6-diphosphatase. • Enhancing synthesis of fatty acids. 1. Increases glycolysis, which increases the formation of pyruvate. Pyruvate is then converted to acetyl-CoA. 2. Stimulates acetyl-CoA carboxylase which converts acetyl-CoA to malonyl-CoA, the rate limiting step in fatty acid synthesis.
Fat	Facilitates glucose entry into cells via glucose transporters, as in muscle. • Glucose is then converted to α-glycerol phosphate, which is used in the storage of fatty acids and triglycerides.
Other tissues	Since brain cells are highly permeable to glucose, insulin has little effect on glucose uptake and use in the brain.

▨▨▨▨	*Effects of Insulin on Fat Metabolism*
TISSUE	ACTIONS
Muscle	No major effect.
Liver	Promotes the synthesis and inhibits the oxidation of fatty acids: • Due to the availability of α-glycerol phosphate, fats are esterified into triglycerides. • Insulin is "antiketogenic." When fatty acid synthesis is occurring in the cytoplasm, the newly made fatty acid chains cannot be transferred into the mitochondria and degraded. Insulin stimulates formation of fatty acids; their main building block is malonyl-CoA. This inhibits carnitine acyltransferase, the enzyme responsible for moving cytoplasmic fatty acids into the mitochondria. Otherwise, the fatty acids would be oxidized to ketoacids.
Fat	Enhances storage and inhibits the mobilization of fatty acids: • Inhibition of hormone-sensitive lipase — decreases the rate of lipolysis of triglycerides and the release of stored fatty acids into the circulation. • Increased glucose transport — metabolism of glucose to α-glycerol phosphate increases the rate of metabolism of fatty acids for storage as triglycerides. • Induction of lipoprotein lipase — splits circulating triglycerides into fatty acids. This breakdown is necessary so they can be transported into fat cells.
▨▨▨▨	*Effects of Insulin on Protein Metabolism*
TISSUE	ACTIONS — The anabolic effects of insulin and growth hormone are synergistic.
Muscle	• Increases muscle cell uptake across the cell membrane of amino acids from the blood. • Increases gene transcription and translation of mRNA. • Inhibits catabolism of proteins, which decreases release of amino acids from muscle.
Liver	• Increases the liver cell uptake across the cell membrane of amino acids. • Increases gene transcription and translation of mRNA.
Fat	Not applicable

OBJECTIVE: List and explain the mechanism by which glucagon and epinephrine affect the blood glucose level.

How does glucagon raise the blood sugar? Whether administered by us, or secreted by the pancreas, glucagon binds hepatic receptors and activates adenyl cyclase. Cyclic AMP (cAMP) is produced and acts as a second messenger, activating protein kinase A. This kinase phosphorylates a number of enzymes, activating them. Glucagon promotes hyperglycemia in several ways:

1. Stimulation of glycogenolysis — via activation of glycogen phosphorylase (which breaks glycogen down into glucose) and simultaneous inhibition of glycogen synthetase (which links glucose into glycogen).

2. Inhibition of glycolysis — via inhibition of phosphofructokinase and pyruvate kinase. Glucose-6-phosphate levels rise, leading to increased glucose release from the liver.

3. Stimulation of gluconeogenesis — increases hepatic extraction of amino acids from plasma; also increases activity of two key gluconeogenic enzymes, pyruvate carboxylase and fructose-1,6-diphosphatase.

An identical set of events takes place when epinephrine stimulates β-1 receptors in the liver and skeletal muscle.

Essentially, the effects of glucagon are *opposite* to those of insulin. As such, glucagon is ketogenic. Glucagon inhibits acetyl-CoA carboxylase (which catalyzes the conversion of acetyl-CoA to malonyl-CoA). This forces the liver to metabolize acetyl-CoA to ketones.

How does epinephrine raise the blood sugar level? Stimulation of β-1 receptors in the liver and skeletal muscle by epinephrine leads to G-protein mediated activation of adenyl cyclase. This enzyme catalyzes the conversion of ATP to cAMP (cyclic AMP). Acting as a second messenger, cAMP catalyzes the activation of protein kinase. From here, a series of events occurs:

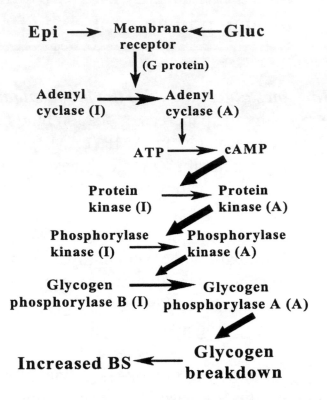

1. Activated protein kinase catalyzes the conversion of phosphorylase kinase to its active form.

2. Activated phosphorylase kinase catalyzes the conversion of glycogen phosphorylase B (inactive) to glycogen phosphorylase A (active).

3. Activated glycogen phosphorylase A breaks down glycogen (glycogenolysis), raising the blood sugar.

Figure 2-3 — Epinephrine (Epi) and glucagon (Gluc) bind membrane receptors in the liver (both) and muscle (Epi). A G-protein mediated reaction activates adenyl cylase, which converts ATP to cAMP. cAMP acts as a second messenger, activating protein kinase. The cascade continues with activation of phosphorylase kinase and glycogen phosphorylase A. Glycogen is then broken down to glucose and the blood sugar rises. (I) = inactive; (A) = activated.

An identical set of events takes place when glucagon stimulates its receptors in the liver. In addition to stimulating glycogen breakdown, activated protein kinase inhibits the action of glycogen synthetase, blocking further synthesis of glycogen. This negative feedback system makes sense — remember, the goal is to break down glycogen and raise the BS level. If the cells just broke down glycogen, while continuing to synthesize it at the same time, the net effect would be nil! **[FIGURE 2-3]**

What does signal amplification by epinephrine and glucagon mean? When either epinephrine or glucagon stimulate adenyl cyclase activity, the binding of one hormone molecule activates several G-protein molecules. Thus, several molecules of cAMP are formed for each molecule of hormone. This process is called **amplification** of signals. A similar set of events also occurs during the initial activation of protein kinase A by cAMP, the first major enzymatic step in glycogenolysis. The result is that very low concentrations of epinephrine or glucagon are required for a significant hormonal effect to occur.

How do glucocorticoids raise the blood sugar level? Glucocorticoids, such as cortisol, have two interrelated modes of action that raise the blood sugar level:

1.   Cortisol increases hepatic gluconeogenesis. During this process, proteins mobilized from peripheral tissues are converted into glucose.

2.   Cortisol also impairs utilization of glucose by peripheral tissues. This "anti-insulin" effect, especially in muscle and fat tissue, tends also to raise the blood glucose level. This is why corticosteroids are considered to be "diabetogenic."

Hypoglycemia

Low blood sugar (BS) is a common problem in a wide variety of circumstances. Though hypoglycemic patients may present with any of a number of symptoms, the most worrisome are those involving altered level of consciousness (LOC). The brain relies on glucose as its sole source of oxidative metabolism. As such, when deprived of glucose for more than a short period of time, "out go the lights." And, as we'll see, if the "lights are off" for more than thirty minutes, the "tungsten filament" of the lightbulb suffers permanent damage!

The normal blood sugar in most laboratories ranges from 80-100 mg/dl. The level at which a given patient becomes symptomatic, however, is totally unpredictable. Diabetics with diabetic ketoacidosis (DKA), for example, may suffer significant hypoglycemic symptoms when their elevated sugar is dropped

REMEMBER — the brain will also utilize ketone bodies for fuel, when these are present. Ketogenesis is *not* a response to acute hypoglycemia but may occur in fasting, dieting, or poor nutritional states.

too rapidly during treatment, even though it is still above normal limits. As a general rule, most patients who are not in DKA become symptomatic at BS levels lower than 60 mg/dl.

HYPOGLYCEMIA

DEFINITION	COMMON CAUSES	HISTORY (SYMPTOMS)	PHYSICAL (SIGNS)	"TESTS"	TREATMENT
Decreased BS level that results in symptoms	Insulin, poor diet, oral diabetic drugs, alcohol	Usually, rapid onset of anxiety, weakness, altered LOC	Adrenergic signs early; altered LOC later; seizures uncommon in adults	BS low, though the value varies from patient to patient	ABCs, IV DW50 (50% glucose in water); thiamine optional; glucagon is an alternative when no IV route possible; oral sugar in conscious patients

OBJECTIVE: Summarize the role of counter-regulatory hormones in the body's "early warning system" for hypoglycemia.

Normal physiology and our "early warning system." To understand the abnormal, it's essential (as always) that we know normal physiology first. Let's assume we take a group of nondiabetics and place their BS level on a "rheostat" so that we can turn it up and down. Don't be surprised — this can actually be done in the laboratory using what is called a "glucose clamp" technique. As we turn the BS down, we all reach a point of starting to develop symptoms, though, as I said earlier, that exact blood sugar level differs from person to person. What are our symptoms? You'd probably say "shaky, sweaty, nauseated, dizzy, etc." What about the signs (objective findings): we look diaphoretic, and our vital signs (pulse, RR) are likely on the high side — agreed?

My question — what is taking place that causes us to develop diaphoresis, tachycardia, and tachypnea? Sure sounds a lot like the typical "flight or fight" response from sympathetic stimulation. And, you're exactly right — the *normal* response to moderate levels of hypoglycemia is the body's release of "stuff" called counter-regulatory hormones (CRHs — and please don't confuse this with "corticotropin releasing hormone," which we *won't* be discussing). Besides glucagon, other CRHs include epinephrine, cortisol, and T4

Hypoglycemia

CRH production (epi, glucagon, cortisol, T4)

Increased hepatic gluconeogenesis + glycogenolysis

Increased BS

Figure 2-4 — The normal response system in hypoglycemia. Production of counter-regulatory hormones.

(thyroxine). Though cortisol and thyroxine take a while longer to act, all of the CRHs lead to increased hepatic gluconeogenesis and glycogenolysis — the liver manufactures new sugar and breaks down its already present glycogen stores into glucose. The net result is a rise in the BS level. [**FIGURE 2-4**]. The sympathetic-like effect of glucagon and epinephrine also causes noticeable signs and symptoms — effectively serving as an "early warning system" when the blood sugar gets too low.

Loss of the normal "early warning system" in diabetics. Now, let's imagine that we continued to turn the BS rheostat down — what would happen? Despite the body's attempt to increase the BS via CRH production, the level would continue to drop. The result — CNS (central nervous system) symptoms. Remember, the central nervous system only "eats" glucose, while the peripheral nervous system (PNS) isn't quite as selective. That's why altered levels of consciousness (LOC) are far more common in significant hypoglycemia than are peripheral neuropathies.

Let's carry our thinking one step further. It should be clear, at this point, that the effects of CRHs serve as the body's normal "early warning system" to alert us and prevent the development of worsened CNS symptoms. And, diabetics with low-grade hypoglycemic reactions are all taught to take sugar (in some form) at this point to avoid loss of consciousness.

Let's imagine, however, what would occur if a person *lost* the "early warning system." As the BS level descended through the range where the patient would normally sense early hypoglycemia, *nothing would happen.* This means that the patient cannot take any measures to prevent severe neuroglycopenia (altered LOC) if the BS drops lower! OK so far? Unfortunately, my example is far from theoretical. You and I both know that the majority of diabetic hypoglycemic reactions we see involve the *late stage*, with altered LOC — often, the patient presents simply with unconsciousness.

Decreased or absent perception of "early warning symptoms" is common in diabetics, particularly those on insulin (whether they are Type I or Type II). This clinical finding is associated with impaired release of glucose counter-regulatory hormones, especially glucagon and epinephrine.

What happens to the normal regulatory system as diabetes progresses?
Biochemists now feel that glucagon is the most significant of the CRHs. Recall that glucagon is made by A cells (also called α-cells) in the pancreas. Within four years of disease onset, most Type I diabetics (and some Type II diabetics on insulin) develop significant glucagon deficiency. At this point, they are totally dependent on the effects of epinephrine secretion as their "early warning system." Depending on various factors (e.g., intensity of insulin therapy, patient compliance, hereditary factors), autonomic neuropathy may develop. When this occurs, patients not only lack glucagon, but also have decreased levels of epinephrine secretion. Low levels of both glucagon and epinephrine, combined, markedly increase the patients' susceptibility to severe hypoglycemic reactions.[2]

Unfortunately, the "tighter" the patient's diabetic control, the more likely the risk of a severe hypoglycemic reaction. And, "tight" control is associated with a significant decrease in diabetic complications. This forces clinician and patient to walk a tightrope, balancing between optimal blood sugar control and avoidance of severe hypoglycemic reactions.[3]

> ### *OBJECTIVE:* Summarize at least one therapeutic strategy that may be tried to improve awareness of early hypoglycemia.

Can we restore the "early warning system?" So, if more severe hypoglycemic reactions occur as a result of loss of the normal CRH mechanism, wouldn't it be neat if there were a way to restore this "early warning system?" You bet — and while you're wondering how, this is a good time to enjoy a cup of coffee. . . whoops, I just gave you the answer!

The pharmacology of coffee. It shouldn't come as any great surprise that coffee (especially with lots of caffeine) is a stimulant. Pharmacologically, caffeine is one of the methylxanthine (MX) drugs, as is aminophylline. The net effect is similar to that of adrenergic stimulation of β-receptors. The exact mechanism of MXs is uncertain, but may involve:

- Translocation of intracellular calcium.
- Increased concentrations of cyclic AMP (cAMP) by phosphodiesterase inhibition (the enzyme that breaks down adenyl cyclase, a main catalyst in cAMP formation).
- Blockade of adenosine receptors.

Though the "classic teaching" was that MXs work primarily via phosphodiesterase inhibition, experimental work indicates that human plasma levels *rarely* reach the necessary level to sufficiently inhibit this enzyme. On the other hand, therapeutic plasma levels *may* enhance the formation of cyclic GMP (cGMP, a guanosine-based nucleotide, similar to cAMP) via an effect on phosphodiesterase.[4] Similar thinking applies to an *in vivo* human pharmacologic effect on intracellular calcium movement. The most likely possibility is antagonism of adenosine receptors.

What does adenosine have to do with sympathetic stimulation? The action of adenosine is mediated by receptors in numerous areas of the body. It:

- Dilates blood vessels, particularly in the coronary and cerebral circulation.
- Slows the discharge rate of cardiac pacemaker cells.
- Slows the discharge rate of CNS neurons.
- Potentiates some α-adrenergic actions of norepinephrine, leading to smooth muscle contraction (e.g., bronchospasm).

Thus, inhibition of adenosine by MXs results in effects *opposite* from those above, similar to administration of epinephrine or glucagon. The initial pathways may differ, but the end result is the same.

Meanwhile, back at the farm . . . It's important to understand that the main "drug" in coffee is caffeine, which is a methylxanthine. Of course, that's why people get a "caffeine buzz." Let's see how this concept might be helpful therapeutically.

Studies in nondiabetics, using the glucose clamp technique, have shown that one or two cups of "average strength" caffeinated coffee *increase* a person's sensitivity to borderline hypoglycemia. The tests went as follows:

1. The glucose clamp was used to determine at which BS level a person started to develop early hypoglycemic symptoms.

2. The subject then drank coffee and was retested with the glucose clamp.

3. A majority of individuals developed signs and symptoms at a BS level significantly *higher* than the level at which they became symptomatic *prior to* drinking coffee.

These results led investigators to conclude that, at least in nondiabetic individuals, caffeine ingestion *increases* one's awareness of BS levels that would otherwise be considered in the "normal" range.

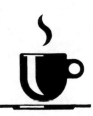

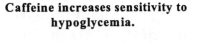
Caffeine increases sensitivity to hypoglycemia.

Hypoglycemia ("the event") normally leads to production of CRHs ("stuff"). Diabetics with severe reactions have lost the ability to make "stuff." Coffee is chemically related to the biological "stuff" (CRHs) and should be the pharmacologic equivalent of restoring some of the missing CRHs. **[FIGURE 2-5]**

Figure 2-5

Several studies show that administration of regular strength caffeinated coffee to diabetics studied with the glucose clamp technique increases their previously lost sensitivity, reducing the incidence of severe hypoglycemic reactions.[5] Even more exciting is a new study evaluating the benefits of coffee in diabetics in a *real-world* setting (out of the laboratory). The investigators found that caffeine consumption (two to four cups of drip-brewed coffee per day) increases the intensity of warning symptoms without having an adverse effect on either glycemic control or plasma lipid levels.[6] Please note that as exciting (and logical) as these findings are, "a coffee a day to keep the 'hypo' away" is *not* considered a standard of care in diabetes treatment.

> *OBJECTIVE:* **Describe the Somogyi Phenomenon — why it occurs; when it should be suspected; potential treatments.**

The Somogyi or "Dawn" Phenomenon. When I teach classes, most students claim to have never heard of either the Somogyi or "Dawn" phenomenon. . . at least until I ask a question: "have you ever seen a patient whose fasting BS is rising and continues to rise despite the fact that you *increase* the

> *REMEMBER*: **Insulin typically *lowers* the BS level. When the level continues to *rise*, despite gradually increasing doses of insulin, something is wrong.**

insulin dose?" The "yeahs" suddenly increase tenfold. Granted, the most common cause for a patient's fasting blood sugar (FBS) to increase is a need for still *more* insulin. And, after raising the dose a few times, only to be met with yet increasing FBS levels, let me suggest you consider an alternative — one that makes good sense based on what you already know about the body's response to hypoglycemia.

Even in normal individuals, hypoglycemia is common during sleep. It's usually asymptomatic and due to circadian changes in CRH release.[7] Actually, a better term for this normal response, rather than hypoglycemia, is "circadian hypoglycemia" or a "transitional low blood glucose state."

Diabetics have this same circadian rhythm — only now, add in diabetes and treatment with insulin. In addition to "circadian hypoglycemia," the diabetic patient on insulin may also develop true nocturnal hypoglycemia. Findings may include: [**FIGURE 2-6**]

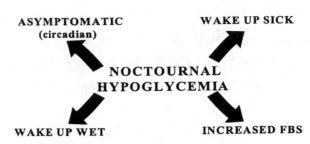

Figure 2-6 — The different types of potential noctournal hypoglycemia. "Circadian hypoglycemia" is sometimes called "transitional low blood glucose state" because it reflects normal circadian variation in counter-regulatory hormone production.

1.   Asymptomatic.
2.   Waking in the middle of the night with symptoms.
3.   Waking in the morning with soaked bed sheets (nocturnal sweats in a diabetic suggest hypoglycemia or infection).
4.   No symptoms but elevation of the morning BS secondary to release of CRHs. This response is termed the Somogyi phenomenon (also called the "dawn phenomenon").

The Somogyi phenomenon is a "classic" example of activation of a normal response system activated under *abnormal* circumstances, resulting in *untoward results*. The patient develops nocturnal hypoglycemia. CRH release is blunted enough to prevent waking up with symptoms in the middle of the night or soaking one's bedsheets. Enough CRHs are present, however, to cause a rise in the BS that is reflected by an elevated FBS.

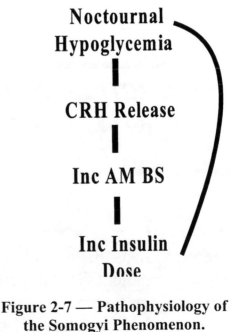

Figure 2-7 — Pathophysiology of the Somogyi Phenomenon.

Of course, our initial response to the elevated FBS is to increase whatever part of a patient's insulin regimen affects the FBS. Mindlessly, insulin exacerbates the nocturnal hypoglycemia even further, and the FBS continues to rise. The cycle continues unless recognized and changes in therapy are made. [see **FIGURE 2-7**]

Though there are several possible therapeutic/diagnostic approaches once you suspect the Somogyi phenomenon, perhaps the easiest is to try *decreasing* the relevant insulin dose and seeing what happens. Within a couple of days, the pattern should start to reverse. Generally, this approach is relatively patient-safe unless the person is extremely "brittle." Don't expect instant changes, however; some of the CRHs have half-lives of up to four days. This is also the reason why some diabetics are very difficult to re-control for up to a week after suffering a severe hypoglycemic reaction.

The advent of fixed mixtures of intermediate and short-acting insulins (70% NPH/30% Regular) may be problematic in patients with the Somogyi phenomenon. With two different insulins in the same bottle, each peaking at different times, it is impossible to decide which (intermediate, short-acting, or both) is responsible for the nocturnal hypoglycemia. Despite widespread thinking that the most likely "culprit" was the intermediate-acting component, recent data have suggested that short-acting (e.g., regular) insulin is responsible in many patients. Substitution of Lispro, an insulin analogue, for regular insulin appears to *decrease* significantly the incidence of nocturnal hypoglycemia, especially in patients on frequent daily insulin injections.[8]

> ## *OBJECTIVE:* Explain the pathophysiological basis for many of the neurological effects of prolonged hypoglycemia.

Prolonged hypoglycemia is harmful. Hypoglycemia sufficient to cause altered LOC is also sufficient to cause permanent CNS damage, especially to the cerebral cortex. The "lightbulb" metaphor I used earlier holds — if the BS level goes low enough, the "lights go out," and

---

PRINCIPLE: Unstopped, damage begets more damage!

---

if it stays low enough for long enough (more than thirty minutes), some of the "tungsten filaments" (ie., neurons) are irreparably damaged. Research has indicated that loss of neuronal tissues during prolonged hypoglycemia is not simply a function of loss of glucose. The lack of energy prevents a cell from performing its usual "activities of daily living," such as oxidative metabolism. The result — production of toxic metabolites ("stuff"), such as free radicals that cause permanent damage.

Free radicals are highly reactive molecules that lack one electron. The chemical tendency of an unstable species, such as free radicals, is to stabilize itself by binding to another substance. Usually, this "lucky" recipient is some type of biological membrane. When the free radical binds to lipids, additional

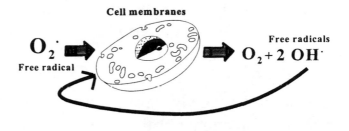

Figure 2-8 — Free radical formation begets more free radical formation, leading to a vicious cycle of increasing cell damage.

free radicals are formed, usually in the chemical form of peroxides, and a vicious cycle ensues. [FIGURE 2-8]

The practical implications of this biochemical oxidation-reduction nightmare are simple — prolonged hyoglycemia is dangerous and likely more harmful, at least over a period of several hours, than hyperglycemia has ever been shown to be! This is the basis for the long-standing recommendation to always assume *hypoglycemia* in a diabetic emergency and to treat empirically with dextrose until proven otherwise. Of course, fingerstick BS determinations have markedly refined our decision making capacity.

Why is thiamine sometimes given along with glucose in the treatment of hypoglycemia? The first step in energy production by the brain is glycolysis of glucose to pyruvate. Pyruvate is then normally converted to acetyl-CoA (by pyruvate dehydrogenase) and enters the citric acid (Krebb's) cycle to produce energy. Pyruvate dehydrogenase is a multienzyme complex of which thiamine is an integral component. Since the brain usually obtains all of its energy from the oxidation of glucose to pyruvate, then to acetyl-CoA, thiamine deficiency may result in severe brain damage by preventing formation of adequate brain ATP. **[FIGURE 2-9]**

The basis for empirically giving thiamine to hypoglycemic patients is that they may be nutritionally deficient, not only in glucose, but in thiamine, as well. Though "classically" thought necessary only in long-standing alcoholics with hypoglycemia, current thinking holds that thiamine may benefit *any* hypoglycemic patient who is also undernourished (as in cancer, AIDS, other chronic disease).

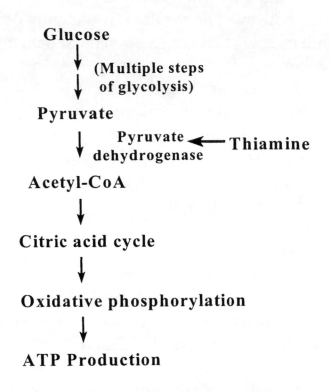

Figure 2-9 — Thiamine is an essential component of the pyruvate dehydrogenase enzyme complex, which converts pyruvate to acetyl CoA. Thiamine deficiency slows this reaction, decreasing the amount of ATP produced. Since the brain relies nearly wholly on this pathway for energy, severe damage may occur.

Though academically sound, routine administration of thiamine is *not* considered a standard of care in most areas. Perhaps the more significant issue is that the *order* of administration is not crucial. Thiamine uptake is far slower than that of glucose. Even if thiamine is given first, glucose will exert its molecular effects first. The bottom line is simple — emergent initial administration of thiamine is not absolutely necessary, though it may be beneficial in therapy once the patient is stabilized.[9]

OBJECTIVE: Describe at least two common situations where unsuspected hypoglycemia may be responsible for a patient's condition.

Atypical presentations of hypoglycemia. When an older person presents with neurological symptoms (e.g., lightheadedness, unsteadiness), the first "tunnel vision" conclusion we come to is stroke (cerebrovascular disease). And, we're often right. Unfortunately, there remains a significant minority of elderly patients with Type II diabetes, even if on oral agents, who may develop hypoglycemia and present with "stroke-like" symptoms.[10] In fact, any altered BS level (too high *or* too low) may cause neurological symptoms.

PRINCIPLE: Patients don't always "read the textbook" before they get sick.

Another potential trap occurs in the trauma victim with an altered sensorium, a focal neurological finding, or bradycardia. Our first (and correct) tendency is to think of head injury. There's nothing wrong with this. Wouldn't it be nice, though, if there were an easily treatable alternative explanation? Hypoglycemia has also been reported to cause respiratory failure in children.[11]

Remember the "Four Fixes" —
always consider hypoglycemia in all
patients with any degree of mental
status abnormality, even when the
findings seem to be explained initially by other etiologies.

OBJECTIVE: Describe the mechanism by which angiotensin converting enzyme (ACE) inhibitors increase a person's risk of hypoglycemia.

ACE inhibitors and hypoglycemia in diabetics. Another potentially significant, but less-well-known, cause of hypoglycemia is angiotensin converting enzyme (ACE) inhibitors. One study reported that as many as 13.8% of all hospital admissions for hypoglycemia might be attributable to use of ACE inhibitors (ACE blockers).[12] These drugs are used widely for many diseases, including hypertension, congestive heart failure, renal failure in diabetics, and myocardial infarction. Most cases of hypoglycemia have been reported in diabetics on either insulin or oral agents (most commonly, sulfonylureas). Enalapril may be more likely to cause problems, though hypoglycemia has been noted with captopril as well.[13] Symptoms may occur after one dose or during chronic therapy.[14]

ACE catalyzes the formation of angiotensin II from angiotensin I. One major effect of angiotensin II is to stimulate the release of norepinephrine (NE), with a resultant increase in renal absorption

REMEMBER: If ACE inhibitors block part of the *normal* sympathetic response system (by inhibiting sympathetic stimulation by angiotensin II), the diabetic "early warning system" for hypoglycemia is impaired.

of fluid and salt due to vasoconstriction. Blocking ACE decreases the amount of available circulating angiotensin II. The effect of lower angiotensin II levels is decreased NE release. **[FIGURE 2-10]** The result is a blunted counter-regulatory hormone response (especially of epinephrine and norepinephrine) to hypoglycemia.[15] There may be a central pituitary effect as well, involving interaction of prolactin releasing hormone and epinephrine.[16]

Why not just stop ACE-inhibitors in diabetics?
Sounds good, in theory, but the chances that this will happen nowadays are extremely unlikely. Numerous studies demonstrate that ACE-inhibitors (blockers) significantly decrease the progression rate of diabetic renal complications. In addition, they also decrease a diabetic's cardiovascular mortality, irrespective of the presence of associated hypertension. These drugs are viewed by many experts as mandatory therapy in any adult diabetic.[17]

ANGIOTENSINOGEN

RENIN (from kidneys)

ANGIOTENSIN I

ACE (in lungs)   **X** (Blocked by ACE blockers)

ANGIOTENSIN II

-**Vasoconstriction**
-**Aldosterone secretion**
-*NE release*
-**Inc Na absorption**
-**Inc ADH secretion**

ACE inhibitors decrease NE release

Figure 2-10 — ACE inhibitors decrease the amount of NE that would normally be released by angiotensin II. This makes some persons more susceptible to severe hypoglycemic spells due to loss of a part of their "early warning system."

Are other drugs associated with hypoglycemia? Other drugs associated with hypoglycemia include alcohol, fluoxetine (Prozac®), and glyburide (Micronase®) when combined with ciprofloxacin (Cipro®). Glyburide, a second-generation sulfonylurea hypoglycemic agent, is metabolized by the P-450 hepatic enzyme system. Ciprofloxacin, a widely used quinolone antibiotic, is a recognized P-450 enzyme inhibitor. Life-threatening hypoglycemia has been reported when the two drugs are used together.[18]

Why does alcohol (ethanol) cause hypoglycemia? Ethanol is metabolized first to acetaldehyde by the enzyme alcohol dehydrogenase. Acetaldehyde is then oxidized to acetate by aldehyde dehydrogenase. Both of these reactions involve the transfer of electrons to NAD^+. The result is a massive increase in the cellular concentration of NADH. This abundance favors the reduction of pyruvate to lactate, and oxaloacetate to malate. Both pyruvate and oxaloacetate are intermediates in the process of gluconeogenesis. So, the net effect is that "resources" are diverted to metabolize ethanol that results in decreased synthesis of glucose. Hypoglycemia may result, especially in individuals who are starved or malnourished.

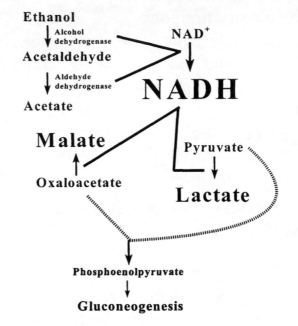

Metabolism of ethanol decreases available oxaloacetate and pyruvate for entry into gluconeogenesis.

Glucagon to treat hypoglycemia. Most of us are aware that besides being one of the CRHs released during hypoglycemia, glucagon is also used clinically to raise the BS, especially when an intravenous route cannot be established easily to give DW50 (dextrose). When I ask students, "How does glucagon work in hypoglycemia?," I usually hear, "It raises the blood sugar." Correct, but not good enough — at least not for a pathophysiology text. As I noted earlier, both epinephrine and glucagon have sympathetic-like effects. They just work via different mechanisms — the end result is the same.

Remember — epinephrine stimulates β-1 receptors, while glucagon stimulates glucagon-specific receptors in the liver. The result of either pathway is an increase in cAMP levels. cAMP then combines with a **G-protein** (see Chapter 1). The "duo" induces enzymes (second messengers) in the liver to catalyze reactions that facilitate hepatic gluconeogenesis and glycogenolysis, raising the blood sugar. cAMP release leads to the clinical warning signs and symptoms (e.g., tachycardia, diaphoresis) by causing adrenergic stimulation.

Can we T&R (treat and release) patients with hypoglycemia? The answer is "sometimes. . ." Think about many of the hypoglycemic patients who are treated, then transported to an emergency department. What happens at the hospital (assuming the patient is now completely awake and alert)? Well, we usually recheck the BS level and offer the patient a rather expensive hospital meal. Then, the patient is sent home with instructions on how to avoid similar episodes in the future.

Fortunately, the trend continues toward identification of patients who really don't need to come to the hospital in the first place — they can be treated and released ("T&R'd") by paramedics, clinic staff, or family. The paperwork and politics of such a policy are beyond the scope of this discussion. Rather than list patients who may be candidates for T&R, let's take a look at those who should *not* be T&R'd — those who need to be observed by someone for several hours. These include (but are not necessarily limited to — nice legal jargon, huh?) persons whose hypoglycemic reactions were due to:

- Oral agents (of any type).
- Long-acting (e.g., UltraLente) insulin.
- Insulin overdose.

Can you tell me the common denominator underlying all of the above conditions? Think about the generic pathophysiology model. If the production or presence of "stuff" causes the original problem, doesn't it make sense that if the "stuff" outlasts the treatment, the patient's still got a problem?

PRINCIPLE: If "stuff" causes the problem, as long as the "stuff's" still around, there's still a problem!

Many oral agents have long half lives (6 to 8 hours; 24 to 36 hours in some of the older preparations such as tolbutamide). UltraLente insulin lasts for 24 to 36 hours; large doses of insulin injected at one time (e.g., a suicide attempt) or "functional insulin overdose" (e.g., a prisoner is kept on 100U NPH insulin BID but fed only one roast beef sandwich per day) cause excess insulin to be absorbed into fat and released erratically over the next several hours. *All* of these patients need to be observed for recurrence of symptoms. The average duration of intravenous DW50 is one and one-half hours. Many health care providers routinely start continuous glucose infusions of D10W to supplement intravenous boluses.

The principle illustrated here for hypoglycemia and the persistence of "stuff" is applicable to a wide variety of medical situations. Remember — if "stuff" causes the problem in the first place, unless

COROLLARY: Some "stuff" outlasts "anti-stuff."

you block, stop, or get rid of that "stuff," the patient's still got a problem!

Diabetic ketoacidosis

Diabetic ketoacidosis (DKA) is a serious and fascinating metabolic condition that illustrates just about every important principle of clinical pathophysiology. Most of us have seen a complex biochemical diagram drawn in an "attempt" to explain what happens. Have no fear — I promise *not* to repeat that sordid performance here. You *will* understand DKA and the why's of treatment, and enjoy doing it. Essentially, DKA results from a combination of insulin *deficiency* and glucagon *excess*.

DIABETIC KETOACIDOSIS

DEFINITION	COMMON CAUSES	HISTORY (SYMPTOMS)	PHYSICAL (SIGNS)	"TESTS"	TREATMENT
Metabolic disturbance caused by insulin depletion and counter-regulatory hormone excess, resulting in hyperglycemia and the production of abnormal ketones and acids in the body	Underlying diabetes (usually Type I); precipitated by infection, usually viral gastroenteritis	12 to 48 hours of progressive weakness, nausea, vomiting; abdominal pain and coffee-grounds emesis in 50% of patients	Kussmaul respirations (hyperventilation); dehydration; mild alteration in LOC; acetone odor to breath (< 50% of patients); inappropriate normothermia; hypothermia associated with increased mortality	Inc BS, positive serum ketones; dec HCO_3^- on electrolytes; UA shows glucose + ketones; degree of acidosis does not correlate with degree of BS elevation or severity of DKA!	Fluids (mainstay of therapy); continuous insulin infusion, potassium. AVOID bicarb!

What insulin normally does. DKA occurs when there is a relative (rare) or absolute (common) lack of insulin, combined with an excess of counter-regulatory hormones (predominantly glucagon). Simply raising the blood sugar, by itself,

PRINCIPLE: **The absence of "good stuff" and/or the production of "bad stuff" leads to disease.**

will *not* lead to DKA, even in the most brittle of Type I diabetics. Glucagon excess is also required. Think of DKA as a great example of NRS (normal regulatory system) imbalance — too little insulin, too much glucagon.

To appreciate the pathophysiology of DKA, we must understand what insulin normally does; then it's easy to predict what would happen when it "doesn't." Then, take those results and magnify them, due to excess glucagon levels (which have the *opposite* metabolic effect of insulin).

Insulin has three main metabolic functions; it:

1. Shifts glucose into cells.
2. Facilitates formation of glycogen by cells to store glucose.
3. Prevents breakdown of fat and muscle tissue (by facilitating formation of triglycerides and proteins from free fatty acids and amino acids)

Metaphorically speaking, insulin reminds me of feeding my children when they were infants. Insulin "feeds" glucose to the cells. By keeping the cells satiated, it prevents cells from resorting to alternative fuel sources, such as fat and muscle (thus, "preventing" their breakdown).

What happens when insulin "doesn't." Let's divide the processes that occur in the absence of insulin into two parts, just for the sake of convenience. Without insulin, sugar can't be transported as effectively into the cells (plain English translation — they get "underfed"). The result:

1. **"Hungry cells"** (intracellular starvation due to the lack of glucose) — since the cells still need nutrition, they turn to other sources. Next in line to be consumed is fat tissue. A lack of insulin activates hormone-sensitive lipase, causing rapid mobilization of fatty acids.[19] When fat is "eaten" by the cells, it is metabolized to its components, glycerol and free fatty acids (FFAs). FFAs are then metabolized by the liver to ketones. Ketones dissociate in serum, resulting in free protons (H$^+$). When enough ketones, thus many H$^+$ ions, are present, acidosis develops. **[FIGURE 2-11]**

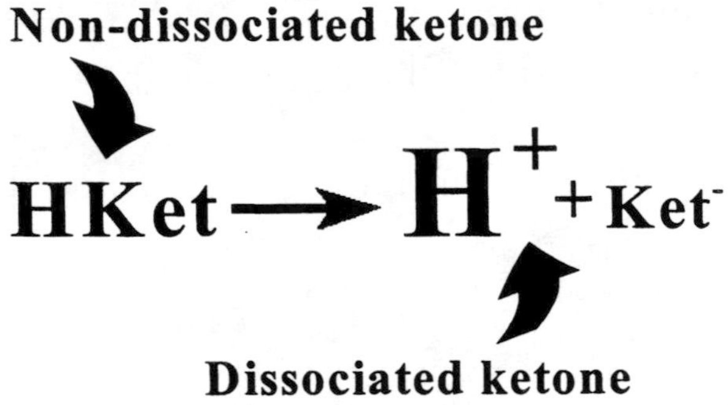

Non-dissociated ketone

$$HKet \longrightarrow H^+ + Ket^-$$

Dissociated ketone

Figure 2-11 — Ketones freely dissociate in serum. When high concentrations of ketones are present, the [H$^+$] is high, leading to a decrease in the pH.

If the process persists long enough without treatment, fat stores are exhausted and the cells start breaking down muscle tissue into its constituent amino acids. Of course, when these run out, the next step is death.

So, metaphorically speaking, cells prefer to eat at the "Glucose Inn." When it's closed, they go to the "Fat Cafe." And, when all else fails, they have a third choice to stay alive — "The Muscle Madhouse."

> ### *OBJECTIVE:* Defend the concept that most patients in DKA are total-body potassium-depleted, regardless of their serum level.

2. **Increased serum glucose** (blood sugar) **levels** occur for two reasons. First, less sugar is being "fed" intracellularly to the cells due to the lack of insulin — the obvious result is an increase in the serum BS level (no big surprise, eh?). The second reason is due to glucagon excess — this results in glycogenolysis, as well as gluconeogenesis in the liver. Both also contribute to elevated blood sugar levels.

    When blood passes through the kidney, sugar crosses the filtration membrane into the urine. Well, sugar is a big molecule and tends to have a significant osmotic effect. The result — sugar draws along with it fluids and electrolytes (especially potassium) across the glomerular filtration membrane. Potassium and sugar "hang together." Where glucose goes, potassium is sure to follow. In DKA, sugar draws fluids into the urine and potassium follows.

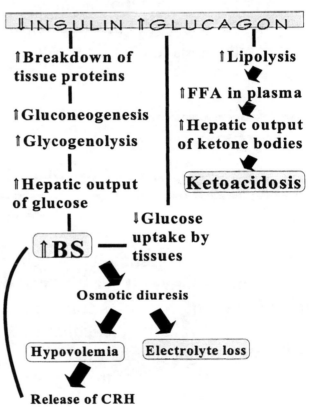

Figure 2-12 — **Pathophysiology of diabetic ketoacidosis**

All factors considered, the end result in DKA is a sick patient with: **[Figure 2-12]**

- Elevated serum BS.
- Ketones and acids in the serum.
- Dehydration due to glucosuria (average fluid deficit in an adult is 6-9 liters!).
- Depleted total body potassium stores, regardless of the measured *serum* K^+ level (potassium shifts readily between intracellular and extracellular compartments, especially during acid-base changes; see "Electrolytes and Acid-Base Disorders," below).
- The resulting hypovolemia also leads to release of counter-regulatory hormones (e.g., epinephrine), which further raises the blood sugar (and contributes to a vicious cycle).

OBJECTIVE: Defend the concept that fluids are often the first and best therapy for DKA.

Now, I'm not suggesting that we eliminate insulin from our treatment algorithm for DKA. It is a vital part of therapy — just remember that maintenance of the ABCs comes first, including adequate replenishment of intravascular volume (the *major* pathophysiological deficit in DKA). Fluids form the basis of therapy in most cases of DKA. Studies have shown that even in patients with severe DKA, giving fluids while

PRINCIPLE: Patients live or die based on the adequacy of Airway, Breathing, and Circulation!

cautiously withholding initial insulin led to significant patient improvement. And, these findings make sense. Rehydration dilutes the blood sugar and increases hepatic perfusion; the liver is then able to clear excess ketones and acids.

Fluid administration in DKA can generally be divided into three successive phases: (i) a short period of rapid isotonic saline infusion, (ii) slower infusion of isotonic saline with potassium chloride, and (iii) glucose-potassium infusion until oral food intake is well established.[20] Initially, most patients will benefit from one or two liters of normal saline, infused as fast as the patient can tolerate. Later, potassium is usually required. Most continuous insulin infusion protocols change to sugar-containing intravenous fluids when the BS reaches 250 mg/dl to prevent development of hypoglycemia (and cerebral edema in children).

Bicarbonate still isn't indicated! When I mention during my classes that I don't often obtain arterial blood gases (ABGs) in DKA, some of the looks from students are incredulous! This is as good as a place as any to give you the uses for bicarb:

- Keeping your refrigerator clean-smelling (after all, isn't it just liquid "baking soda?").
- Treatment of hyperkalemia.
- Treatment of tricyclic antidepressant poisoning.

Routine use of bicarb in other conditions, including metabolic acidosis from any cause (e.g., DKA), is usually more risky than helpful. The reason is simple — remember the oxyhemoglobin dissociation curve that we all learned early in school?

If we plot hemoglobin O_2 saturation versus pO_2 (partial pressure of oxygen) the result is a sigmoid-shaped ("S-shaped") curve. [**FIGURE 2-13**] The position of this curve is a good reflection of the hemoglobin's affinity for oxygen. The sigmoid shape of the curve is due to stronger binding of oxygen to hemoglobin as more oxygen molecules become bound (the **Haldane effect**).

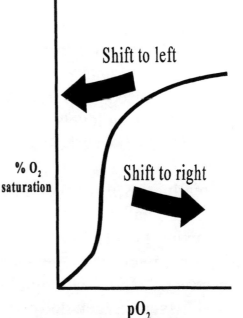

Figure 2-13 — Oxyhemoglobin desaturation curve: shifts to the *right* increase tissue oxygen delivery by *decreasing* the affinity of hemoglobin for oxygen. Shifts to the *left* decrease tissue oxygen delivery by *increasing* the affinity of hemoglobin for oxygen.

2-37

Hemoglobin is capable of binding four molecules of oxygen. After binding one oxygen molecule, the affinity of Hg for the second oxygen molecule increases, and so on. As you'd suspect, the affinity for the fourth oxygen molecule is greatest.

Factors that shift the curve to the right *decrease* the affinity of hemoglobin for oxygen, while those that shift it to the left *increase* the affinity of hemoglobin for oxygen (the **Bohr effect**; see immediately below). While increased affinity for oxygen may be great for hemoglobin, it doesn't do much for the tissues — the result is a *decrease* in tissue oxygen delivery. And isn't that really what happens in shock — decreased tissue O_2 delivery?

The following factors shift the curve to the right, leading to a decrease in the affinity of hemoglobin for oxygen and an increase in tissue oxygen delivery:

- Increased temperature.
- Increased levels of 2,3-diphosphoglycerate (2,3-DPG).
- Acidosis (decreased pH).

And those that shift the curve to the left, resulting in opposite effects (decreased tissue oxygen delivery), include:

- Decreased temperature.
- Decreased levels of 2,3-diphosphoglycerate (2,3,-DPG).
- *Alkalosis* (increased pH).

Normally, the pH of blood in the lungs is 7.60; in the tissues, it is 7.20. This difference naturally favors release of oxygen by hemoglobin into the tissues. By raising the pH, even on a localized level, bicarb shifts the oxyhemoglobin dissociation curve to the *left*. This results in *increased* affinity of hemoglobin for oxygen. Since hemoglobin now "holds on" to oxygen more strongly than usual, tissue oxygen delivery *decreases*.

In light of this, it should come as no surprise to you that patients in an ICU setting fare far *worse* with alkalosis (pH = 7.60) than with mild acidosis (pH = 7.20). Data in patients with DKA shows that they get better *without* bicarbonate, anyway. In addition, bicarb administration augments ketone production and promotes a selective build up of acetoacetate.[21]

How do chronic diabetic complications, such as renal failure and retinopathy, fit into the overall picture? There are two leading theories that link the degree of blood sugar elevation to complications:

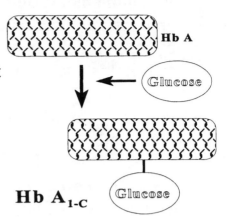

Figure 2-14 — The glycosylated hemoglobin level (Hb A$_{1-C}$) gives an estimate of the "average" blood sugar over the past one or two months.

1. Glycosylation of proteins — Elevated serum glucose levels lead to the attachment of glucose to cell proteins. This process is known as **glycosylation**. The higher the blood sugar over a period of time, the more protein that is glycosylated. Laboratory tests currently exist for glycosylated hemoglobin (HbA1-c). This level reflects the average blood sugar level over a period of one or two months. **[FIGURE 2-14]** Experts hypothesize that similar glycosylation of other proteins in the kidneys, nerves, and eyes may lead to chronic complications.

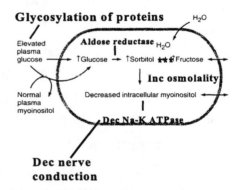

DIABETIC COMPLICATIONS

*** Sorbitol dehydrogenase is lacking in eye, nerve, kidney; trapping of sorbitol in cell increases osmolality, leading to tissue dysfunction.

Figure 2-15

2. Accumulation of sorbitol — Sugar that enters the cell may either undergo glycolysis or be converted to sorbitol. Normally, sorbitol is then converted to fructose by the enzyme **sorbitol dehydrogenase**. Fructose moves freely in and out of cells. **[FIGURE 2-15]** Tissues of the lens, kidney, and nerve lack sorbitol dehydrogenase.

When the blood sugar is persistently elevated, such as in diabetes, large amounts of sugar enter the cells and are converted to sorbitol. The lack of sorbitol dehydrogenase effectively traps sorbitol within the cell. Sorbitol is a large molecule and exerts a significant osmotic effect, drawing water into the cells. The resultant swelling is thought to contribute to the formation of diabetic cataracts, nephropathy, and neuropathy.

DKA versus hyperosmolar hyperglycemic nonketotic coma (HHNC). Since patients with DKA often have significant elevations of their BS, their serum becomes hypertonic, at least to some degree. For this reason, some confuse HHNC with DKA. HHNC is a very different disease, though still considered one of the "diabetic emergencies." Though the serum is hypertonic in DKA, calculated or measured osmolality is close to normal. In HHNC, the serum osmolality is markedly elevated.

HHNC occurs in elderly patients with underlying cardiovascular, pulmonary, and renal disease. They may or may not be known diabetics. In the face of stress, often pneumonia or genitourinary tract sepsis, the patient becomes relatively insulin resistant. The result is a *marked* increase in blood sugar (often greater than 1000 mg/dl) and a significant elevation of serum osmolality. The normal level is 290 mOsml/kg.; in HHNC, osmolality averages 350 mOsml/kg. Despite the relative insulin deficiency and blood sugar elevation, the patient has no measurable degree of ketosis or acidosis. The reasons for this are unknown — some hypothesize that sufficient insulin activity remains to prevent development of ketoacidosis.

As you might expect, elevations of the blood sugar lead to glucosuria, potassium, and volume loss. Part of the reason for the associated 40% mortality is likely related to the mean 12-16 liter deficit (versus 6-9 liters per day in DKA). Imagine your mission — this degree of fluid replenishment over 24-36 hours to an elderly patient with pre-existing heart, lung, and kidney disease! Hemodynamic monitoring in an intensive care unit is mandatory.

HYPEROSMOLAR HYPERGLYCEMIC NONKETOTIC COMA (HHNC)

DEFINITION	COMMON CAUSES	HISTORY (SYMPTOMS)	PHYSICAL (SIGNS)	"TESTS"	TREATMENT
Syndrome of marked hyperglycemia, dehydration, and coma with markedly increased (> 350) serum osmolality; minimal (if any) ketosis or acidosis	Severe underlying medical illnesses; often in elderly persons without history of significant diabetes (diet controlled Type II DM); usually precipitated by infection (pneumonia in women; urosepsis in men)	Progressive dec in LOC over days; polyuria may occur	Dec LOC; neuro findings (may mimic stroke); significant dehydration	BS markedly elevated; serum osmolality inc (normal ~ 290; pt often ~ 350); inc BUN/Cr due to hypovolemia; mild lactate elevations possible, due to tissue hypoperfusion from massive hypovolemia	Critical care unit; IV fluids, oxygen, potassium replenishment; insulin is a secondary treatment; treat underlying or precipitating causes

Electrolytes and acid-base disorders

Typically, the mere thought of "lytes" or acid-base puts terror into the most hardened of health care providers. Trust me (and *not* because I'm a doctor), it's really not that bad. To make our journey even easier, I've left out arterial blood gases (ABGs) until later, because what we're going to cover here is *independent* of blood gas results! And, I promise that ABGs will be *easier* than you ever thought, as well!

OBJECTIVE: **Summarize the primary roles of sodium, potassium, chloride, and bicarbonate in the body.**

A tale of four lytes. Regardless of the names our many labs choose for multipanel testing (e.g., "SMA"), the "contents" of each varies widely throughout the country. The good news — at least four of the values are relatively constant. These are the electrolytes: sodium (Na^+), potassium (K^+), chloride (Cl^-), and bicarbonate (HCO_3^-). We'll spend most of this section on potassium and bicarbonate. But first, a general summary of the role of each:

1.   **Sodium** (Na^+) — The primary role for Na^+ is regulation of osmotic balance between the extracellular and intracellular compartments of the body. It also plays a vital role in neural transmission (ie., intracellular communication), especially in the brain and the heart. The bulk of the body's Na^+ is in the extracellular space and is reflected by the serum Na^+ concentration. Fluids and drugs can rapidly affect the Na^+ level, but changes can also occur slowly. Though changes in the Na^+ concentration may lead to sudden osmotic imbalance, acute life-

> ***REMEMBER:*** **Sodium is the major extracellular fluid electrolyte.**

threatening symptoms are not common. Don't get me wrong —
seizures and dysrhythmias *can* occur with an acute change in the Na⁺
level, but our concern should rest more with rapidly-changing
potassium levels.

When Na⁺ levels change, they alter
osmotic balance; depending on the
time span during which the level was
abnormal, the "osmostat" may or may
not reset to the new Na⁺
concentration. The new setting is *not*
"normal," but is *baseline* (balanced)
for the *abnormal* circumstances.
Sometimes, the "osmostat" doesn't
change much at all (e.g., after rapid
changes in Na⁺ level, as during heat
exhaustion). On the other hand, the
"osmostat" may reset radically if the
Na⁺ level has been too high or too
low for more than a few hours. In
this case, a new (though "abnormal")
level of balance (homeostasis) is
reached. OK so far?

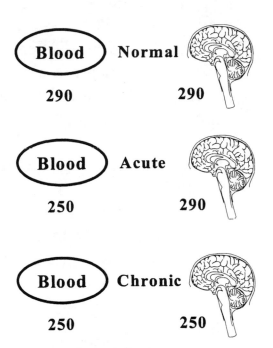

Figure 2-16 — When the sodium level
changes quickly, a marked difference
between the extracellular and
intracellular osmolality develops. If
hyponatremia persists for more than a
few hours, the "osmostat" resets, so
that the extracellular and intracellular
osmolalities are more similar, though
neither is truly "normal."

Make certain you are comfortable
with the concept that *rapid* changes
in Na⁺ levels have a different effect
on osmotic balance than do *slower*
ones. When the level changes
quickly, a marked difference between the extracellular and intracellular
osmolality develops. If hyponatremia persists for more than a few
hours, the "osmostat" resets so that the extracellular and intracellular
osmolalities are more similar, though neither is truly "normal."
[FIGURE 2-16]

This leads to the most important consideration in treatment of either hyper- or hyponatremia: correct the Na⁺ level over the same span of time that it took to become abnormal. So, if the [Na⁺] is 165 meq/L in a patient with acute heat exhaustion, our mission is to replenish fluids and salt (IV saline) as soon as possible. On the other hand, if a patient's [Na⁺] is 105 meq/L a week after receiving daily IV fluids consisting only of D5W at 150 cc/hr, we can assume that (though abnormal) the "osmostat" has reset. The last thing this person needs is to have us come along with hypertonic saline, diuretics, and the like to try and raise the [Na⁺] over minutes to hours! See why? In this case, we'd re-alter the altered osmotic balance, likely precipitating status epilepticus and death. If it took a week to develop the full-blown abnormality, we need that much time to allow the "osmostat" to reset back to normal.

> **REMEMBER**: "Fix" sodium level abnormalities over the time period it took for them to develop. . .

2. **Chloride** (Cl⁻) — Most Cl⁻ is also extracellular and accurately reflected in the serum Cl⁻ level. Cl⁻ is more of a "hitchhiker," in that it passively follows other positively charged electrolytes and rarely, if ever, is the isolated cause of a problem. An exception is in renal tubular acidosis, where the kidney's handling of Cl⁻ is impaired and the patient develops a hyperchloremic acidosis. This situation is beyond the intended scope of this text and won't be discussed further here.

> **REMEMBER**: Potassium is the major intracellular fluid electrolyte.

3. **Potassium** (K⁺) — The clout's in the K⁺, or something like that. K⁺ levels are probably the *most* important of the four electrolyte tests, because they can change rapidly, leading to cardiac membrane toxicity (EKG changes, arrhythmias, or both) within seconds. Please understand

that the majority of the body's K^+ ions "live" within the cells (150 - 300 meq/L); the serum level that we measure on the lab panel (approximately 3.5 - 5.0 meq/L) doesn't really reflect *total body potassium stores*. On the other hand, it's

REMEMBER: It's the *serum level*, not the intracellular level, of potassium that rapidly affects the cardiac membrane potential.

the *serum level* that, whether too high or too low, can rapidly lead to problems. Since that level is subject to rapid change for a number of reasons, we'll explore K^+ in depth in a bit.

Summary of Major Serum Electrolytes

Electrolyte	Major Functions	Comments
Sodium (Na^+)	• Osmotic balance • Neural transmission	Major extracellular electrolyte; correct abnormalities over the time span it took for them to develop.
Chloride (Cl^-)	• "Hitchhiker" • Electrical balance	Majority is extracellular
Potassium (K^+)	• Electrical stability of excitable tissues	Majority is intracellular
Bicarbonate (HCO_3^-) [see immediately below]	• Acid-base balance • Metabolic *base* • Regulated by kidneys	Don't confuse with calculated HCO_3^- or pCO_2 on ABGs.

4. **Bicarbonate** (HCO_3^-) — The serum HCO_3^- level confuses many of us because it goes by other names, depending on the lab (total CO_2, TCO_2, bicarbonate, or HCO_3^-). For simplicity's sake, I will use "HCO_3^-" throughout this section. Remember, what I am going to tell you here is correct and clinically applicable *regardless* of the patient's pH on an ABG. In fact, let's just assume that ABGs aren't available at this point. The reason — the ABG report usually contains a calculated HCO_3^- value; like many of the other calculated parameters on the report, it is potentially more confusing than helpful to the average health care professional. Take my advice — there are only *four* things worth looking at on an ABG report, and the patient's name is one of them (and the calculated HCO_3^- isn't — more on this later.).

   For now, please ignore the pH because the following is correct, *regardless* of the patient's pH. HCO_3^- represents *metabolic base*, and might simply be called the "serum baking soda level." It is regulated primarily by the kidneys and, as such, takes hours to days to change. It has absolutely *nothing* directly to do with the pCO_2 measurement or the pH on ABGs. As we'll see later, pCO_2 reflects *respiratory acid* and is rapidly changed and controlled by the lungs — totally different customer, so to speak.

   Back to the basics. Our choice of lab results is normal or abnormal (too high, too low). If the HCO_3^- level is *too high*, then we have excess metabolic base in the blood. This defines a *process* known as a metabolic alkalosis. Note that the suffix "sis" connotes a process rather than the net pH. It's possible to have several competing and possibly compensating acid-base processes underway at once, each contributing to the net pH. That's why it's important at this stage to look only at the HCO_3^- level on the electrolyte panel. If the HCO_3^- is elevated, regardless of the pH, the patient has (at a minimum) a *metabolic alkalosis*. Similarly, if the HCO_3^- if too low, there's too little base ("baking soda") and the patient has a *metabolic acidosis*. Again, the *process* is present regardless of total serum pH. Make certain you understand this concept — a *process* (metabolic alkalosis, metabolic acidosis) is different from a *result* (the net pH). **[FIGURE 2-17]**

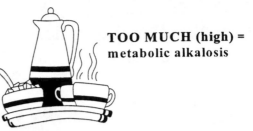

TOO MUCH (high) = metabolic alkalosis

$HCO_3^- =$ Serum Baking Soda = metabolic BASE; regulated by kidneys...

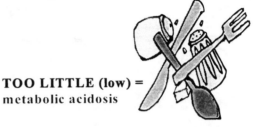

TOO LITTLE (low) = metabolic acidosis

Figure 2-17 — HCO_3^- is metabolic base and is regulated by the kidneys.

Metabolic acidosis — Based on the above information, it should be clear to you that simply looking at an electrolyte panel immediately tells you if there is a metabolic alkalosis or metabolic acidosis present:

- If the HCO_3^- is elevated, there is a metabolic alkalosis (too much "baking soda").

- If the HCO_3^- is low, there is a metabolic acidosis (too little "baking soda").

And, both the above statements are correct, regardless of the pH.

In clinical "challenges," metabolic alkalosis is less common than metabolic acidosis. The remainder of this portion of the discussion will center on a physiologically-based approach to a patient whose electrolyte panel shows metabolic acidosis. Of course, you'd immediately recognize the metabolic acidosis by the *low* serum HCO_3^- level, right?

Once you've recognized the presence of metabolic acidosis (and assuming stability of the ABCs, of course), the approach is two-pronged:

1. What are the implications for potassium?
2. Is the patient "SLUMPED?"

Let's deal with each of these important questions separately.

OBJECTIVE: Summarize the kinetics of potassium in the presence of a metabolic acidosis.

What are the implications for potassium? K^+ moves easily between the extracellular fluid (ECF) and the intracellular fluid (ICF). Factors that influence these movements include:

- Adrenergic stimulation — β-1 stimulation, primarily via epinephrine, stimulates K^+ ion channels, causing intracellular movement of potassium and reducing the serum level. This movement is thought to explain at least some episodes of sudden death — adrenergic stimulation leads to acute hypokalemia, which causes life-threatening dysrhythmias. The beneficial role of β-blockers in dysrhythmias and in acute myocardial infarction is likely related to a similar mechanism.

- Glucose — We mentioned earlier that K^+ and glucose "hang together." In DKA, glucose lost in the urine results in dehydration as well as loss of potassium. Similarly, in hyperkalemia, we give glucose and insulin. Insulin forces glucose intracellularly, drawing K^+ with it.

- Acid-base balance — Administration of bicarbonate in hyperkalemia causes a localized alkalosis that forces potassium into the ICF, lowering the serum level. The underlying physiology has far wider applications, however (see immediately below).

Metabolic acid-base changes affect serum potassium levels — When a person develops a metabolic acidosis, for just about any reason, there is a transient increase in the ECF acid concentration. The acid moves rapidly into the ICF, resulting in an intracellular *acidosis*. It is the ICF acid-base milieu that results in problems. So far, so good?

Realize that when the acid shifts to the intracellular compartment, it also carries with it an electric charge, usually positive. So, in addition to the intracellular acidosis, the ICF has a transient *excess* of positive charges. Since we need to remain electrically neutral within each fluid compartment (ECF and ICF), the ICF compensates (to maintain electrical neutrality) by shifting positively-charged K^+ ions into the serum. As a result, the serum K^+ level rises and electrical neutrality is maintained.

Of course, when the acidosis is corrected, acid shifts *out* of the ICF and is excreted by the kidneys. Transiently, the ECF now has too many cations; to compensate, K^+ is shifted *back* into the ICF. And, the serum K^+ level decreases. So, in summary: **[Figure 2-18]**

REMEMBER: Metabolic acidosis causes an *intracellular* shift of acid and an *extracellular* shift of potassium to maintain electrical neutrality. The reverse occurs during correction of the acidosis.

---

1. When metabolic acidosis develops (remember, *independent* of the pH), acid moves into the ICF.

2. The positively charged acid transiently increases the ICF positivity.

3. To compensate electrically, K^+ shifts from the ICF to the ECF.

The net result is an intracellular acidosis and an elevated serum K^+ level (by "elevated," I mean higher than it was prior to the acidosis).

When the ICF acidosis has been corrected, the acid then shifts back to the ECF and is excreted by the kidneys. As a result:

1. Acid in the ECF results in a transient increase in positive charge. To compensate, K^+ shifts back into the ICF.

2. The serum K^+ level drops.

Acidosis also decreases renal potassium secretion, by inhibiting the sodium-potassium ATPase pump. This also contributes to increased serum potassium levels.

Though not always correct, it's a helpful initial assumption in approaching a patient with a metabolic acidosis (regardless of the net pH) that the measured serum K^+ level is *higher* than it would have been prior to the development of the metabolic acidosis. And, as the metabolic acidosis is being corrected, it's another safe initial assumption that with treatment, the serum K^+ level will *decrease*.

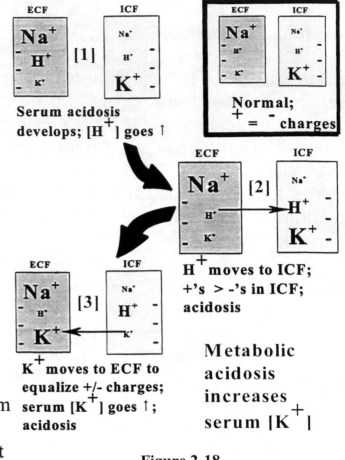

Figure 2-18

So, let's put this all together. By understanding the predictable inter-relationship of acid-base balance and K^+ kinetics, it's easy to understand why the following set of serum electrolytes is potentially life threatening:

* Na^+ = 135 meq/L
* K^+ = 3.5 meq/L
* Cl^- = 105 meq/L
* HCO_3^- = 16 meq/L

None of these lab values are particularly exciting. Other than a mild decrease in the HCO_3^- level, many of us may note the results and do nothing further. Admit it — the trap here is that the above lytes just aren't *abnormal enough* to really get your attention. The potassium level is normal; or isn't it?

Remember, the patient also has a metabolic acidosis, as evidenced by the low serum HCO_3^- (normal, in most labs, averages around 25 - 30 meq/L). This implies that whatever the serum potassium level, it is likely to be *higher* than if the acidosis were not present. And, with treatment, it's going to fall.

If the potassium were 6.0 or 3.0, the scenario might be different (and, perhaps, more obvious):

- As long as there is no evidence of cardiac membrane toxicity (e.g., EKG changes or dysrhythmias), a mildly elevated potassium level, such as 6.0 meq/L, in the face of metabolic acidosis, is not surprising. And, with treatment, this level is likely to fall well into the normal range. Simply treating the metabolic acidosis, without further "potassium-directed" therapy, may be all that is required.

- The level of 3.0 meq/L, by itself, isn't all that dangerous. Except — if the level is due to metabolic acidosis, we can assume that the measured level of 3.0 is *higher* than it would have been in the *absence* of metabolic acidosis. And, it's bound to decrease even further after treatment. I doubt anyone would disagree that a serum potassium level below 3.0 meq/L *is* dangerous.

- Even more worrisome is when the patient has diabetic ketoacidosis as the source of the acidosis. Everything we already said regarding the potassium level remains correct; add to this the fact that the *total body* potassium level is likely to be severely depleted due to the loss of potassium with sugar in the urine. As a result, the patient's "reserves" of potassium are even lower than

> **REMEMBER**: Patients with DKA are usually total body potassium-depleted, *regardless* of the measured serum potassium level.

those of a patient with a level of 3.0 meq/L and a metabolic acidosis for another reason. Not only must we assume that the K⁺ level will fall, but that the fall may be precipitous. Translation — these patients require cardiac monitoring and, often, need supplemental potassium *earlier than usual* in the course of treatment.

Why do small changes in the serum K⁺ level potentially lead to significant changes in the cardiac membrane potential? There are significant differences between the electrical charge inside and outside of cardiac cells. Electrically, the difference is measured in millivolts and referred to as the **cardiac membrane potential**. When calculated (see immediately below), the interior of the cell is significantly more negatively charged than outside of the cell. The resting or baseline cardiac membrane potential, then, is - 90 millivolts (mV).

Small (0.1 - 0.2 mEq/L) changes in the serum K⁺ level have far greater effect on the resting cardiac membrane potential than do changes in the intracellular level, even if these are significantly higher (50 - 100 mEq/L). The reason involves some fairly complex mathematical formulas but is easily summarized. The electrical potential (difference between inside and outside the cell) is determined by three factors for *each* major electrolyte (sodium, potassium, chloride):

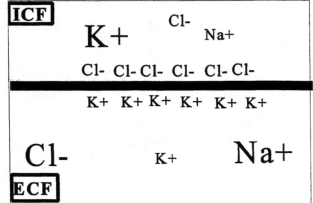

Figure 2-19 — The resting membrane potential is a result of potassium movement from ICF to ECF *without* concomitant movement of chloride. The ICF remains relatively negative compared to the ECF, resulting in a negative potential.

● Concentration.
● Electrical charge.
● Cell membrane permeability.

The cell membrane is 100 times more permeable to potassium (in both directions) than it is to either sodium or chloride. Remember, there is a large concentration gradient between the intracellular fluid (ICF) and the extracellular fluid (ECF). This, combined with the great membrane permeability of potassium, favors a small "leak" of potassium from ICF to ECF. Cells lose a few positively-charged potassium ions into the ECF, but the chloride (negatively charged) remains within. The result is like a capacitor — at the cell membrane is a "row" of "escaped potassium ions" in the ECF that are electrically attracted to the chloride anions remaining in the cell. **[FIGURE 2-19]** The excess negative charge inside the cell leads to generation of a negative membrane potential of -90 mV.

Since only a few potassium ions actually participate in the generation of this electrical gradient, changes in the intracellular potassium concentration have little effect. The leak (and the resulting electrical difference) continues due to the concentration gradient and permeability of potassium, even with significant changes (50 - 100 meq/L) in ICF potassium concentration.

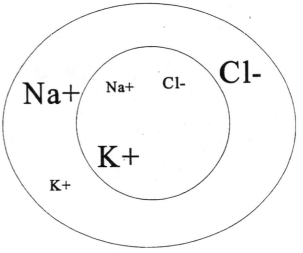

Due to the large number of potassium ions in the ICF, only a small number need diffuse into the ECF to establish a significant electrochemical gradient. So, large changes in ICF potassium concentrations have essentially no effect on membrane potential. Because of the small number of potassium ions in the ECF to begin with, any change in number may have a significant change in membrane potential. **[FIGURE 2-20]**

Figure 2-20 -- Due to the large number of potassium ions in the ICF, only a small number need diffuse into the ECF to establish a significant electrochemical gradient. Because of the small number of potassium ions in the ECF to begin with, any change in number may have a significant change in membrane potential.

Now, back to the original question: Why is the following set of electrolytes potentially life threatening?

- Na^+ = 135 meq/L
- K^+ = 3.5 meq/L
- Cl^- = 105 meq/L
- HCO_3^- = 16 meq/L

Recall that because this pattern is "less abnormal" than the alternative situations discussed above (K^+ of either 3.0 meq/L or 6.0 meq/L), we're far more likely to "blow it off." The K^+ of 3.5 meq/L is normal, but on the low side of normal. Of course, in the face of metabolic acidosis, we know that the level of 3.5 is *higher* than if the metabolic acidosis weren't there in the first place. And, it's going to fall into "abnormally low" territory as the acidosis is corrected. The result — because of the apparently unexciting appearance of these electrolytes, the patient may be treated without proper attention paid to the possibility of life-threatening hypokalemia's developing during treatment.

Remember that even small changes in the serum potassium level may change the cardiac membrane potential enough to result in significant dysrhythmias. These are the circumstances under which your understanding of acid-base and potassium kinetics may be life-saving.

Now, there's a second consideration. After dealing with any potential potassium problems, we next look into potential causes of the metabolic acidosis.

Is the patient "slumped?" "SLUMPED" is an acronym for potentially easily-treatable causes of metabolic acidosis. These include:

S — **Salicylates**
L — **Lactate**
U — **Uremia, underfed**
M — **Methanol**
P — **Paraldehyde**
E — **Ethanol, ethylene glycol**
D — **Diabetes**

OBJECTIVE: Defend the statement: "The anion gap, as performed in most clinical laboratories, is of no benefit and may be dangerously misleading."

Actually, many of us were taught that "SLUMPED" was the differential diagnosis of a "widened anion gap" metabolic acidosis. The anion gap is a calculation done either by us or by the lab based on this equation:

$$AG = [(Na^+ + K^+) - (Cl^- + HCO_3^-)]$$

The normal value for this calculation is less than 16.

I felt obligated to define "anion gap," since I brought it up in the first place, but its current utility is limited. In days of old, we assumed that an elevated anion gap indicated excess *unmeasured acids* in the blood, resulting in a **widened anion gap metabolic acidosis**. If the anion gap was normal, the metabolic acidosis was classified as a **non-widened anion gap metabolic acidosis**. Most non-widened anion gap acidoses are due to renal tubular acidosis, or another cause of a hyperchloremic acidosis — not much acutely (other than hemodialysis in rare circumstances) we can do. If the patient is "SLUMPED," the diagnostic and therapeutic options are wide open.

This differentiation sounds logical but is *unreliable* clinically. Recent data show that *regardless* of the calculated anion gap, patients may have a metabolic acidosis from any of the "SLUMPED" causes.[22] And, in DKA, the urine ketone dip test is a far better screening test than the anion gap.[23]

It's *dangerous* to assume that because the calculated anion gap is "normal," that the patient can't have a metabolic acidosis from the "SLUMPED" causes — and vice versa. Hence, my strong recommendation that we *always* think of "SLUMPED" in the differential diagnosis of *any* patient

> **REMEMBER**: "Anion gap" calculations are usually more confusing than helpful; current data also suggest they are unreliable in differentiating the causes of a metabolic acidosis!

with a metabolic acidosis. This doesn't mean, of course, that we order salicylate, lactate, methanol, ad nauseam . . . levels on everybody — just that we think about it and consider the most likely "culprits.".

How I nearly blew it . . . Take the set of lytes we talked about earlier:

- Na^+ = 135 meq/L
- K^+ = 3.5 meq/L
- Cl^- = 105 meq/L
- HCO_3^- = 16 meq/L

> **PRINCIPLE**: "Borderline abnormal" lab results are the *most* dangerous for the patient because they encourage us to become complacent.

Say they belong to a 17 year old white female with one day of right upper quadrant abdominal pain, nausea, and vomiting. And her "ob-gyn" work-up is completely negative. Other than her age, it's tempting to think about gall bladder disease — at least, that's what I thought when I saw her as a third-year medical student. As many of us might, I "blew off" the electrolytes above and was ready to send her home with a diagnosis of the "flu" (which really means I didn't have a clue!).

Enter the attending, who noted the metabolic acidosis and suggested (undoubtedly thinking of "SLUMPED") getting a blood sugar level. Great suggestion — it came back at 750 mg/dl. This was this girl's first presentation of DKA; had we not pursued the "SLUMPED" algorithm, it may well have been her last.

Abdominal pain is a common initial presentation of DKA, especially in teenagers, due to acute abdominal neuropathy. For some reason, the presentation tends to mimic acute cholecystitis (RUQ [right upper quadrant] pain, nausea, vomiting) but the gallbladder is normal. I learned an unforgettable lesson that day — by understanding "subtle" changes in light of pathophysiology, we provide better patient care and may even save a life.

Hypothermia

Hypothermia, its causes, and treatments are fairly well known (see Table). The underlying pathophysiology of cold exposure, however, is rarely discussed. An understanding of the "cold diuresis," described below, assures a sound approach to patient care.

PRINCIPLE: A *normal response* to an *abnormal situation* may lead to problems.

OBJECTIVE: **Enumerate the body's typical physiologic response to cold exposure; what are the implications of this response for the health care provider regarding volume therapy?**

What really happens when we get "too cold?" The "classic" picture of early (mild) hypothermia portrays a patient who is "hyperactive." He or she is tremulous, tachycardic, and tachypneic. Sure sounds like the sympathetic nervous system at work again, eh? Exactly right — cold "sensors" in the body stimulate the release of epinephrine ("stuff"). Epinephrine causes peripheral vasoconstriction, shunting some of the peripheral blood flow to the central circulation. This is why testing capillary refill isn't really helpful when the patient is cold — refill is slow in everyone, including the health care provider. Now, a side effect of peripheral vasoconstriction is an increase in the central blood volume. Receptors in the carotids and kidneys sense "fluid overload" in the central circulation and try

REMEMBER: Assume that all hypothermic patients are also hypovolemic until proven otherwise.

to fix it. Of course, the result is a diuresis. It's safe to assume that most hypothermic individuals have undergone at least a partial "cold diuresis," whether there is obvious evidence or not! The bottom line — assume that hypothermic patients are also hypovolemic.

> **OBJECTIVE:** Describe the implications of the body's physiologic response to cold exposure for rescue and movement of hypothermic patients, especially from cold water situations.

Rescue implications. The cold diuresis has extremely important implications in rescue work, particularly in cold water near-drownings. Remember, hypothermic patients are assumed to be hypovolemic. When *anyone* is removed from water, the effect on the body is like quickly removing a MAST suit (pneumatic anti-shock garment) — the hydrostatic pressure of the water makes us appear lighter in water than out (if I were a fish, I wouldn't be overweight!). Leaving the water rapidly removes this external pressure and we return to our "land mass."

REMEMBER: The body's normal response systems don't always "communicate" with each other prior to functioning. Diuresis is a *normal* response to perceived central volume overload.

Now, let's apply these principles to *hypothermic* patients who are in water. The additional factor here is that they are probably hypovolemic due to the cold diuresis. The physiological effect on the body during water rescue in a hypothermic patient is like quickly cutting off a MAST garment (poor form!) in a patient who is already hypovolemic. To add insult to injury, if the patient is taken vertically from the water, an orthostatic stress complicates things.

Now, we can't eliminate the need for rescue, nor should we "float" people around the water in MAST suits. Common sense simply dictates that these patients *must* be removed from the water in a *horizontal* position. Be sure you are convinced why the underlying pathophysiology of cold diuresis, combined with the hydrostatic effects of water, makes this mandatory! "Understanding *is* owning!"

Why doesn't aspirin cause hypothermia or lower the temperature in normal people? The presence of bacteria or viruses activates white blood cells, tissue macrophages, and killer lymphocytes. These cells release interleukin-1, which induces the formation of prostaglandin E_2. Prostaglandin E_2 acts on the hypothalamus to produce fever. Aspirin blocks prostaglandin formation, reducing the temperature. Since a normal individual does not have interleukin-1 released in the first place, no prostaglandin E_2 is made to be blocked. Therefore, the hypothalamus is not affected in the absence of interleukin-1 or prostaglandin E_2. Very logical, eh? (Wish I'd thought of it first!)

HYPOTHERMIA

DEFINITION	COMMON CAUSES	HISTORY (SYMPTOMS)	PHYSICAL (SIGNS)	"TESTS"	TREATMENT
Decrease of core temperature below 95° F or 35° C	Environmental; cold water; sepsis; endocrine disease	Depends on circumstances	Early = hyperactive (tachycardia, tachypnea, tremor); moderate = more lethargic; severe = looks dead	Core temperature!! Cold alters many laboratory measurements; may also affect blood clotting	Core re-warming; treatment of underlying causes (endocrine problems, infection)

Jaundice

The biochemistry of bilirubin, urobilinogen, and their interrelationship with liver function tests (LFTs) is confusing, if not downright threatening, to many of us. When I originally prepared my Lab Tests course, I asked myself a simple question: "What are the kinetics of bilirubin and where does urobilinogen come from?" Of the nearly 600,000 students I've asked, few would feel comfortable trying to answer the question, including "yours truly!" I figured that the solution must lie in my friendly collection of medical, nursing, lab, and allied health professions books. Was I ever wrong. I couldn't find the whole picture nicely summarized in any single volume I searched. After about a week, I finally put this material together — I'm very proud of it, though also quite frustrated that my thousands of dollars worth of reference books were basically worthless in this endeavor. Hopefully, you'll have the opportunity to "get it right" the first time, and understand this elegant system so you'll remember it forever.

What are the normal metabolic functions of the liver? The liver plays a major role in the metabolism of carbohydrates, fat, and proteins. In carbohydrate metabolism it:

1. Stores large quantities of glycogen.
2. Converts galactose and fructose to glucose.
3. Acts as the primary site for gluconeogenesis.

Most cells of the body play a role in fat metabolism, though the liver has a primary role in:

1. Oxidation of fats to acetyl-coenzyme A (acetyl-CoA).
2. Synthesis of cholesterol, phospholipids, and lipoproteins.
3. Fat synthesis from carbohydrates and proteins.

The liver is vital in numerous steps of protein metabolism. These include:

- Deamination of amino acids — amino acids cannot be used for energy or converted into carbohydrates or fats until they have been deaminated (ammonia removed).

- Formation of urea — large amounts of ammonia are formed during the deamination process, as well as produced by the metabolism of protein by colonic bacteria. The liver converts ammonia to urea, which is then excreted in the urine.

- Formation of plasma proteins — all plasma proteins, except for gamma globulins, are made in the liver. Gamma globulins are made in the lymphoid tissues.

- Metabolism of amino acids and synthesis of compounds from amino acids — the liver synthesizes nonessential amino acids and converts all the amino acids into other metabolically significant compounds.

Other functions of the liver include:

- Storage of vitamins and iron.
- Production of clotting factors II, VII, IX, and X.
- Detoxification and excretion of drugs and hormones.
- Conjugation and secretion of bilirubin into the bile.

My jaundiced opinion. Jaundice is common in a wide variety of disease states. For now, we'll limit ourselves to adults with all of their "innards" intact. Neonatal jaundice, hereditary conjugation defects, asplenia, and persons without a gallbladder make the picture more confusing than it needs to be.

Basic facts ("simple yet true!"). In this section, I want to outline a simple but elegant pathophysiologically-based approach to the "yellow fellow" — a patient with clinical jaundice. The bottom line is simple, but to understand, rather than memorize, I respectfully *beg* you to follow the steps, and not jump ahead. Just so you don't lose any precious sleep, I'll mention that the "bottom line" is "Give 'em a cup. . ." When we're done with the details, the beauty of this will *prove* to you that the dip UA is the single *best* liver function test in a jaundiced patient!

This approach is based on certain facts:

***REMEMBER*: The bilirubin system is a *normal* excretory mechanism for hemoglobin breakdown products. Jaundice is seen during a *normal response* to an *abnormal situation*.**

1. Red blood cells (RBCs) live 120 days; at that time they undergo a normal apoptotic death. Dead RBCs are then "recycled" by the reticuloendothelial system (RES), primarily the tissue macrophages and spleen.

2. When RBCs are recycled by the RES, hemoglobin is broken down into its constituents, heme and globin.

3. Globin is a vital plasma protein and is recycled to the protein pool of the body.

4. Heme is broken down and prepared for excretion. First, iron is removed and "recycled" by binding to transferrin (iron transport protein). This replenishes the body's iron stores and provides iron for

new hemoglobin synthesis. Interestingly, carbon monoxide (CO) is made in the process and acts as a chemical messenger, causing the conversion of GTP to cyclic GMP (cGMP). CO is then excreted in the lungs. The remnants of heme are then eliminated from the body (described in detail immediately below).

5. The entire purpose of the bilirubin system is to *eliminate* heme from the body via a series of metabolic steps.

The main reason people get confused is because they lose track of the reason for the entire system — to *metabolize* heme and *eliminate* it in either the stool (first choice) or the urine (second choice).

> ***REMEMBER*: The main purpose of the bilirubin system is to *metabolize* heme and *eliminate* it in either the stool (first choice) or in the urine (second choice).**

The "bilirubin factory tour." It's easiest to separate out the steps in space and time, though we all know that *in vivo*, there is some overlap. The areas of our "factory" are: **[Figure 2-21]**

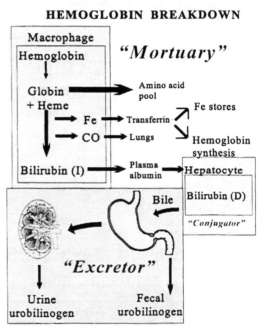

Figure 2-21 — The "Bilirubin Factory Tour"

1. The "mortuary" — the reticuloendothelial system, primarily tissue macrophages and the spleen, is essentially a mortician, preparing the dead RBC for recycling and excretion of non-recyclable components (e.g., heme).

2. The "conjugator" — the liver; converts heme into an excretable form.

3. The "excretor" — the GI tract and kidneys.

Of course, all three sections of the bilirubin "factory" are interconnected by blood vessels. In a nutshell, the process goes something like this:

1. The RES recycles iron and globin, and converts heme to a nonwater-soluble form of bilirubin.

2. The liver conjugates nonwater-soluble bilirubin to a water-soluble form so it can be secreted into the bile.

3. Bile drains into the duodenum via the common bile duct; bilirubin "hitchhikes" along.

4. Bilirubin is converted to "urobilinogens" in the colon, and either excreted in the stool or filtered by the kidneys and excreted in the urine.

    REMEMBER: The main purpose of the bilirubin system is to *metabolize* heme and *eliminate* it in either the stool (first choice) or in the urine (second choice).

5. Either way, the end product of heme breakdown, urobilinogens, are excreted from the body.

Now, let's observe the process in more detail and add in the many names for the two forms of bilirubin. Like it or not, this is potentially confusing, so watch out — you and I didn't create this mess, we just have to deal with it!

PART I: In the "mortuary" (RES). The RES sequesters the dead RBCs, and enzymes break down their cell walls. Hemoglobin is separated into globin, which is recycled into the plasma protein pool, and heme (an iron-containing protoporphyrin, for those of you *really interested* in biochemistry), which must be prepared for excretion. Iron from heme is recycled by binding to transferrin in an energy-requiring reaction that also produces carbon monoxide (CO). CO is excreted via the lungs.

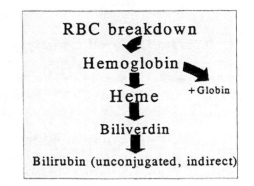

RBC breakdown

Hemoglobin

Heme + Globin

Biliverdin

Bilirubin (unconjugated, indirect)

The RES converts heme to **biliverdin**, then to **unconjugated bilirubin**. The latter, an early form of bilirubin, is not water-soluble. (Though I strongly believe that the only two terms for bilirubin should be "water-soluble" and "nonwater-soluble," it's a battle I won't win.) Early, nonwater-soluble bilirubin goes by one of two names, depending on the laboratory — **unconjugated** or **indirect**. Remember, the whole purpose of our tour is to see how *early, nonwater-soluble (i.e., unconjugated, indirect) bilirubin is made water-soluble so it will dissolve in bile to be excreted into the GI tract and eliminated from the body*! Pretty straightforward, eh?

The "yellow taxi" ride to the liver. Bilirubin is converted to a water-soluble form in the liver, but first it needs to get there. Remember that this early form isn't going to dissolve by itself in the blood (nonwater-soluble). To get to the liver, via the blood, unconjugated bilirubin (which we'll abbreviate as BU) binds to albumin (BU-A). This is a common way that nonwater-soluble molecules become temporarily soluble in liquid. Albumin acts as the "yellow taxi" and carries BU to the liver. Like any good cab driver, the albumin taxi drops BU off and returns

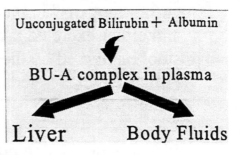

to the cab stand (plasma) to await further passengers. Don't forget — we *still* want to get rid of BU, regardless of what name we call it. When we measure unconjugated (indirect) bilirubin levels in the lab, we're essentially determining how many "passengers" (BU) are in "yellow taxis" on their way to the liver to be conjugated. In more formal terms, the unconjugated bilirubin test measured albumin-bound unconjugated bilirubin levels. Keep this in mind, and consider which non-hepatic problem would lead to jaundice and an elevation of indirect (early, nonwater-soluble, etc.) bilirubin. The answer in a bit. . .

PART II: In the "converter" (liver). The hepatocyte performs two separate, though related, actions on early, nonwater-soluble bilirubin (BU). The first is **conjugation**, the process of chemically adding two glucuronide molecules, resulting in the formation of

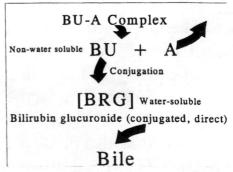

bilirubin diglucuronide (BRG). BRG is a long word, so I find it easier to call it "late," or water-soluble, bilirubin. The lab people use somewhat different terms — **conjugated** or **direct**. So, the liver conjugates BU to a water-soluble form. Second, the hepatocyte then *secretes* the conjugated (direct, late, water-soluble) bilirubin, via the bile

REMEMBER: Once early bilirubin (nonwater-soluble, indirect, unconjugated) reaches the liver, it *will* be converted to late bilirubin (water-soluble, direct, conjugated).

canaliculi, into the biliary drainage system (i.e., bile ducts, hepatic ducts, gallbladder).

It's important to understand that conjugation and secretion, though both carried out by the hepatocyte, are *separate* processes. As such, various diseases may damage one function (e.g., secretion) but leave the other (e.g., conjugation) intact. In fact, this is usually the case. Conjugation isn't completely impaired until late hepatic failure — by then, the patient has "flapping" (sign language for "I need a transplant") and numerous other stigmata of severe liver failure. Secretion, on the other hand, is impaired (but seldom completely blocked) at a much earlier stage. Diseases causing hepatocellular damage, such as hepatitis, will affect *secretion* and rarely alter *conjugation* unless they progress to end-stage liver failure. In most cases, it's safe to assume that once unconjugated bilirubin (early, nonwater-soluble, indirect) reaches the liver, it *will* be converted to conjugated bilirubin (late, water-soluble, direct).

The *conjugated* (*direct*) bilirubin level that we measure in the lab reflects the very small amount of conjugated bilirubin that "backs up" normally in the serum. The *total bilirubin* level is the mathematical sum of unconjugated plus conjugated (indirect + direct) bilirugin levels. Most experts recommend that you measure only two of the three, and calculate the remaining value. If you rely on separate lab tests to measure each, the math never works out, and outside reviewers have a picnic!

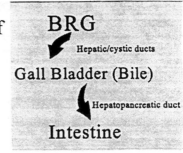

BRG
Hepatic/cystic ducts
Gall Bladder (Bile)
Hepatopancreatic duct
Intestine

PART III: The "hitchhiker." Once in the bile, conjugated bilirubin flows through the sphincter of Odi into the duodenum. Bilirubin has *no* digestive functions; it's merely a passive follower, or "hitchhiker," taking the shortest direct and "physiologically-legal" route to the intestine. Remember — our body's "mission" is to excrete heme!

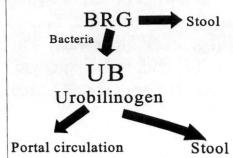

In the intestines. Water-soluble bilirubin passes through the duodenum and small intestine unchanged. In the colon, normal enteric bacteria convert it to **urobilinogens (UBs)**, the final breakdown product of heme and the form in which "heme" is finally excreted normally (at last!). Most of the urobilinogen mixes with fecal material, imparting the normal brownish color of stool to it. Some physiologists refer to this portion of urobilinogen as stercobilin. Thus (and this is gross, but memorable!), urobilinogen (stercobilin) is essentially "brown dye #2." It passes in the stool and is eliminated from the body, which is what we wanted to do in the first place — right?

NOTE: Some experts use the term "urobilinogens" as a generic term for conjugated bilirubin broken down by the colonic bacteria. Others use stercobilin *to refer to the portion that "colors" the stool, and* urobilinogen *as the remnant that is excreted in the urine and lends a golden hue to the urine color. The concept of elimination of bilirubin breakdown products, first in the stool, then in the urine (if any is left over) is more important than specific names. The term "urobilinogens" will work for both — and the "bottom line" is unchanged, since the dip UA indeed measures "urobilinogen" in the urine, as well as bilirubin. For simplicity's sake, I use the term "urobilinogens" to refer to both compounds, regardless of their location in the stool or urine.*

> **REMEMBER: Assume if conjugated bilirubin reaches the bowel (via the bile), it *will* be converted to urobilinogens.**

In the "beans" (kidneys). The quanity of urobilinogens that leave the body in the stool is dependent on the bilirubin load thrust upon the liver. If there is more unconjugated bilirubin than usual to conjugate, more conjugated bilirubin is made. More enters the intestine and more urobilinogens are made by the colonic flora. Remember, regardless of the amount, we *still* want to excrete urobilinogens from the body.

REMEMBER: Under normal circumstances, bilirubin leaves the body as urobilinogen — most in the stool, the rest in the urine.

The urobilinogen that doesn't pass in the stool is reabsorbed into the blood (portal circulation) and transported to the kidneys. Being water-soluble, it freely crosses the glomerular filtration membrane and is excreted in the urine. Normally, the dip urinalysis (UA) contains "zero to trace" urobilinogen, because most is excreted in the stool. Whatever appears in the urine represents the "colonic overload" that wasn't excreted via the stool. So, the "beans" are the "back door" or secondary route for final heme breakdown product excretion.

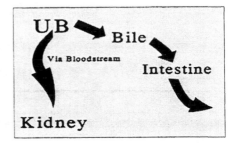

Make certain you're comfortable at this stage that:

1. Colonic bacteria manufacture urobilinogens from conjugated bilirubin.

2. Urobilinogens "color" the stools brown, and to some extent, the urine yellow.

3. If there is complete hepatobiliary obstruction (e.g., common duct stone, pancreatic cancer, choledocal cyst), *no bilirubin* enters the GI tract.

REMEMBER: the main purpose of the bilirubin system is to *metabolize* heme and *eliminate* it in either the stool (first choice) or in the urine (second choice).

4. If there is *no bilirubin* in the gut, there can be *no urobilinogen* made by the colonic bacteria.

5. The presence of *any* urobilinogen in the urine virtually excludes *complete* hepatobiliary obstruction.

6. Stool without "brown dye #2" can't be normal color.

7. The body *still* wants to get rid of the bilirubin!

I know these tenets seem almost insultingly simple — trust me, and NOT because I'm a doctor. As obvious as they may seem during a casual reading, most students lose sight of this simple elegance at some point.

OBJECTIVE: Defend the statement: "the dip UA is the single best initial screening test for the jaundiced patient."

The meaning of jaundice. The presence of clinical jaundice means that a patient's serum *total* bilirubin level is elevated (usually 2.5 - 3.0 mg/dL). This is true regardless of whether the elevation consists primarily of conjugated, unconjugated, or (rarely) both types of bilirubin. In fact, we could argue that measuring the actual total bilirubin level in adults, other than to follow a patient's progress, is academic.

In adults, the absolute "peak" of the bilirubin level isn't as much of a concern as it is in newborns. Bilirubin doesn't cross the blood-brain barrier, which is fully developed in adults. So, the risk of kernicterus and brain damage is absent. We could argue that once we visually observe jaundice, we *already know* that the total bilirubin level is up. Remember — once you see yellow, you already *know* the bilirubin level is "too high." In fact, we can often predict from the dip UA which fraction (direct or indirect) predominates.

Generically speaking, there are only two causes of jaundice (if we exclude congenital conjugation defects) — hemolysis or "liverolysis." Intravascular hemolysis is *not* a liver problem and requires a totally different lab and clinical approach than does "liverolysis." Of course, I invented the term "liverolysis," yet the concept is very helpful. Once we've determined that the patient has "liver jaundice," we can use our understanding of bilirubin kinetics to differentiate between the two types of liver problems — **obstructive jaundice** (e.g., common duct stone, pancreatic tumor) and **hepatocellular jaundice** (e.g., hepatitis, toxins such as carbon tetrachloride, acetaminophen, or alcohol). And here's how we do it. **[FIGURE 2-22]**

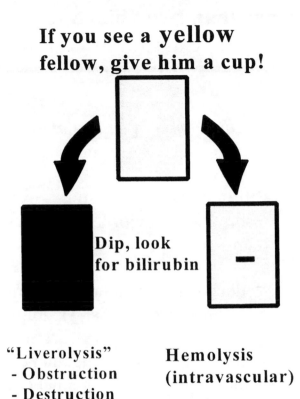

If you see a yellow fellow, give him a cup!

Dip, look for bilirubin

"Liverolysis"
- Obstruction
- Destruction

Hemolysis (intravascular)

Figure 2-22 — The generic approach to jaundice.

Liver problems, regardless of whether primarily obstructive or destructive (hepatocellular injury), result in a backup of conjugated bilirubin in the blood. Though the causes are different for each type of jaundice, the bottom line effect is the same. The backup causes jaundice and an elevation of the serum total and direct bilirubin levels. Remember that the body *still* wants to get rid of bilirubin (heme) — what doesn't get to the bowel (due to failure of hepatic secretion or due to hepatobiliary obstruction) is excreted in the urine. Thus, the appearance of bilirubin in the urine *always* means a liver problem — either obstruction or "destruction."

What are the common causes of **unconjugated** *hyperbilirubinemia?* There are three generic causes of unconjugated hyperbilirubinemia:

1. Bilirubin overproduction — excessive hemolysis of red blood cells; resorption of major hemorrhages; ineffective erythropoiesis in the bone marrow.

2. Reduced hepatic uptake of bilirubin formed peripherally — Gilbert syndrome (see number 3); drugs (rifampin).

3. Impaired hepatic conjugation of bilirubin — neonatal jaundice; Crigler-Najjar syndrome (congenital decrease or absence of bilirubin uridine duiphosphate-glucuronosyltransferase (UGT); Gilbert syndrome (congenital mutation in the UGT gene resulting in mild, fluctuating unconjugated hyperbilirubinemia).

What are the common causes of **conjugated** *hyperbilirubinemia?* Three common causes are:

1. Dubin-Johnson syndrome — congenital defect resulting in defective secretion of bilirubin due to absence of canalicular plasma transport protein.

2. Rotor syndrome — asymptomatic, genetic form of conjugated hyperbilirubinemia.

3. Cholestasis — due to hepatocellular dysfunction (failure of hepatocyte secretion of bile) or biliary obstruction.

A simplified (and still correct) approach. If we exclude neonatal jaundice and congenital defects (e.g., Dubin-Johnson, Gilbert syndromes) the causes of jaundice boil down to two: increased bilirubin production or decreased bilirubin excretion. By "excretion," I mean failure of conjugated bilirubin to reach the bowel and undergo conversion to urobilinogen.

Decreased bilirubin excretion occurs due to some type of hepatobiliary dysfunction, either hepatocellular damage ("destruction," with failure of the hepatocyte to secrete bile into the ductal system) or obstruction (partial or complete). Either results in an accumulation of *conjugated* bilirubin.

The only cause of increased bilirubin production is intravascular hemolysis. And, this results in an increased level of *unconjugated* bilirubin, which is then metabolized normally. **[FIGURE 2-23]**

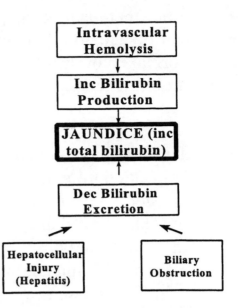

Figure 2-23 — Excluding neonatal jaundice and congenital defects, there are two causes of jaundice: increased bilirubin production (hemolysis) or decreased bilirubin excretion (hepatocellular damage, biliary obstruction).

Obstructive jaundice. Let's assume that the entire system works well until we get to the common bile duct. Mentally, let's tie it off with a nice yellow ribbon and determine what would happen. Clinically, we see this as complete obstructive jaundice due to common duct stones, tumor, cysts, or (less commonly) long-standing inflammation. Since the GI tract is "closed for business" to the liver and its ducts, no bilirubin can enter the bowel. Think about what happens at this point:

1. No conjugated bilirubin enters the intestines — it *must* back up into the blood. The patient becomes jaundiced and the elevated serum bilirubin is primarily conjugated.

2. Since there is no conjugated bilirubin entering the colon, the bacteria can't make urobilinogens. Without "brown dye #2," the stool loses its normal color, leading to acholic (clay-colored) stools. Since no urobilinogens can be made, there can't be any excess in the bowel to "back up" into the urine, can there?

3. Though obstruction has caused virtually all of the conjugated bilirubin to back up into the blood, don't lose sight of the body's primary mission — it *still* wants to get rid of the stuff. Since the usual route (GI tract) isn't available, all of the conjugated bilirubin is excreted (eliminated) in the urine. Thus, we see bilirubinuria and *LOTS* of it. Of course, since none of this conjugated bilirubin finds its way to the colon to be made into urobilinogen, the hint is a jaundiced patient with high urine bilirubin levels (3-4+) and *no* urobilinogen in the urine.

> **REMEMBER**: the presence of *any* urobilinogen in the dip UA excludes complete hepatobiliary obstruction.

At that point, I recommend that the next test be a CT scan or ultrasound looking for pancreatic cancer, a common duct stone, or a choledochal cyst (cyst of the biliary tree). The only other test we might need is an ALT or AST level. In pure obstruction, these enzymes aren't usually elevated more than twice normal. The only time these ALT or AST levels rise greater than twice normal during obstruction is if there is concomitant ascending cholangitis. This is unusual and these patients are incredibly ill. Most people with purely obstructive jaundice, unless they have a common duct stone, have painless jaundice. And, even those with an impacted stone may not have pain.

Hepatocellular jaundice. "Destructive" jaundice means that the hepatocytes are injured, for any of a number of reasons. This generic process is called **hepatocellular injury**. They contain enzymes, such as ALT and AST, that are normal cellular components to catalyze day to day chemical reactions. That's why there are *normal* levels of these enzymes in the serum — this reflects normal cell turnover. Only when the hepatocytes are injured significantly do their membrane walls become abnormally permeable, allowing more enzymes to leak into the serum. Thus, elevations of ALT or AST greater than twice normal imply hepatocellular damage.

Remember that secretion of bilirubin into the bile by the hepatocyte is lost relatively *early,* but that conjugation continues until end stage hepatic failure. Patients with hepatocellular jaundice, such as hepatitis, conjugate all the indirect bilirubin that reaches the liver (as long as they don't develop end-stage hepatic failure). The problem is that they don't *secrete* it into the bile as well as they normally would. It's a safe bet that some conjugated bilirubin will back up, due to loss of hepatic secretion, and need to be excreted in the urine.

As a general rule, there is less bilirubin "backed up" in hepatocellular damage than in complete obstruction. The reason: Some conjugated bilirubin enters the bowel (since a portion is secreted normally), and some urobilinogens are made. Typically, the urine bilirubin levels are not as high as in complete obstruction. If the UA shows some bilirubin (which *must be* conjugated, since it's dissolved in the urine!), as well as urobilinogen, that patient is very unlikely to have complete biliary obstruction. Why? Of course — some bilirubin *must* have entered the colon for urobilinogen to be made and, thus, to "back up" into the urine.

Hemolytic jaundice. In intravascular hemolysis, the defect lies not in the hepatobiliary system, but in the red blood cell (RBC). Essentially, the "mortuary" is overloaded with prematurely lysed RBCs. As such, there is more heme to excrete. Assuming the rest of the system is OK (which is usually a safe assumption), all the unconjugated bilirubin that gets to the liver will be conjugated. The patient is jaundiced due to the load of early, unconjugated bilirubin taking the "yellow taxi" to the liver to be excreted. Again, regardless of the cause, don't forget that the body's "mission" is to get rid of heme! And, if we measure serum bilirubin levels, the total *and* indirect (unconjugated) fractions are elevated.

Once unconjugated reaches the liver, it is conjugated as in the normal patient. The amounts of conjugated bilirubin made are just *increased*. Not a problem, as the hepatobiliary system has great functional reserve. Once conjugated, conjugated bilirubin is secreted into the bile. In hemolysis, there is *more* than usual. Thus, the colonic bacteria make *more* urobilinogens. Since the whole purpose of the system is *still* to eliminate urobilinogens, chances are excellent that more of them will back up in the blood and require excretion by the kidneys. So, we'd expect to find elevated levels of urobilinogen in the urine, but *no* bilirubin of any kind.

The clue here is a jaundiced patient (implies elevated bilirubin), no bilirubin, but *lots* of urobilinogen in the urine. The UA is telling us that "extra" urobilinogen has overloaded the GI tract and is being eliminated via the kidneys. Since there is no backup of bilirubin, the liver must be OK. So, our conclusion — hemolysis. The next series of "tests" should involve the blood cells (e.g., Coombs, Hgb, Hct), *not* the liver.

The bottom line. By now it should be clear that of the common types of jaundice, only liver problems result in bilirubinuria; hemolysis does not. So, when you see a "yellow fellow," give him a cup — meaning obtain a dip UA. Look first for one thing — bilirubin. Remember, to appear in the urine, bilirubin must be water soluble; thus, *only* conjugated bilirubin is detectable on the dip UA. Then: **[FIGURE 2-24]**

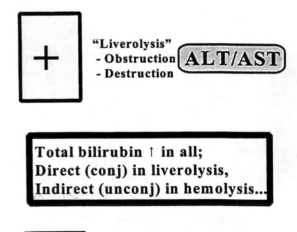

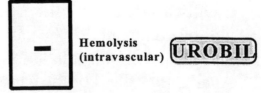

- If there is any bilirubin in the urine, you are dealing with "liverolysis."

- Large urine bilirubin levels with absolutely no urobilinogen suggest complete hepatobiliary obstruction.

Figure 2-24 — Summary of the lab approach to jaundice. (+) and (-) refer to the presence or absence, respectively, of bilirubin on the dip urinalysis (UA).

- A mixed picture (some bilirubin, some urobilinogen) suggests hepatocellular damage (or partial obstruction).

- Regardless of the presence, absence, or amount of urobilinogen in the dip UA, the presence of any bilirubin means a liver problem.

- Use ALT or AST (GPT/GOT) to confirm hepatocellular damage (elevated greater than twice normal). Then you can judiciously consider the next step (e.g., hepatitis antigen testing).

> *REMEMBER*: the main purpose of the bilirubin system is to *metabolize* heme and *eliminate* it in either the stool (first choice) or in the urine (second choice).

- If there is no bilirubin on the dip UA, the problem is most likely hemolysis; elevated urobilinogen levels in the *absence* of bilirubin strongly support this conclusion. Congenital abnormalities of bilirubin metabolism will *not* increase the amount of urobilinogen made. Only hemolysis actually increases the "workload" on the RE system ("mortuary").

Summary

Hypoglycemia is common and often occurs in diabetics, due to loss of the normal counter-regulatory hormone response or "early warning system." Some evidence suggests that simple means, such as drinking coffee, may help to restore it. Reducing the number and duration of significant hypoglycemic spells is important, because with each, the potential for permanent brain damage arises, due to release of free radicals and other "stuff."

Diabetic ketoacidosis occurs when there is insufficient insulin to "feed" the cells; in addition to insulin depletion, something occurs that results in an excess of counter-regulatory hormones. Elevated blood sugar, by itself, will *not* lead to diabetic ketoacidosis. By understanding the actions of insulin, it is relatively easy to predict what happens — cells starve and turn to other sources of food, such as fat and muscle. Fat and muscle metabolism lead to production of ketoacids. Elevation of the serum glucose level causes an osmotic diuresis with 5-6 liters of fluid being lost in the average adult. Since potassium follows glucose, it is also lost in the urine. Thus, most DKA patients are total body potassium depleted,

PRINCIPLE: **Many diseases arise from *loss* of a normal response system (NRS), or *normal activation* of a NRS under *abnormal* circumstances, with untoward results.**

PRINCIPLE: **Unstopped, damage begets more damage!**

PRINCIPLE: **The absence of "good stuff" and/or the production of "bad stuff" leads to disease.**

PRINCIPLE: **Patients don't always "read the textbook" before they get sick.**

PRINCIPLE: **Always think sugar!**

regardless of the measured serum level. The mainstay of DKA treatment is fluids, then insulin. Without fluids, patients fare poorly. Hyperosmolar coma (HHNC) differs from DKA in many ways, including a distinct absence of ketones and acids.

Though all serum electrolytes are important, changes in the potassium level result in nearly-instantaneous effects in the cardiac membrane potential. As a result, dysrhythmias may occur suddenly and with only small changes in the serum potassium value. The serum bicarbonate level is integrally related to the potassium level — metabolic acidosis (low bicarbonate) raises the serum potassium level, while the reverse occurs during metabolic alkalosis (or during the correction of metabolic acidosis). In approaching any patient with a metabolic acidosis, regardless of the pH, the clinician must always:

- Carefully consider implications of the measured potassium level.
- Ask if the patient is "SLUMPED."

Hypothermia results in activation of the adrenergic nervous system. This normal response leads to the "cold diuresis," causing most hypothermic patients to be hypovolemic. This fact must always be kept in mind,

PRINCIPLE: A *normal response* to an *abnormal situation* may lead to problems.

especially when considering patient body position during cold water near-drowning rescue.

Jaundice is a common patient problem. A thorough understanding of the bilirubin system, based on the premise that the body "just wants to get rid of heme," leads to a simple, yet elegant bottom line: If you see a yellow fellow, give him a cup!

Crossword Puzzle Review

Path Chap 2 -- Endocrine/Metabolic

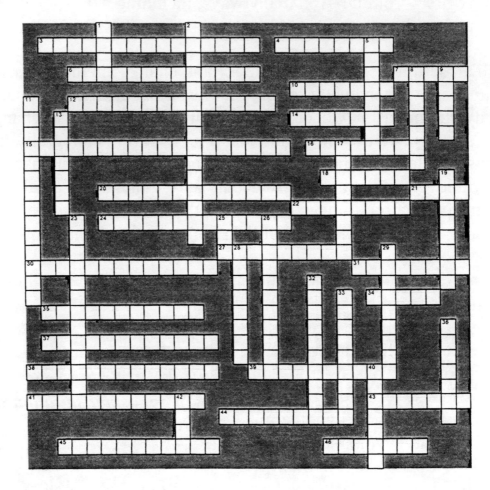

Across

3. Unconjugated (indirect) bilirubin is _____.
4. Chronic complications of diabetes probably occur from a combination of protein glycosylation and accumulations of intracellular _____.
6. Epinephrine leads to the G-protein mediated activation of _____.
7. The _____ potassium exerts a major effect on membrane electrical potential.
10. Other drugs associated with hypoglycemia include _____, fluoxetine (Prozac), and glyburide (Micronase) when combined with ciprofloxacin (Cipro).
12. Caffeine is a _____ drug, much like aminophylline.
14. The main role of sodium is to maintain _____ balance between the extracellular and intracellular compartments of the body.
15. Diabetics who have lost part of their _____ _____ _____ (3 words) are more likely to have severe hypoglycemic spells.
16. Acidosis results in an _____ in the serum potassium level.
18. The major initial treatment in DKA.
20. Sodium is the major _____ fluid electrolyte.
21. Compared to DKA, _____ (abbrev) results in significant elevations of serum osmolality.
22. Exposure of the body to cold usually results in a cold _____.
24. Mechanism by which very low concentrations of epinephrine or glucagon are required for a significant hormonal effect to occur.
27. Many important biochemical reactions involve the addition or removal of _____ to or from a substance.
30. Potassium is the major _____ fluid electrolyte.
31. A low serum bicarbonate level indicates a metabolic _____.
34. The presence of bilirubin on the dip UA indicates a _____ or hepatobiliary problem.
34. Unconjugated (indirect) bilirubin is converted to conjugated (direct) bilirubin by the _____.
35. Second most important counterregulatory hormone of glucose metabolism.
37. Conjugated (direct) bilirubin is _____.
38. Bilirubin is converted to _____ in the colon and either excreted in the stool or filtered by the kidneys and excreted in the urine.
39. Bilirubin is a normal breakdown product of _____.
41. One major source of brain damage after prolonged hypoglycemia is _____ _____ (2 words).
43. Acronym for common causes of metabolic acidosis.
44. A high serum bicarbonate level indicates a metabolic _____.
45. Glucose move into cells by either _____ transport or cotransport.
46. Rapid changes in the serum sodium level should be corrected _____.

Down

1. Bicarbonate represents metabolic _____.
2. Glucagon stimulates glycogenolysis, inhibits glycogenesis, and stimulates _____.
2. Ethanol causes hypoglycemia by diverting resources from the process of _____.
2. Cortisol increases hepatic _____.
5. The effects of glucagon are _____ to those of insulin.
8. In hepatocellular damage, liver _____ are elevated greater than two times normal.
9. Conjugated bilirubin that does not enter the bowel leaves the body in the _____.
11. ACE blockers increase the likelihood of hypoglycemia in diabetics by decreasing the production of _____.
13. Prolonged hypoglycemia is _____.
17. The resting membrane potential occurs as a result of potassium movement with movement of _____.
19. Insulin has _____ effects while counterregulatory hormones have catabolic actions.
23. The blood sugar level at which a given patient becomes symptomatic from hypoglycemia is _____.
25. Thiamine deficiency leads to formation of inadequate brain _____.
26. Patients with total _____ jaundice have absolutely no urobilinogen in their urine.
28. Ketones dissociate in serum, resulting in free _____ ions.
29. The presence of visible clinical jaundice means that the patient's _____ level is elevated.
32. Insulin does not act through second _____.
33. Red blood cells die every 120 days via the normal process of _____.
36. The _____ a person's diabetic control, the greater the risk of hypoglycemic spells.
40. Facilitates intracellular transport of ingested nutrients.
42. Bicarbonate causes the oxyhemoglobin desaturation curve to shift to the _____.

References

1. Swain, DP. *The beaver pond analogy of blood glucose control.* Am J Physiol (Adv. Physiol. Educ 21) 1999; 276: S69-S73.

2. Bolli, GB. *Counterregulatory mechanisms to insulin-induced hypoglycemia in humans: relevance to the problem of intensive treatment of IDDM.* J Pediatr Endocrinol Metab 1998 Mar; 11 Suppl 1:103-15.

2. Edelman, SV. *Importance of glucose control.* Med Clin North Am; 1998 Jul; 82(4);665-87.

4. Pearl, RG, et al. *Aminophylline potentiates sodium nitroprusside-induced hypotension in the dog.* Anesthesiology 1984; 61:712-15.

5. Debrah, K, et al. *Effect of caffeine on recognition of and physiological responses to hypoglycaemia in insulin-dependent diabetes.* Lancet 1996 Jan 6; 347(8993):19-24; Kerr, D, et al. *Effect of caffeine on the recognition of and responses to hypoglycemia in humans.* Ann Intern Med 1993 Oct 15; 119(8):799-804.

6. Kerr, DD, et al. *Caffeine consumption increases intensity of hypoglycemic warning symptoms.* Diabetes Care 2000; 23:455-59.

7. Jones, TW, et al. *Decreased epinephrine responses to hypoglycemia during sleep.* N Engl J Med 1998 Jun 4; 338(23):1657-62.

8. Heller, SR, et al. *Effect of the fast-acting insulin analog lispro on the risk of nocturnal hypoglycemia during intensified insulin therapy.* U.K. Lispro Study Group. Diabetes Care 1999 Oct; 22(10):1607-11.

9. Feske, SK. *Coma and confusional states: emergency diagnosis and management.* Neurol Clin 1998 May; 16(2):237-56.

10. Jaap, AJ, et al. *Perceived symptoms of hypoglycaemia in elderly type 2 diabetic patients treated with insulin.* Diabet Med 1998 May; 15(5):398-401.

11. Luber, S, et al. *Hypoglycemia presenting as acute respiratory failure in an infant.* Am J Emerg Med 1998 May; 16(3):281-4.

12. Herings, RM, et al. *Hypoglycaemia associated with use of inhibitors of angiotensin converting enzyme.* Lancet 1995 May 13; 345(8959):1195-8.

13. Thamer, M, et al. *Association between antihypertensive drug use and hypoglycemia: a case-control study of diabetic users of insulin or sulfonylureas.* Clin Ther 1999 Aug; 21(8):1387-400.

14. Moore, N, et al. *Reports of hypoglycaemia associated with the use of ACE inhibitors and other drugs: a case/non-case study in the French pharmacovigilance system database.* Br J Clin Pharmacol 1997 Nov; 44(5):513-8.

15. Madsen, BK, et al. *The influence of captopril on the epinephrine response to insulin-induced hypoglycemia in humans. The interaction between the renin-angiotensin system and the sympathetic nervous system.* Am J Hypertens 1992 Jun; 5(6 Pt 1):361-5; Worck, RH, et al. *AT1 and AT2 receptor blockade and epinephrine release during insulin- induced hypoglycemia.* Hypertension 1998 Jan; 31(1 Pt 2):384-90.

16. Winer, LM, et al. *Effect of angiotensin-converting enzyme inhibition on pituitary hormone responses to insulin-induced hypoglycemia in humans.* J Clin Endocrinol Metab 1990 Jul; 71(1):256-9.

17. Kshirsagar, AB, et al. *ACE inhibitors slow progression of nephropathy.* Am J Kid Dis 2000; 35:695-707.

18. Roberge, RJ, et al. *Glyburide-ciprofloxacin interaction with resistant hypoglycemia.* Ann Emerg Med. August 2000; 36:160-3.

19. Guyton, AC and Hall, JE. Pocket Companion to Textbook of Medical Physiology, Sixth Edition. WB Saunders: Philadelphia, 1999; p. 600.

20. Hamblin, PS, et al. *Practical management of diabetic ketoacidosis and hyperosmolar coma.* Aust N Z J Med 1990 Dec; 20(6):836-41; Bratton, SL, and Krane, EJ. *Diabetic ketoacidosis: pathophysiology, management, and complications,* J Intensive Care Med 1992; 7:199-211.

21. Morris LR, et al. *Bicarbonate therapy in severe diabetic ketoacidosis.* Ann Intern Med 1986 Dec; 105(6):836-40; Gamba, G, et al. *Bicarbonate therapy in severe diabetic ketoacidosis. A double blind, randomized, placebo controlled trial.* Rev Invest Clin 1991 Jul-Sep; 43(3):234-8; Green, SM, et al. *Failure of adjunctive bicarbonate to improve outcome in severe pediatric diabetic ketoacidosis.* Ann Emerg Med 1998 Jan; 31(1):41-8; Okuda, Y, et al. *Counterproductive effects of sodium bicarbonate in diabetic ketoacidosis.* J Clin Endocrinol Metab 1996 Jan; 81(1):314-20.

22. Balasubramanyan, N, et al. *Unmeasured anions identified by the Fencl-Stewart method predict mortality better than base excess, anion gap, and lactate in patients in the pediatric intensive care unit.* Crit Care Med 1999 Aug; 27(8):1577-81.

23. Schwab, TM, et al. *Screening for ketonemia in patients with diabetes.* Ann Emerg Med 1999 Sep; 34(3):342-6.

CHAPTER 3
CARDIOVASCULAR PROBLEMS

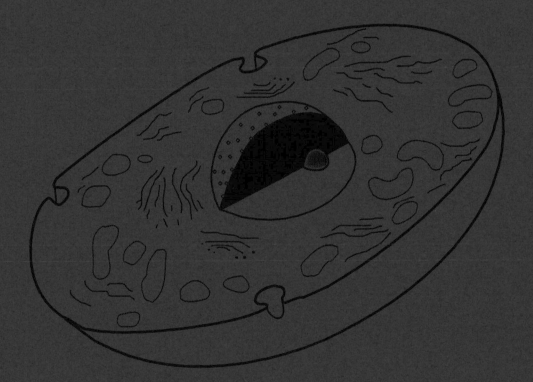

CHAPTER 3 — CARDIOVASCULAR PROBLEMS

Contents

Objectives

After reading this chapter, you'll be able to:

Explain Starling's Law of Fluid Flux into and out of "biological tubes."
Apply Starling's Law of Fluid Flux directly to normal fluid kinetics in the pulmonary circulation.
Using Starling's laws, define the difference between hydrostatic and hypo-oncotic (permeability) pulmonary edema.
Using Starling's laws, describe the reasons for the typical chest x-ray appearance of progressive left-sided systolic congestive heart failure.
Define and describe ventricular remodeling; explain its contribution to already-poor cardiac function in congestive heart failure.
Define the zones of the lung, based on different ventilation-perfusion ratios; explain the zones' practical significance as the basis for cephalization of flow in congestive heart failure.
Explain the anatomical basis for the fact that an isolated right sided pleural effusion, under the appropriate clinical circumstances, is due to left-sided congestive heart failure until proven otherwise.

Based on the pathophysiology, describe why each of the following therapeutic modalities or agents may be effective in acute pulmonary edema: positive pressure breathing, nitrates, morphine, and furosemide.

Defend the statement: "Congestive heart failure is a disease characterized by neuroendocrine dysfunction and sympathetic excess with hemodynamic manifestations."

Describe the molecular mechanisms of action of aldosterone; summarize the most recent data concerning use of spironolactone in chronic congestive heart failure.

Define the term "escape phenomenon" and explain its role in normal fluid balance, as well as in the pathogenesis of congestive heart failure.

Summarize the newly-discovered interrelationships between inflammation, infection, and rupture of atherosclerotic plaques; describe at least two potential therapeutic implications of these findings, in addition to reperfusion therapy (e.g., bypass, thrombolysis, angioplasty).

Describe the role of cerebral autoregulation in the decision whether or not to treat acutely elevated blood pressure levels.

Illustrate the pathophysiological basis for an anaphylactic reaction. Describe the anatomical basis for the most common symptoms of anaphylaxis.

Defend the statement: "Antihistamines, such as Benadryl® or H_2-blockers, by themselves, may be dangerous in the treatment of low-grade anaphylactic reactions, such as progressive urticaria."

Explain the statement: "Many patients with anaphylaxis should be observed in a medical facility for 4 to 6 hours, even if they completely respond to initial therapy."

Summarize recent evidence regarding the absorption of IM versus SQ epinephrine; formulate a rational approach to treatment.

Introduction

Nowhere is it more obvious to me that a fundamental understanding of normal physiology and disease states has a *direct* impact on patient care as in cardiovascular medicine. Coronary artery disease and congestive heart failure comprise a significant percentage of both acute and ongoing patient care challenges. We'll share many exciting new

PRINCIPLE: You must appreciate the *normal* to understand the *abnormal*.

revelations on the pathophysiology of both of these potentially deadly diseases and place them into a useful clinical perspective.

In addition, we'll explore relevant aspects of hypertensive emergencies and cerebral autoregulation and learn why sometimes the best treatment is none at all. Finally, we cover anaphylaxis — a disease with a broad spectrum of findings, all of which are potentially deadly.

Fluid movement in and out of "tubes"

> ## *OBJECTIVE:* Explain Starling's Law of Fluid Flux into and out of "biological tubes."

What is the Starling equation? The Starling equation is a mathematical relationship that expresses the net direction of fluid flow inward or outward through the wall of a biologic tube. And, I mean *any* type of tube — capillary, lymph vessel, or kidney tubule. If you understand this principle, then all kinds of concepts become obvious including:

○ Congestive heart failure (CHF).
○ Edema.
○ Ascites.
○ Pleural effusions.
○ Normal and abnormal kidney function

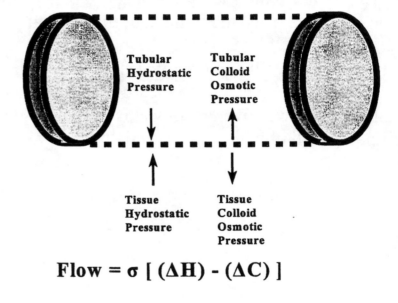

$$\text{Flow} = \sigma \, [\, (\Delta H) - (\Delta C) \,]$$

Figure 3-1

Starling's Law states that there are three forces determining the net flow direction of fluid into or out of a tubule: **[FIGURE 3-1]**

Hydrostatic forces — Usually called "hydrostatic pressure," this refers to the "water pressure" either in the tubule, the surrounding tissue, or both.

Oncotic forces — Usually called "oncotic pressure," this refers to the osmotic load (usually due to protein, but not necessarily) or oncotic pressure either in the tubule, the surrounding tissue, or both.

- **Permeability** — the permeability of the tubule; Starling used the Greek letter, sigma (σ), to refer to the permeability of the tubule. "σ" is formally called the *capillary filtration coefficient* and is equal to the product of tubular permeability and surface area of the tube. For our purposes, the concept of "leaky tubes" is far more important than the mathematical particulars.

There are hydrostatic and oncotic forces both in the tissues as well as in the "tubules." Taking into account the capillary permeability, Starling formulated the **Starling Equation**, which describes the *net* direction fluid flow through the wall of a "biological tube":

Flow = σ [(Tubular hydrostatic pressure - tissue hydrostatic pressure) - (Tubular oncotic pressure - tissue oncotic pressure)]

I thought that Starling's Law was good only in CHF and pulmonary edema. Not so — it's a very generic relationship that we can use to understand a wide variety of states, both normal and abnormal. For example, the entire ability of the kidney to concentrate or to dilute the urine is based upon this relationship. When the osmolality of the renal medulla changes (the equivalent of changing osmotic pressure), fluid is either drawn back into the body from the collecting tubules or allowed to leave as urine (see **"Normal Renal Function," Chapter 7**). Analogous changes occur during the formation of ascites in the peritoneal cavity or of peripheral edema in the extremities:

- Ascites — Altered liver function leads to decreased protein production. In turn, oncotic pressure in the blood vessels is decreased. Combined with increased portal pressures (hydrostatic forces in the vessels), the result is extravasation of fluid from the abdominal vessels into the peritoneal cavity, or ascites.

- Peripheral edema — Various mechanisms, both systemic and local, can lead to alterations of the Starling pressure relationships and then, to edema. Starvation leads to a generalized decrease of intravascular oncotic pressure and "leaky capillaries." Venous obstruction or stasis may lead to increased venous hydrostatic pressures, causing edema formation. Alterations in lymphatic return may also lead to increased pressure and fluid extravasation.

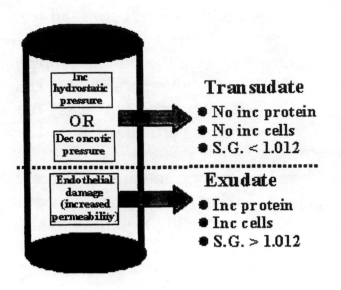

Simply put, edema is the production of excess fluid in the interstitium or body cavities. It may result from either inflammatory damage to blood vessels (inflammatory edema) or abnormalities or the normal hydrostatic or oncotic pressures that affect blood vessels (noninflammatory edema). Edema fluid produced by inflammation is called an **exudate**. Fluid produced by noninflammatory mechanisms is called a **transudate**.

What "safety features" are built-in to our bodies to minimize the risk of edema? The major compensatory mechanism is increased lymphatic flow. Lymph vessels are able to dilate and increase their fluid carrying capacity up to fifty times normal! Thus, they are able to carry away large amounts of fluid and proteins in response to an increased capillary fluid leak into the interstitium. For example, patients with chronic mitral stenosis sometimes have capillary pressures of 40 to 45 mm Hg (normal 10 - 12 mm Hg) with *no* sign of significant pulmonary edema.

Isn't Starling's Law just a mathematical expression of an experiment we all did in elementary school? Yes — remember when we took two beakers of water, separated by a semipermeable membrane? Think about what happened if we put salt into one beaker . . . Water crossed the membrane to the "salty side." And, if we increased the height of the water column on one side, the increased pressure caused some water to pass to the other side. Finally, if we cut tiny slits in the membrane, water flowed freely between both sides. Our memories are summarized in **Figure 3-2**.

Now, let's just rename each part of **Figure 3-2** (see **Figure 3-3**). As you can see in **Figure 3-3**, I've labeled each set of beakers with a variable from the Starling equation. The implications of this entire experiment, whether thought of on a "first grade" level or one more advanced, are:

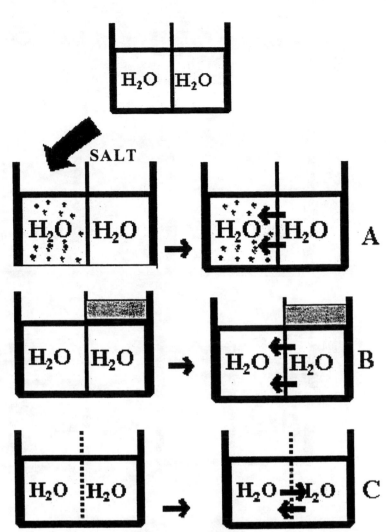

1. Putting salt into one side (and causing fluid to flow in that direction) is the "first grade" equivalent of increasing the oncotic (osmotic) pressure of that side.

2. Increasing the volume of water on one side (causing fluid to flow in the opposite direction) is the equivalent of increasing the hydrostatic pressure of that side.

Figure 3-2 — In "A," salt placed in the left-hand beaker causes water to flow from right to left across the semipermeable membrane. In "B," additional water ("pressure") in the right-side beaker causes the movement of water to the left. In "C," slits in the membrane allow free flow of water from side to side.

3. Cutting slits in the semipermeable membrane is the equivalent of altering the permeability.

FLOW ∝

$$\{ \sigma [(\Delta H) - \Delta C)]\}$$

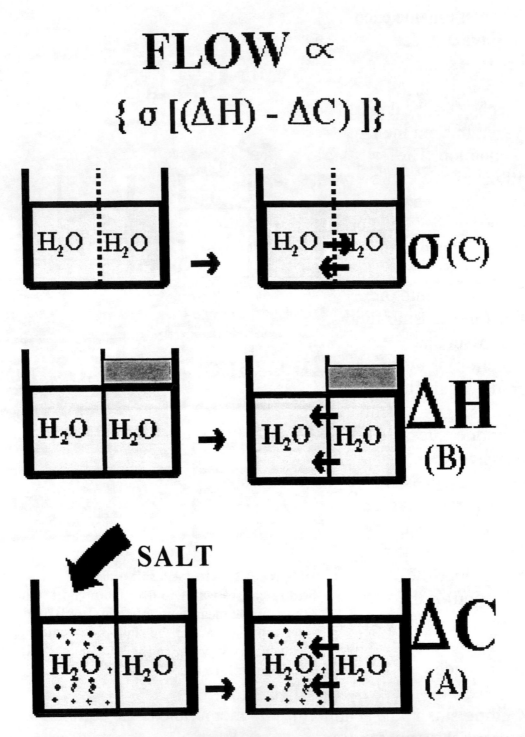

Figure 3-3 — Putting salt into one side (and causing fluid to flow in that direction) is the "first grade" equivalent of decreasing the oncotic (osmotic) pressure (C). Increasing the volume of water on one side (causing fluid to flow in the opposite direction) is the equivalent of increasing the hydrostatic pressure (B). Cutting slits in the semipermeable membrane is the equivalent of altering the permeability (A).

Pulmonary edema and congestive heart failure

Pulmonary edema means "fluid in the lungs" — the interstitium, the air spaces (alveoli), or both. Many of us use the *wrong* terms. Acute pulmonary edema (APE) is not simply "cardiogenic" or "noncardiogenic." The proper, physiologically-based classification of APE is "hydrostatic" and "hypo-oncotic." Cardiogenic pulmonary edema is the most common form of "hydrostatic" pulmonary edema and adult respiratory distress syndrome (ARDS) is the most common form of "hypo-oncotic" pulmonary edema, but many other disease states may lead to APE via one or both of these mechanisms.

OBJECTIVE: Apply Starling's Law of Fluid Flux directly to normal fluid kinetics in the pulmonary circulation.

Enter Dr. Starling. Nearly a hundred years ago, the physiologist Starling did some incredible studies that form the basis for our current-day understanding of CV physiology. **Starling's Law of Fluid Flux** (explained above) "tells it all," regarding the classification of APE. He described, in a mathematical format, the interplay of various forces in the capillaries that determine the net flux (flow) of fluid (in or out) through the capillary walls. Recall, the main Starling forces are:

1. Capillary integrity or permeability (σ) — keeps fluid in vessels.
2. Oncotic (protein) pressure within the capillary — keeps fluid in vessels.
3. Hydrostatic pressure within the capillary — tries to push fluid out, as well as through the lumen of vessels.

There are hydrostatic and oncotic forces both in the tissues and in the vessels. Taking into account the capillary permeability, Starling formulated the **Starling Equation** that describes the *net* fluid flow into or out of a capillary through its wall:

Flow = σ [(Capillary hydrostatic - tissue hydrostatic) - (Capillary oncotic - tissue oncotic)]

All you really need to understand in order to use the Starling Equation in patient care are the following principles:

1.   There are three sets of forces that affect flow through capillary walls.

2.   Two of these forces, (capillary integrity [σ] and oncotic pressure) try to keep fluid *in the vessels*.

3.   One (hydrostatic pressure) pushes fluid through the lumen of the capillaries, but also tries to push fluid *out* through the capillary walls.

4.   There are hydrostatic and oncotic forces in the surrounding tissues that have the opposite effects of those within the capillaries.

What does the Starling calculation look like in normal pulmonary capillaries? Thought you'd never ask — and you might be just a little bit surprised. Here are the numbers:

Capillary hydrostatic pressure	7 mm Hg
Tissue hydrostatic pressure	-8 mm Hg
Capillary oncotic pressure	28 mm Hg
Tissue oncotic pressure	14 mm Hg

If we take permeability (σ) to be a constant (1), we get the following:

- **Flow = σ [(Capillary hydrostatic - tissue hydrostatic) - (Capillary oncotic - tissue oncotic)]**

- **Flow = 1 [(7 - {-8}) - (28 - {14})]**

- **Flow = 1 [(15) - (14)] = + 1 mm Hg**

So, all Starling factors considered, there is a net flow gradient pressure of one mm Hg from the inside of the vessels to flow through the wall to the interstitium. We all have "leaky" pulmonary capillaries. Remember, this calculation represents an *average* since the hydrostatic pressure within the vessels varies, depending on the distance from the arterial side of the circulation. Now, why aren't we in pulmonary edema?

The "missing link" is the final normal structure, the lymphatics — remember the old acronym "NAVL" — nerve, artery, vein, lymph? Whatever tissue fluid isn't returned back into the capillaries by the plasma colloid osmotic pressure is channeled into the lymphatic drainage of the lungs and "recycled" to the blood vessels by either the thoracic duct (on the left) or the lymphatic duct (on the right). Thus, our lungs normally remain "high and dry."

Be sure you are comfortable with this normal cycle [**FIGURE 3-4**]. Many of us were not taught correctly the first time around and, as a result, have trouble with what should be a simple concept!

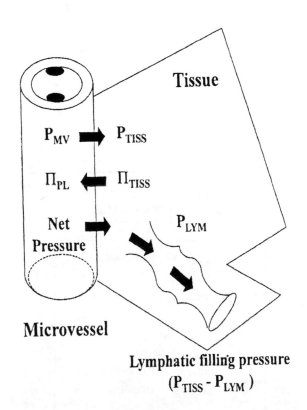

Figure 3-4 — Hydrostatic pressure forces fluid from the capillaries; the plasma oncotic pressure "sucks up" some, but not all. The remainder is "recycled" by the lymphatic channels into the central circulation. Thus, the lungs normally remain "dry" despite a normal "leak" from the capillary lumen to the interstitial tissues.

3-11

OBJECTIVE: Using Starling's laws, define the difference between hydrostatic and hypo-oncotic (permeability) pulmonary edema.

Classification of pulmonary edema based on the Starling Equation. There are three mechanisms by which fluid could abnormally leave the capillaries and accumulate in the lung (leading to APE) — leaky vessels (abnormal permeability), low oncotic pressure, or increased hydrostatic pressure. Agreed?

The *physiologically correct* classification of acute pulmonary edema, based on the Starling Equation, is:

* **Hydrostatic** (capillary hydrostatic pressure increased, regardless of the reason).
* **Hypo-oncotic** ("leaky vessels" whether due to low oncotic pressure, abnormal permeability, i.e., leaky vessel walls, or both).

There are numerous causes for each type, as illustrated in the **Table** below:

INCREASED HYDROSTATIC PRESSURE	DECREASED ONCOTIC PRESSURE	INCREASED CAPILLARY PERMEABILITY
• Left-sided heart failure • Mitral stenosis • Volume overload • Pulmonary vein obstruction • High altitude (?) • Early neurogenic (?)	• Hypoalbuminemia (nephrotic syndrome, liver disease, protein-losing enteropathy)	• Infection • Toxic inhalation • Liquid aspiration • Drugs and chemicals • Shock, trauma, sepsis • Radiation • Acute pancreatitis • Fat embolism • DKA • DIC • Neurogenic

The most common form of hydrostatic pulmonary edema that we see is "cardiogenic," due to acute loss of left ventricular contractility (secondary to ischemia), with backflow of the increased pressures (hydrostatic pressure) to the lung. Remember, though, that mitral stenosis can also cause elevation of the left atrial filling pressure, resulting in APE — isn't this also a form of "cardiogenic pulmonary edema?" Other disease states may also result in an elevation of the pulmonary capillary hydrostatic pressure and APE. These include scorpion bites, early neurogenic pulmonary edema, and over-pressurization accidents (e.g., diving accidents). They are all far less common than typical "ischemic cardiogenic pulmonary edema."

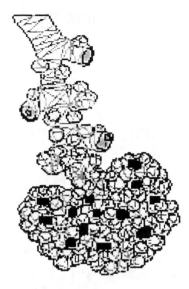

Figure 3-5 — ARDS is a specific constellation of clinical findings:

●**Pulmonary edema in the** *absence* **of any cardiogenic or other contributing component.**
●**Increased capillary permeability.**
●**Numerous underlying causes.**
●**Inability to adequately oxygenate the patient** *despite* **an FIO$_2$ of 100%.**

Similarly, adult respiratory distress syndrome (ARDS) is the most common form of "leaky vessel" (hypo-oncotic) pulmonary edema. ARDS is a distinct clinical entity with the following diagnostic features: **[FIGURE 3-5]**

1. Pulmonary edema in the *absence* of any cardiogenic or other contributing component.
2. Increased capillary permeability.
3. Numerous underlying causes.
4. Inability to adequately oxygenate the patient *despite* an FIO$_2$ (percentage of inspired oxygen concentration) of 100%.

Note that *all* of the above criteria are required to properly make a diagnosis of ARDS. There are also specific microscopic features of ARDS visible to the pathologist:

●   Pink membranes (hyaline membranes) that line the alveolar septa.
●   Damage to type I pneumocytes with replacement by type II pneumocytes.

Many clinicians incorrectly assume that if it's not "from the heart," it's ARDS. Other diseases besides ARDS lead to hypo-oncotic pulmonary edema (e.g., smoke inhalation, chlorine gas exposure, heroin, sepsis . . . and the list goes on!).

For now, let's limit our discussion to ischemic cardiogenic pulmonary edema (what most of us used to call "cardiogenic pulmonary edema"), since it's potentially deadly and seen commonly in primary care practice.

The underlying lesion. The triggering event in APE (now specifically referring to *ischemic cardiogenic pulmonary edema*, just so we're on the same frequency!) is usually acute myocardial ischemia. APE can develop as the end stage of progressive chronic congestive heart failure as well, but in many cases, the picture is more dramatic, with the patient getting into trouble rapidly, as if someone "flipped a switch."

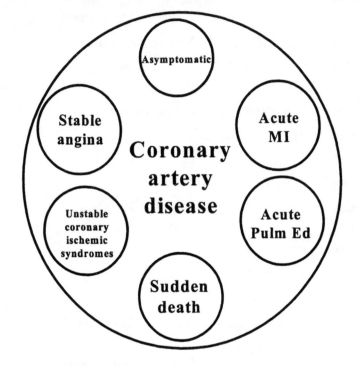

Figure 3-6 — Coronary artery disease presents as a spectrum of findings, ranging from no symptoms (asymptomatic) to sudden death. These findings include myocardial infarction and acute pulmonary edema.

A "myth" of medicine is that patients with APE have had a myocardial infarction (MI) at the same time. This is the *exception* rather than the *rule*. Less than half of the patients with APE turn out to have concomitant MI. On the other hand, nearly *all* patients with acute MI do have something in common with nearly *all* APE victims — severe underlying coronary artery disease. Surprised? Consider the following:

Coronary artery disease (CAD) presents as a *spectrum of findings*, ranging from no symptoms (asymptomatic) to sudden death. In the "middle" [**FIGURE 3-6**] are angina, unstable coronary ischemic syndromes (formerly known as "unstable angina"), myocardial infarction (transmural and nontransmural), and APE. Thus, in patients with the same degree of CAD, one patient might be asymptomatic, while another may have an MI, and still another may go in and out of APE. In each patient, the degree of underlying

---
REMEMBER: The common denominator underlying both APE and acute MI is coronary artery disease.

CAD is similar but the *manifestation* is different. It's important to appreciate this concept, since the work-up for acute MI (though it should be done) is usually negative in patients with APE.

A study published several years ago showed that in patients who never had acute MI but did suffer recurrent APE, the degree of angiographic CAD was similar. These findings led to the recommendation that recurrent APE, even in the absence of MI, is an indication for cardiac catheterization and potential revascularization (bypass, stenting, etc.).[1]

Water pressure rises . . . APE develops in response to an acute decrease in left ventricular (LV) compliance ("stretchability"), as a result of coronary ischemia. Essentially, the LV becomes "stiffer" than normal, leading to increased end diastolic pressure. Other synonyms for end diastolic pressure (some more scientific than others) include pulmonary artery wedge pressure, LV

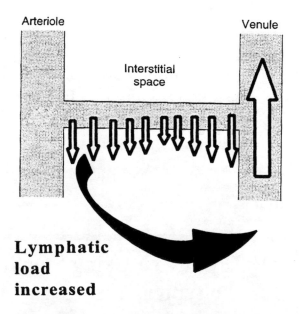

Figure 3-7 — As the venous (hydrostatic) pressure in the lungs rises, fluid leaks from the vessels into the interstitium. Initially, lymphatic flow compensates for the leak but after a while, the patient develops interstitial, followed by alveolar, edema.

filling pressure, preload, water pressure, and hydrostatic pressures. These excess pressures are transmitted retrograde (back up) into the pulmonary capillaries. The end result, regardless of the name, is that the hydrostatic pressure is *increased* within the pulmonary capillaries. Starling's Equation tells you the rest. **[FIGURE 3-7]**

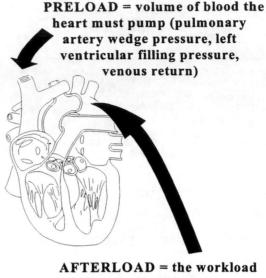

PRELOAD = volume of blood the heart must pump (pulmonary artery wedge pressure, left ventricular filling pressure, venous return)

AFTERLOAD = the workload against which the heart must pump the blood (systemic vascular resistance)

Figure 3-8

Preload and afterload — *Preload* refers to the load (blood volume) that the heart must pump out, while *afterload* reflects the resistance against which it must pump. Increasing the preload or the afterload often impairs cardiac function, but not always. Though the concept of preload and afterload are used in many different settings, the "formal" use of these is often as follows: **[FIGURE 3-8]**

- **Preload** — left ventricular filling pressure, pulmonary artery wedge pressure (PAWP), left ventricle end diastolic pressure (LVEDP).

- **Afterload** — systemic vascular resistance (SVR).

OBJECTIVE: **Using Starling's laws, describe the reasons for the typical chest x-ray appearance of progressive left-sided systolic congestive heart failure.**

Radiographic manifestations of progressive APE reflect underlying anatomic changes. Often, patients go directly into fulminant APE. It's instructive, however, to trace the natural progression, rapid as it may be, of

CHF from early stages to APE. Just remember that the patient hasn't always "read the book" before getting sick.

There are two types of CXR changes in progressive CHF:

1. Enlargement of the cardiac silhouette (heart shadow) — reflects changes in the shape of the heart. In early CHF and acute pulmonary edema, this is due to dilation of the heart by the Starling mechanism as an attempt to compensate for decreased cardiac output. In later states of CHF, changes in the heart shadow reflect ventricular remodeling.

2. Vascular changes — reflect increasing hydrostatic pressures and hypoxia. Progress from redistribution of flow (cephalization) to the upper lobes, to interstitial, then mixed interstitial-alveolar edema.

Cardiac dilation — a common initial response in early CHF is for the left ventricle to *dilate*, an attempt to *increase* cardiac output (contractility) via the **Starling mechanism**. Starling showed that, to a point, stretching an isolated muscle fiber prior to stimulating it to contract (resulting in increased "preload") led to increased contractility, hence, greater cardiac output. You may remember diagrams in old physiology books showing how he hung an isolated cat papillary muscle from a hook and then gradually added weight to the bottom portion. After adding each weight, he applied an electrical current and measured the rate of contraction. **[FIGURE 3-9]** By plotting the weight ("preload") versus contractility (dv/dt, slope of the line, "oomph of contraction," cardiac output, and contractility have all been used to convey the concept), he found that:

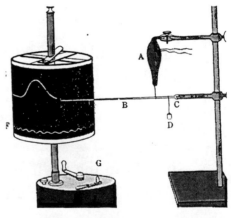

The Starling "Gizmo"

Figure 3-9 — The "Starling Gizmo"

1.   Increasing the weight *increases* contractility, to a point.

2.   After a certain point, further increases in weight led to a *decrease* in contractility. **[FIGURE 3-10]**

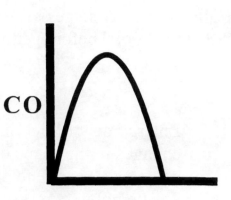

Preload

Figure 3-10 — Starling's Law of the Heart — to a point, increases in preload lead to increased velocity ("oomph") of cardiac contraction. This normal response system to decreased cardiac function soon reaches a point of diminishing returns, however.

Note that **Starling's Law of the Heart** (also called the **Frank-Starling mechanism**) really describes a "normal regulatory system." This NRS is designed to assure that, within limits, the heart pumps all the blood that comes to it, without allowing excess "damming of blood" in the veins, in normal persons *and* in those with CHF. The mechanism is as follows:

1.   Increased venous return stretches the heart.

2.   Anatomically, the extra "stretch" of the muscle causes actin and myosin to become more optimally aligned.

3.   As a result, the force of contraction is increased.

4.   Stretching the right atrium also causes a reflex increase in the heart rate of 10 to 20 percent, also helping increase the cardiac output.

Let's go back in time and relive Dr. Starling's original description:

"The energy of contraction is a function of the length of the muscle fibres . . . up to a certain optimum length, the energy of contraction increases with every increase in initial length of the fibres. Beyond this point it requires considerable tension to cause a further increase in length, but this is associated with a diminution in the effectiveness of the contractions."[2]

In CHF, dilation is often helpful initially; at some point, however, diminishing returns are achieved and contractility decreases. Reasons for this include the following:

- Unlike some other body systems (e.g., endocrine), there is no intrinsic negative feedback loop that tells the heart "enough is enough" and to stop dilating. Once the process is triggered, it continues until *we* help the patient improve. Though dilation is a normal response to increased left ventricular load, this is *transient* under normal circumstances. In CHF, volume overload and, thus, dilation, persists.

- Anatomically, muscles (including the heart) contract because of the crawling or sliding of actin and myosin filaments over each other — the so-called "sliding filament model."

  In the nonstretched state, the filaments overlap and are unable to increase their rate and strength of contraction. With dilation, however, the filaments are separated. It is thought that this stretching more optimally aligns the actin and myosin filaments, and facilitates better contraction . . . at least, to a point. **[FIGURE 3-11]**

- There comes a stage where the filaments are *so far* apart that contractility actually *decreases*. It was originally thought that the human heart could stretch so much as to fall on this "descending limb" of the curve (see **Figure 3-10**). Though possible, it is unlikely that heart failure ever progresses to a stage in humans where the fibers are actually completely separated. Death usually comes first. Failure to understand this formed the incorrect basis for for phlebotomy treatment in APE. If too much volume stretches the muscle too much, reducing its contractility, removing excess volume should improve the situation. It just didn't work out that way clinically.

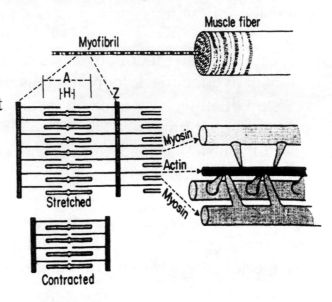

Initially, dilation is a viable compensatory mechanism. The dilated heart is manifested on the CXR as increased width of the cardiac silhouette (also called "heart shadow"). Dilation occurs *in conjunction with* the vascular stages of cephalization, interstitial, and mixed alveolar-interstitial edema. These are findings of *acute* congestive heart failure. In chronic CHF, an enlarged cardiac silhouette occurs for different reasons.

Figure 3-11 — The anatomic basis for Starling's Law of the Heart — dilation initially *optimizes* the alignment of actin and myosin filaments, increasing the rate and strength of contraction. There comes a point, though, where the filaments are *too far apart* to continue to contract effectively, and contractility decreases.

What happens when the atria are stretched, such as with increases in venous return? Three separate and complementary responses are triggered:

1. Stretching of the sinus node causes a ten to fifteen percent increase in heart rate.

2. Stretching of the right atrium elicits the *Bainbridge reflex*, which sends impulses to the vasomotor center in the brain. Return signals via the sympathetic and vagus nerves lead to an increase in heart rate. Epinephrine is the major sympathetic mediator of this response.

3. Stretching of both atria leads to production of atrial natriuretic protein (ANP). The effects of ANP are more important in prolonged atrial stretching (more than a few minutes) than during acute volume changes (e.g., changing body position).

The net effect is an increase in cardiac output to compensate for increased venous return. Of course, these mechanisms work in conjunction with stretching of the ventricles and subsequent increases in cardiac contractility via the Frank-Starling mechanism.

OBJECTIVE: Define and describe ventricular remodeling; explain its contribution to already-poor cardiac function in congestive heart failure.

Ventricular remodeling — As noted above, the enlarged cardiac silhouette in chronic heart failure does *not* usually represent pure ventricular dilation. More commonly, it occurs as a result of anatomical changes in cardiac architecture, known as **ventricular remodeling**. This potentially reversible process occurs as a result of mediator release, most likely **α-tumor necrosis factor** (TNF). TNF is thought to be released by sympathetic stimulation (i.e., epinephrine), explaining the beneficial role of beta-blockade in CHF.[3] TNF is a normal inflammatory mediator. In CHF, however, it has deleterious effects on the myocardium:[4]

● It induces premature apoptosis in myocytes.
● It down-regulates (makes *less sensitive* to stimuli) cardiac receptors for nitric oxide synthetase and for creatine transport protein.

As a result of these changes:

1. Cardiac cells die and are replaced by scar tissue.

2.   Nitric oxide, a vasodilator, is made at a far slower rate, leading to decreased delivery of oxygen to the failing myocardium.

3.   Myocardial cells are unable to incorporate creatine, an essential component of muscle tissue, into the cells. Essentially, the cells starve or develop so-called "cardiac cachexia."

In addition, the renin-angiotensin system is involved — activation of angiotensin II promotes scar tissue formation.[5]

These anatomic changes cause the heart to change shape from a cylinder (normal) to a sphere (abnormal). Geometrically speaking, for a cylinder and sphere to have the *same* volume, the radius of the sphere must be *larger* by a factor of 1.33 (one and one-third). **[FIGURE 3-12]** The change in shape has significant hemodynamic consequences that further worsen an already-bad situation.

What's wrong with the spherical configuration? By itself, nothing — it is the change in the radius that causes problems. Remember, the heart's normal regulatory systems want to maintain the same intra-ventricular volume and ejection fraction.

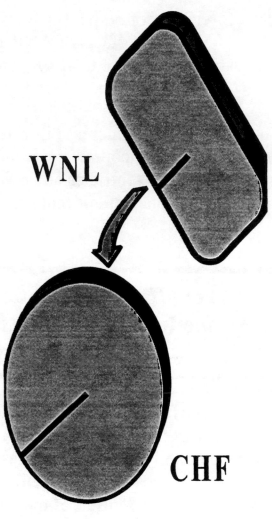

Figure 3-12 — In a sphere and a cylinder of equal volumes, the radius of the sphere is 1.33 times greater than that of the cylinder. This relationship is derived by equating the geometric formulae for each. If all other factors are kept equal, the radius of the sphere is 4/3 times the radius of the cylinder of equal volume.

LaPlace's Law (somewhat paraphrased for comprehension) states that the pressure generated during cardiac contraction equals the wall tension divided by the ventricular radius:

Pressure = Wall Tension/Radius

Do the math — if we increase the denominator (radius), such as by changing shape from a cylinder to a sphere (bigger radius), the pressure *decreases*. The only way to keep the pressure constant is to also *increase* the wall tension. And, this is precisely what the body does, at least initially. The effect of *increasing the wall tension*, however, is an increased workload on an already failing heart. [FIGURE 3-13].

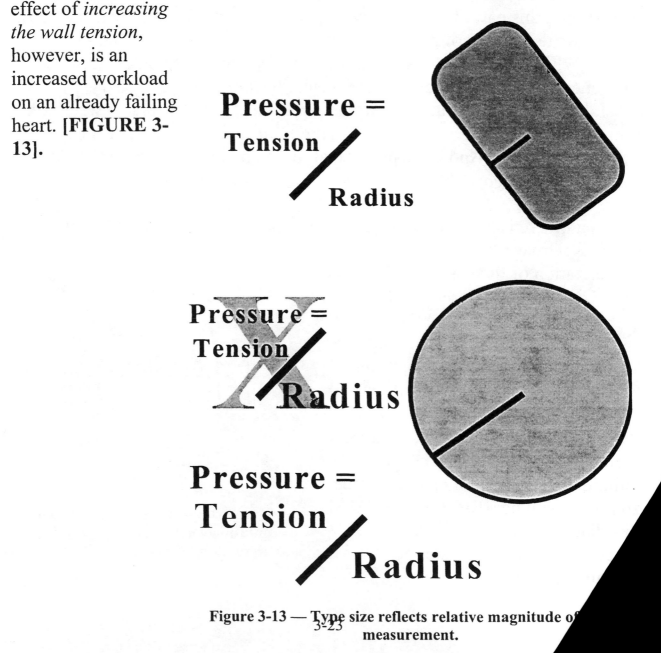

Figure 3-13 — Type size reflects relative magnitude of measurement.

> ## OBJECTIVE: Define the zones of the lung, based on different ventilation-perfusion ratios; explain the zones' practical significance as the basis for cephalization of flow in congestive heart failure.

Cephalization of flow — Law of the Apple. The reason most people have trouble with this part of cardiovascular and respiratory physiology is that they try to rewrite the laws of physics! Remember Sir Isaac Newton and the apple? Why did it fall — gravity, of course (silly me!). If you're OK with this concept, then a lot of otherwise potentially confusing pulmonary physiology should be straight forward. Apply the "apple law" to a waterfall. Why does water fall down (*Please* — humor me and play along, it'll be worth it!) Gravity. And if we place an air hose underwater, what happens? Air rises. *Water goes down and air goes up* — everybody OK?

That's all there is to understanding the concept of *hypoxic vasoconstriction*, which is why we see "deer antlers" or cephalization of flow as one of the best early CXR signs of CHF. I promise to translate every word — just remember, "water goes down and air goes up" and accept that this isn't going to change anytime soon in our lifetimes.

Zones of the lung — Many of us recall ~ a confusing and rather ~ diagram illustrating three ~ [**FIGURE 3-14**] All ~ is what we ~ goes down

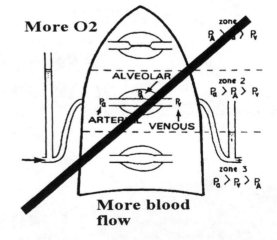

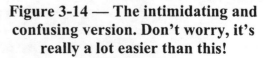

Figure 3-14 — The intimidating and confusing version. Don't worry, it's really a lot easier than this!

Assuming the patient is in an upright position (though the model applies in any position), gravity pulls relatively more fluid to the pulmonary vessels in the lower portions of the lungs, agreed? (I sure hope so, since "water goes down, etc."). Thus, the main pulmonary vessels are fuller and more distended with blood in the inferior parts of the lung. This physiologic truism translated into "x-ray talk" means that the lower vessels are more distended than the upper ones. Therefore, they absorb *more x-rays* than the upper hilar vessels. *Less x-raya* hits the film in the lower zones, resulting in a more prominent ("whiter") shadow of the lower (inferior) hilar vessels than of the upper ones. This is true in any normal, upright CXR [See Chapter 1 for a review of the basics of "more of me, less of me" and XR if you need to — it's OK!]. So far so good? Then, let's move on to our "user-friendly" zone diagram. **[FIGURE 3-15]**

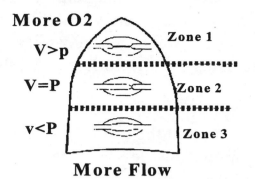

FIGURE 3-15 — The "user-friendly" version — alveolar ventilation is higher in the upper zone (ventilation > perfusion) and perfusion is greater in the lower zone (ventilation < perfusion). The two are relatively equal in the middle zone. Averaged together, once oxygen crosses the alveolar capillary barrier, net total arterial oxygen saturation is normal. *Reason*: "water goes down, air goes up!"

Since water goes *down*, air must go *up*, right? Now, let's consider *alveolar oxygenation* — not total arterial saturation, just the concentration of oxygen in the alveolar air *before* it crosses the alveolar-capillary membrane into the red blood cells. Because "air goes up," the upper part of the lung *must* have a higher oxygen concentration than the lower part. Again, don't get confused thinking about *net* arterial oxygenation, just focus on the O_2 present on a *local* alveolar level.

Remember that blood *flow* to the lower part of the lung is greater than to the upper part. And, at the same time, *oxygenation* of the lower part is *less* than of the upper part. The opposite holds true for upper portions of the lung — *less flow*, yet *greater oxygenation*. Formally stated, there are differing ventilation-perfusion ratios in the upper and lower parts of the lung.

Now, back to the diagram. It divides the lung into three "zones" or areas; each has a different ventilation (oxygenation, or "air goes up") - perfusion (flow, or "water goes down") ratio. In the midzone, ventilation and perfusion are equal — since this is a "wash," we'll leave it out of the discussion for now.

Think about the top zone — more oxygen, less flow. And the bottom zone — more flow, less oxygen. The top and bottom have *opposite* ventilation-perfusion ratios. Add them together and consider the contribution to arterial saturation: they equal each other. Where one is overperfused (lower zone) it has less oxygen and vice versa (upper zone). Also consider that the middle portion has a 50-50 ventilation-perfusion ratio and the bottom line should be clear. Despite differing ventilation-perfusion ratios in the different zones, the *net* arterial oxygenation saturation is normal. And it's all because "water goes down and air goes up!" That's what the diagram's all about. This phenomenon also explains why we don't turn "blue" when we change positions — the rules of physics *still* hold! (Some persons with pulmonary artery stenosis or tetralogy of Fallot are unable to redistribute their pulmonary blood flow properly and *do* demonstrate positional cyanosis.)

So, what does that have to do with hypoxic vasoconstriction? Everything. Realizing that the lower zones of the lung are *normally* relatively hypo-oxic (on the "low end of normal"), it makes sense to us that "hypoxia alarms" that are triggered early in CHF "go off" in the lower zones first, yes? So, it's the *lower zone vessels* that do what pulmonary blood vessels do first in the face of hypoxia — constrict.

The effect of hypoxic vasoconstriction? Redistribution of a portion of the pulmonary circulation to the *upper* zones, which also happen to have *higher* levels of alveolar oxygenation (remember "air goes up"?). The net effect, physiologically, is to "push" some of the lung blood flow into areas of the lung that are better oxygenated (the upper zones). Radiographically, this is seen in the upper lobes as fuller vessels that absorb more x-rays than normal. Less x-rays hit the film and the upper hilar vessels become as visible and discernable as the lower ones — "cephalization," "redistribution of flow toward the top," "top same as bottom," or "deer antlers." **[FIGURE 3-16]**

A helpful hint — in an upright chest film the upper hilar markings should virtually *never* be as discernable as the lower ones ("fluid goes down . . . "). If you see redistribution, cephalization, or whatever other term you choose, the *most likely* explanation (***clinical correlation strongly suggested, of course!***) is CHF. If the clinical picture fits, go for it. This finding has been systematically studied and shown to be extremely accurate *when present*. However, a patient may still have significantly elevated pulmonary wedge pressures and a relatively *normal* chest film.[6]

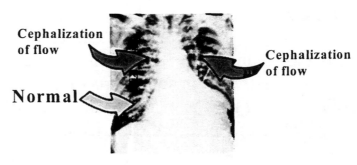

Figure 3-16 — Cephalization of flow ("deer antlers") is an early and clinically-reliable radiographic sign of CHF (assuming the clinical picture fits). Anatomically, it represents hypoxic vasoconstriction in the lower lung zones with redistribution to the better-oxygenated upper zones. Note that the cardiac shadow is also enlarged.

Isn't the response of the pulmonary vessels to hypoxia the opposite of that of the peripheral circulation? Absolutely. If a portion of my hand needs more oxygen, what do I want my blood vessels to do? Of course, to *dilate* and bring in more oxygen. Now, what if a portion of my lung is hypoxic — will the same thing happen? I sure hope not . . .

Remember, the lower zone of the lung is normally hypo-oxic, so when the "hypoxia alarms" go off, they "sound" there first. If these gravitationally-dependent vessels dilated, what would happen? We'd just increase the blood flow to an area of the lung that is *already on the low side* in terms of oxygenation (remember — fluid goes down, air goes up). Fortunately, the Master Architect anticipated this problem and drew different plans for the pulmonary vessels. Instead of *dilating* in response to hypoxia, they *constrict*. This has the effect of forcing blood

REMEMBER: The response of the pulmonary vessels to hypoxia, vasoconstriction, is the *opposite* of that of the systemic vessels (vasodilation).

into the upper zones of the lungs, which are better oxygenated to start with (since "air goes up"). The response of the pulmonary vessels to hypoxia is the *opposite* of those of the systemic circulation.

Does hypoxic vasoconstriction play a role in high altitude pulmonary edema? Though experts are uncertain, it appears that the hypoxia of altitude causes random constriction of pulmonary arterioles. The reasons this constriction is different in some parts of the lung than in others is unclear. Regardless, blood flow is increased in the unconstricted vessels. As a result, capillary hydrostatic pressure rises, leading to local edema formation.

Why not just memorize "deer antlers, butterflies, and snowballs?" I feel strongly that simply memorizing that "deer antlers" progresses to "butterflies" and finally to "snowballs" is worthless *unless* you really know what these cute little terms stand for. Thus, the prolonged explanation — plus, this *is* a text of pathophysiolgy, isn't it ☺?

Interstitial edema. Now, think about the *normal* fluid flow (á la Starling) that we discussed earlier and review it if you need to. Remember, the only way to really understand the abnormal is to have a good "grip" on the normal, first! Again, let's consider what happens pathophysiologically in anatomical terms, and then "translate" this into x-ray anatomy (really, that's all we do whenever reading *any* type of x-ray, isn't it?).

Normally, the capillary hydrostatic pressure *already wins*, in the sense that there is a net efflux of fluid into the interstitial tissue. Recall that this occurs despite the contribution of plasma oncotic pressure to "suck" fluid back in. Our lungs stay "dry" because lymphatics carry away the excess fluid that has seeped into lung interstitial tissue.

As the LVEDP (left ventricular end diastolic pressure, "hydrostatic pressure") rises, pressure backs up into the lungs, leading to a rise in capillary hydrostatic pressure. (We're assuming that the events of ventricular dilation and cephalization of flow have already taken place, which is usually the case, but not always.)

As the capillary hydrostatic pressure increases, the *already present normal "leak"* into the pulmonary interstitium continues. Remember that the plasma protein (oncotic) pressure within the vessels is already normally working at near maximum efficacy, and can offer little to improve the situation by reabsorption of additional fluid. As the interstitial "leak" continues:

- Fluid accumulates in the interstitial tissues, between the vessels.

- Pulmonary stretch receptors sense increased resistance to lung expansion, often (but not always) causing dyspnea that may be out of proportion to the degree of "lung water." *NOTE: there are actually indicator techniques to measure "lung water," though these are somewhat controversial, and not widely available. I have chosen to avoid this debate here, since all you* really *need is a good understanding of pathophysiology and the ABCs to take care of patients, anyway!*

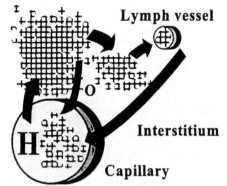

Figure 3-17 — After cephalization, interstitial fluid begins to accumulate; as a result, lymphatic channels become distended.

- The lymphatic "load" increases as the amount of interstitial fluid to "recycle" into the blood vessels increases.

So, anatomically speaking, we've got fluid in the interstitium that normally wouldn't be there, as well as a greater than normal volume of fluid in the lymphatics — agreed? [**FIGURE 3-17**]

Radiographically, a common sign of interstitial edema is increased haziness of the perihilar vessels. Remember, the normal markings have now become "deer antlers" as a reflection of hypoxic vasoconstriction and redistribution of blood to the upper zones of the lung. The next step is that fluid fills in the tissue (interstitial) spaces between these vessels. Typically, these changes progress outward from the hilum. If you mentally fill in the spaces with "white," the "deer antlers" take on a "butterfly" configuration. **[FIGURE 3-18]**

Simultaneously translating between anatomy-speak and x-ray-speak, this means that the fluid that leaks out of the vessels (and has the *same* radiographic density as

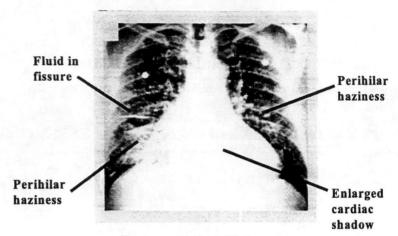

Interstitial Edema

Figure 3-18 — Interstitial edema

the fluid-filled vessels) now absorbs as many x-rays as do the vessels. If both the vessels and the interstitium now absorb the *same* amount of x-rays, the amount hitting the film will be similar and the "colors" (degree of whiteness) now the same. Thus, there will no longer be the nice black and white shadows contrasting the hilar vessels. The whole area has acquire similar radiographic density due to the presence of interstitial fluid, leading to the "butterfly" appearance.

OBJECTIVE: Explain the anatomical basis for the fact that an isolated right sided pleural effusion, under the appropriate clinical circumstances, is due to left-sided congestive heart failure until proven otherwise.

Lymphatic overload. This is a great time to discuss the clinical and radiographic implications of lymphatic overload, regardless of the cause. Remember the role of the lymphatic system in "clearing up" whatever interstitial fluid is normally "left over" after the plasma protein pressure has "sucked in" its portion (metaphorical, but correct). Let's add another crucial concept — the lymphatic drainage of the chest.

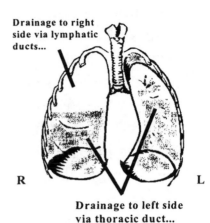

Drainage to right side via lymphatic ducts...

R   L

Drainage to left side via thoracic duct...

Figure 3-19 — Nearly three-fourths of the lungs' lymphatic drainage is on the left side, into the thoracic duct.

Roughly three-quarters of the lung, chest, and all of the left upper extremity are drained by interconnecting lymphatics that enter the circulatory system at the junction of the left subclavian and jugular veins via the **thoracic duct**. [**FIGURE 3-19**] The upper quarter of the right lung, the chest, and the right upper extremity are drained by separate lymphatic channels that empty into the right brachiocephalic vein via the smaller **lymphatic duct**, on the right side of the upper mediastinum.

Thus, the lymphatic drainage for most of the chest enters the central circulation via the left-sided thoracic duct. The left drainage system has nearly three-times the capacity of the smaller right-sided system that enters via the lymphatic duct. Though the lymphatics drain the lungs, lymphatic "overload" does not directly "back up" into the lungs. Rather, it spills over into the pleural space, including the interlobar fissures.

Normal pleural lymphatic flow. The blood supply of the parietal pleura is via the intercostal arteries, branches of the systemic circulation. The visceral pleura is predominantly supplied by the low-pressure pulmonary circulation. Accounting for equal osmotic pressures in both the parietal and visceral vessels, as well as changes in intrapleural pressure, normal fluid flow is from the parietal surface (high pressure) to the pleural space. Fluid is then reabsorbed by the visceral pleura. [**FIGURE 3-20**] Anything that changes these interrelationships may lead to abnormal fluid accumulation.

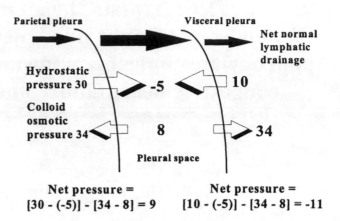

Net pressure =
[30 - (-5)] - [34 - 8] = 9

Net pressure =
[10 - (-5)] - [34 - 8] = -11

Figure 3-20 — Normally, Starling forces favor lymphatic fluid flow from the parietal pleura to the pleural space, then to the visceral pleura, where it is reabsorbed (pressures are in cm H$_2$0).

So, the presence of fluid in a fissure or of a pleural effusion may indicate lymphatic overload for *any* of a number of reasons (e.g., obstruction, fluid overload). As we'll soon see, the same is true for Kerley lines.

Many of us have been taught, but never understood (I just memorized it), the adage: "An isolated right sided pleural effusion is due to CHF until proven otherwise." And, the statement is correct — at least, statistically speaking. Rather than simply memorize, I urge you to understand. Trust me — it will be worth it, as this rule is *very helpful* clinically.

REMEMBER: Lymphatic overload may occur from a variety of causes, *not* just CHF.

Lymphatic overload in CHF. The lymphatic system becomes overloaded in CHF, *regardless* of whether we see it radiographically or not. Absence of a finding on a test doesn't necessarily *exclude* anything — only the *presence* of certain finding helps to establish a diagnosis. If the entire lymphatic drainage system of both lungs were equally overloaded, which side would "back flow" into the pleural space first? Since the "pipes" on the right side (which drains only one-quarter of the lung) are much smaller than those on the left, it seems a sure bet that they will fill first.

Since CHF results in an equal overload to *all* the lymphatics that drain the lungs, logic dictates (and anatomy agrees) that CHF would *first* cause an isolated right-sided effusion, since that part of the system will "back flow" first (because the right-sided "pipes" are much smaller than those on the left). So:

1. An isolated right-sided pleural effusion is due to CHF (assuming the clinical picture matches) until proven otherwise.

REMEMBER: The right-sided lymphatic "pipes" are one-third the size of the left-sided ones. When lymphatic overload is present, the right side "overflows" first (e.g., pleural effusion).

2. It is extremely unlikely that CHF, by itself, would lead to an isolated left-sided pleural effusion, assuming that the patient has normal lymphatic anatomy.

3. Bilateral pleural effusions may be due to anything, including CHF.

4. Findings of fluid in the interlobar fissures (these are *not* Kerley lines — see immediately below) often follow the same three rules listed above.

So, is it "Kerley to B" or not? Most of us are taught at some time that Kerley B lines (KBLs) are a sure-fire sign of CHF. Unfortunately, that's only true if the patient is in a textbook or on a test. Statistically, the presence of KBLs is a *rare* finding in CHF, though certainly helpful *if* present. I guarantee that if you wait to see KBLs to "diagnose" CHF, you'll hurt a lot of patients.

With this caveat in mind, we *still* need to talk about this "mysterious" finding. KBLs *are* a great sign, when present, of lymphatic distension due to many differernt conditions. Understanding the anatomical-pathophysiological-radiographical (whew!) correlation of KBLs will help you, as a primary care provider, in many circumstances *besides* CHF. Read on . . .

KBLs represent a fortuitous occurrence, when a "packet" of x-rays happens to hit perpendicular to a distended lymphatic vessel that lies on the outer surface of the lung. [**FIGURE 3-21**] The result is greater than usual absorption of x-rays by the distended lymphatic. Fewer x-rays hit the film in that area, resulting in "white lines" we know of as Kerley B lines.

Acknowledging that KBLs simply are a *finding* of lymphatic distension, the next question is simple — is CHF the only cause of lymphatic distension? Of course not. Tumor and infection are at least as likely. And, in the

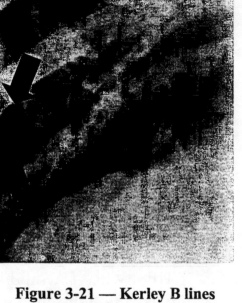

Figure 3-21 — Kerley B lines appear as linear white densities on the edge of the lung fields and represent filled lymphatics.

typical primary care practice, you are more likely to see KBLs as a sign of early lymphatic metastasis, especially in either breast or ovarian carcinoma, than you ever will as a sign of CHF.

Radiographic signs of lymphatic distension. Based on the above discussion, it should be clear that many different disease processes may result in lymphatic distension. Often, it is not visible on x-ray and may not be obvious clinically.

Radiographic signs of lymphatic distension include:

REMEMBER: Kerley B lines show where x-rays hit fluid-filled lymphatics (and are absorbed) in the peripheral portions of the lung.

- Normal.
- Pleural effusions.
- Fluid in the fissures.
- Kerley B lines.

Now, let's continue with our discussion of CHF. After cephalization of flow and interstitial edema accumulation, fluid starts to fill in the alveoli (air spaces).

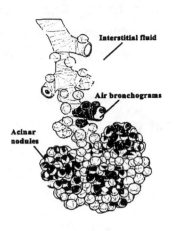

Alveolar filling with mixed alveolar-interstitial edema. Once the interstitium is "saturated," fluid starts to fill in the alveoli. Rather than flood them in any uniform pattern, alveolar filling is typically random and scattered. The result is scattered filling of a few adjacent alveoli, resulting in "splotchy" infiltrates, much as if someone had thrown at the "butterfly." [**FIGURE 3-22**] This random filling of contiguous alveoli is sometimes referred to as "acinar nodules," radiographically. Whether you call them "splotchy" infiltrates, "alveolar nodules," or "snowballs," the concept is the same: scattered alveolar filling. As you'd predict, the degree of filling depends on the severity of the disease.

Figure 3-22 — Late stages of CHF — mixture of interstitial and alveolar filling. Radiographically, these may be seen as perihilar haziness (interstitial), acinar nodules ("snowballs," alveolar filling), or air bronchograms (air-filled terminal bronchioles surrounded by fluid-filled alveoli.

On an anatomical basis, scattered acinar nodules occur due to random rupture of alveolar walls in various **acini** (terminal respiratory bronchioles and their associated alveoli). Within an acinus, each alveolus interconnects via pores of Kohn. Different acini, however, do not interconnect at this anatomical level. The result — if *one* alveolus fills with fluid, the *entire* acinus becomes "flooded," without affecting contiguous acini. As capillary hydrostatic pressure increases, the amount of interstitial fluid increases, resulting in increased

***PRINCIPLE*: Patients live/die due to adequacy/failure of Airway, Breathing, and Circulation!**

interstitial pressure. It is simply a matter of time before the thin alveolar walls start to rupture randomly. In addition to "snowballs," you sometimes see "air bronchograms." Anatomically, they are areas of alveoli that are completely fluid-filled and abut air-filled small respiratory or terminal bronchioles. The result on x-ray is that you see a "white-dark-white" pattern, reflecting the opposite radiographic densities of fluid and air. Though the correlation between *any* of these x-rays signs that suggest alveolar filling and the actual "body-part" (clinical) anatomy is less than perfect (less than 50%)[7], air bronchograms are often helpful. [**FIGURE 3-23**]

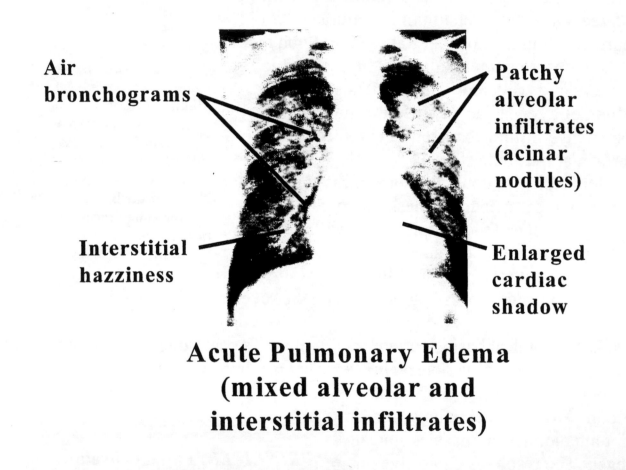

Air bronchograms

Patchy alveolar infiltrates (acinar nodules)

Interstitial hazziness

Enlarged cardiac shadow

Acute Pulmonary Edema (mixed alveolar and interstitial infiltrates)

Figure 3-23 — Acute pulmonary edema or advanced chronic congestive heart failure. Note alveolar infiltrates that appear as "snowballs" superimposed on the butterfly-like configuration of the hilum.

OBJECTIVE: Based on the pathophysiology, describe why each of the following therapeutic modalities or agents may be effective in acute pulmonary edema: positive pressure breathing, nitrates, morphine, and furosemide.

Pathophysiologically-based treatment of APE — By understanding the pathophysiology of CHF and APE, it's easy to understand the way that many of the common treatment modalities we use work. Of course, always keep in mind that the *most important* treatment for any condition is maintenance of the ABCs. Just about everything we do for patients with APE nicely relates back to those goals.

Positive-pressure breathing may really help. The claustrophobia caused by O_2 masks usually makes a bad situation worse, because it heightens anxiety (i.e., the patient feels smothered). This increases catecholamine release, increasing the work of an already overloaded heart.

Now, enter some neat pathophysiology to save the day. If an increase in capillary hydrostatic pressure causes fluid to *extravasate* into the lungs, wouldn't an increase in intrathoracic (pleural) pressure "push" it *back in*? Makes sense and it works. Now, I'm not talking about anything fancy (e.g., nasal BiPAP), though the data for noninvasive ventilation in APE appears promising (see immediately below).

> **REMEMBER:** Positive pressure breathing increases intrathoracic pressure and may counteract elevated hydrostatic pressure in the pulmonary capillaries.

The original studies, now several years old, looked at the old demand valve resuscitator. If this is all you have available and you can convince patients to try one or two "puffs," the improvement is likely to be significant enough that they will be willing to use the mask, despite the claustrophobic feeling.

Noninvasive ventilation. The same concept (i.e., positive pressure breathing) has been employed successfully in intubated patients using PEEP (positive end expiratory pressure), CPAP (continuous positive airway pressure) via both nasal mask and endotracheal tube, and most recently, nasal BiPAP (biphasic positive airway pressure). Nasal BiPAP has been studied in APE, asthma, and exacerbations of COPD. Rather than discuss the technique separately under each section, here's a generic summary (and some references):

- Patients who benefit most are clinically in the "midground" — not so mildly ill that one wonders "whether they needed to be there in the first place," and not "fixin' to die" (or to be intubated!). It is this "middle of the road patient" in whom nasal BiPAP may eliminate the need for invasive mechanical ventilation.

REMEMBER: Noninvasive ventilation is most beneficial in patients with moderately severe disease.

- Good results in the above group of patients have been reported in APE, asthma, and COPD exacerbations. Several studies tout the potential utility of this technique even in the out-of-hospital setting.[8]

- Only one study has commented on potentially *harmful* effects from nasal BiPAP. Investigators found an *increased* risk of myocardial infarction occurring in APE patients who received nasal BiPAP.[9]

Drug therapy — what's old, what's new, what's in the (very near) future? "Standard treatment" for APE has included nitroglycerine (NTG), furosemide (Lasix®), and morphine sulfate (MS). Despite the various studies over the years that have suggested reasons why and why not to include these "standard agents," they remain relatively mainstream.

Nitrates dilate systemic *and* coronary vessels, leading both to a decrease in preload and a dircct increase in myocardial oxygenation, at least theoretically.

The mechanism of action of all the commonly used nitrates involves increasing synthesis of the vasodilator, **nitric oxide** (NO). NO was formerly called endothelial-derived relaxation factor (EDRF) because it is also produced by vessel endothelium as a natural vasodilator. Nitrates provide an exogenous source of NO in vascular cells, inducing coronary vasodilation even when production of NO is impaired by coronary artery disease. Some evidence also suggests that nitrates offer a myocardial protective effect via a different, yet undefined, mechanism.[10]

REMEMBER: "Standard" drug therapy for acute pulmonary edema includes:

- **Nitroglycerine**
- **Morphine**
- **Furosemide**

Nitrates and a potentially deadly drug interaction. Though release of NO and subsequent vasodilation is a beneficial effect of nitrates, it may also result in a potentially deadly interaction with the drug sildenafil (Viagra®), used for erectile dysfunction in both men and women. The physiologic mechanism of erection of the penis involves release of nitric oxide in the corpus cavernosum during sexual stimulation. NO then activates the enzyme guanylate cyclase, which results in increased levels of cyclic guanosine monophosphate (cGMP), producing smooth muscle relaxation in the corpus cavernosum and allowing inflow of blood. Similar mechanisms are thought to occur in the clitoris of a woman.

REMEMBER: Sildenafil (Viagra®) increases cGMP levels, leading to increased levels of the vasodilator nitric oxide.

Sildenafil has no direct relaxant effect on the isolated human corpus cavernosum, but enhances the effect of nitric oxide (NO) by inhibiting phosphodiesterase type 5 (PDE5), which is responsible for degradation of cGMP in the corpus cavernosum. When sexual stimulation causes local release of NO, inhibition of PDE5 by sildenafil causes increased levels of cGMP in the corpus cavernosum, resulting in smooth muscle relaxation and inflow of blood to the corpus cavernosum. Sildenafil at recommended doses has no erectile effect in the absence of sexual stimulation.

The latest FDA package labeling for sildenafil states that nitrates are contraindicated in any person who has taken the drug within the past 24 hours. And, sildenafil is contraindicated in patients who are on any type of nitrate preparations, regardless of the reason. The implications for potential "double-dosing" of NO in a patient, and severe hypotension, shock, or even death, are clear.

So, what about furosemide (Lasix®)? Furosemide (F) has been around a long time and is still considered a first-line drug (at least by most) in the treatment of APE. Most of us would quickly state that the main effect of F is as a diuretic — correct, and not the *full* picture. F actually works, at least early on, in anephric (kidneys or nonfunctioning) patients with APE. Obviously, this finding suggests additional mechanisms of action. Most studies (though not all) have shown that the earliest hemodynamic effect of F is venodilation, with a subsequent reduction in the left ventricular preload.[11] The diuretic effect may take ten to fifteen minutes to occur.

But wait, there's more! Both animal and human data suggest that (at least in some patients) F *increases* efferent lymphatic flow. Think about it — by increasing lymphatic flow *away* from the lungs, the normal "fluid removal" function of the lymphatic system would be magnified. Experimental data show that when patients go into APE, their hematocrit, hemoglobin, plasma oncotic pressure and serum sodium levels all increase, suggesting contraction of the vascular space.[12] Of course, this makes perfect sense, since fluid leaves the intravascular compartment to enter the interstices of the lungs.

Actions of Furosemide in CHF:

- **Venodilation**
- **Diuresis**
- **Inc efferent lymphatic flow**

Administration of F causes a decrease in these aforementioned parameters, as the amount of lung water (pulmonary edema fluid) decreases by shifting back into the intravascular compartment. Then, in combination with its diuretic effect, furosemide results in an *increase* in plasma colloid osmotic pressure, decreasing the efflux of fluid into the interstitial spaces.[13] No other diuretic agent, oral or parenteral, can make this claim.

Why MS? Morphine sulfate (MS) is one of the *best* cardiovascular agents ever discovered, a fact not always appreciated by those unaware of its full spectrum of pharmacologic actions. Like other narcotic agents, it allays anxiety, reducing catecholamine output, and helping reduce cardiac work. *Unlike any other narcotic agent*, however, it has a central nervous system effect that decreases left ventricular preload and, to some extent, afterload. A portion of the mechanism is attributable to histamine release, common in many narcotic agents. MS, though, also appears to have some type of central α-blocking effect that independently enhances vasodilation.[14] Of course, in the presence of pre-existing hypovolemia, MS-induced vasodilation may result in significant hypotension.

Actions of Morphine in CHF:

- **Anxiolytic**
- **Preload and afterload reduction**
- **Histamine release**
- **Central α-blocking effect**

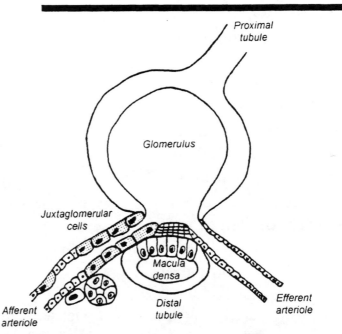

The Juxtaglomerular Apparatus

Figure 3-24

OBJECTIVE: Defend the statement: "Congestive heart failure is a disease characterized by neuroendocrine dysfunction and sympathetic excess with hemodynamic manifestations."

The renin-angiotensin-aldosterone system (RAAS). The physiological purpose of the entire RAAS system is to maintain intravascular volume in states of actual or *perceived* (e.g., CHF) hypovolemia. Receptors in the macula densa region of juxtaglomerular apparatus of the kidney, as well as in the carotid artery (sympathetic nervous system), monitor intravascular volume and serum sodium concentration. **[FIGURE 3-24]** When decreases are noted (again, let's ignore whether these are "real," as in bleeding and dehydration, or "perceived," as in CHF), they stimulate the juxtaglomerular cells to produce **renin**. Renin catalyzes conversion of **angiotensinogen** to **angiotensin-I** (AT-I), which has no pharmacologic or biologic activity. **Angiotensin-converting-enzyme** (ACE), mainly from the lungs, then catalyzes the conversion of AT-I to **angiotensin-II** (AT-II) which *does* have significant biologic activity (see next). **[FIGURE 3-24A]**

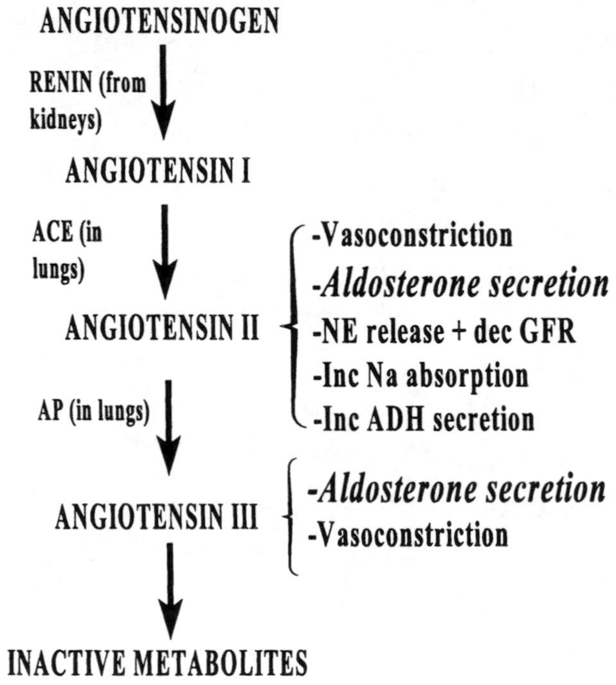
ANGIOTENSINOGEN
RENIN (from kidneys)
ANGIOTENSIN I
ACE (in lungs)
ANGIOTENSIN II
-Vasoconstriction
-Aldosterone secretion
-NE release + dec GFR
-Inc Na absorption
-Inc ADH secretion
AP (in lungs)
ANGIOTENSIN III
-Aldosterone secretion
-Vasoconstriction
INACTIVE METABOLITES

Figure 3-24A — The RAAS is a normal regulatory system whose main purpose is maintenance of intravascular volume and normotension.

AT-II is rapidly (its half-life in the circulation is only one to two minutes) converted to **angiotensin-III** (AT-III) by the enzyme **aminopeptidase** (AP). Regardless of the production pathway, AT-III also has biologic activity. Via unknown mechanisms, AT-II and AT-III are then converted to inactive metabolites.

The major actions of angiotensin-III are:

> Stimulation of aldosterone production and secretion by the adrenal glands.

> Vasoconstriction.

The molecular mechanisms (e.g., receptors, G proteins, second messengers) of AT-III's action are currently unknown. Since so little is known about AT-III, we'll not discuss it further at this time.

Angiotensin-II is the "star" of the CHF show. The major actions of angiotensin-II include:

> Vasoconstriction — AT-II is one of the most potent vasoconstrictors known.
> Stimulation of aldosterone production and secretion by the adrenal glands.
> Norepinephrine (NE) release, contributing to systemic vasoconstriction and renal vasoconstriction (decreases glomerular filtration rate or GFR).

> *PRINCIPLE*: Activation of the **RAAS in CHF is a** *normal response* **to perceived hypovolemia by the juxtaglomerular apparatus in the kidneys!**

> Increased sodium absorption in the renal tubules.
> Increased production of antidiuretic hormone (ADH).
> Stimulates drinking water (dipsogenic action) — this is both by stimulating secretion of ADH and via an independent CNS effect.

3-43

Though all of these actions are significant, the most important are vasoconstriction and stimulation of aldosterone production by the adrenal glands. ADH, by itself, contributes relatively little to the pathogenesis of CHF.

REMEMBER: In CHF, the kidney "thinks" that we are hypovolemic when, in reality, we are *fluid overloaded*!

AT-II works by binding receptors. Two AT-II receptors have been described:

1. **AT_1 receptors** are coupled by a G protein to phospholipase C. Stimulation leads to an increased intracellular calcium concentration, which activates other enzymes.

    Some of the newer antihypertensive drugs specifically block AT_1 receptors, with a somewhat lower incidence of side effects (particularly cough) than ACE inhibitors. These include irbesartan (Avapro®), losartan (Cozaar®), and valsartan (Diovan®).[15] Collectively, this group of drugs is referred to as the **sartans** or **ARBs** (angiotensin receptor blockers).

2. **AT_2 receptors** are coded in humans by the X-chromosome and do not operate via G proteins. The second messengers by which they act are unknown. There are no AT_2 receptor blockers available commercially at this time.

*AT-II binds both AT_1 and AT_2 receptors, with **opposite** results* — the effects of AT-II's binding to AT_1 and AT_2 receptors are opposite, much like the α versus β actions of epinephrine. AT-II preferentially binds the AT_1 receptors, as long as any are unbound. It only binds AT_2 receptors if all AT_1 receptor sites are occupied or blocked. This selective binding of AT-II is also favored by the fact that AT_1 receptors significantly outnumber AT_2 receptors, especially in the heart, kidneys, and blood vessels.

When AT-II binds AT_1 receptors, it stimulates vasoconstriction and aldosterone release, as discussed above. In addition, at least with chronic stimulation, AT-II stimulation of AT_1 receptors has a pro-growth effect. It causes the formation of connective tissue. This tissue is thought to contribute to atherogenesis, kidney dysfunction, and ventricular remodeling.[16] **[FIGURE 3-25]**

Administration of ACE blockers does not eliminate completely the production of AT-II. It is also made, in lesser amounts, by different non-ACE dependent pathways in peripheral tissues.[17] **[FIGURE 3-26]** Blockade of AT_1 receptors with the sartans allows any AT-II present to selectively bind the AT_2 receptors. Unopposed AT-II stimulation of AT_2 receptors, as would be expected, causes vasodilation, blocks aldosterone release, and has "anti-growth" effects. It promotes regression of scar tissue by stimulating premature apoptosis.[18]

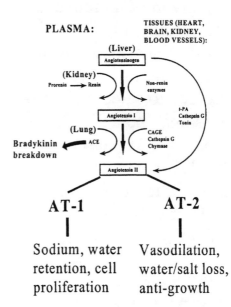

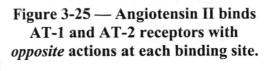

Figure 3-25 — Angiotensin II binds AT-1 and AT-2 receptors with *opposite* actions at each binding site.

Potential benefits of the sartans beyond control of hypertension.
The sartans are relatively mild anti-hypertensive agents; ACE blockers typically reduce the blood pressure more effectively. However, the sartans may have effects independent of blood pressure lowering that make them highly attractive in patients with cardiovascular problems.

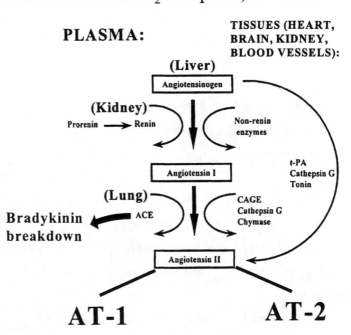

Figure 3-26 — Angiotensin II is manufactured in the lungs by the action of ACE, as well as in peripheral tissues, utilizing other enzymes.

3-45

Recent data have shown that sartans lead to regression of left ventricular hypertrophy in both human and animals, presumably by causing regression of scar tissue formed during remodeling. Thus, AT-II, when forced to selectively bind AT_2 receptors, may actually be

> **REMEMBER:** If AT_1 receptors are blocked, all available AT-II binds AT_2 receptors.

beneficial in CHF. Sartans also appear to have an anti-atherogenic effect.[19] This has led investigators to study whether the sartans should replace ACE blockers in CHF to promote stimulation of AT_2 receptors.[20] Current thinking, despite relatively few clinical studies, is that the combination of sartans *and* ACE-blockers may be the best alternative.[21] Experts cite the following reasons:

1. ACE inhibitors reduce sodium and water retention by the kidney.

2. ACE inhibitors increase bradykinin levels, leading to vasodilation.

3. Sartans force any angiotensin II present to selectively stimulate AT_2 receptors, leading to regression of fibrotic (scar) tissue and, thus, ventricular remodeling.

Why do ACE blockers (inhibitors) cause cough? In addition to catalyzing the conversion of angiotensin I to angiotensin II, ACE catalyzes breakdown of the vasoactive substance bradykinin. So, when ACE is inhibited, not only is production of much of the body's angiotensin II blocked, but so is the breakdown of bradykinin. **[FIGURE 3-27]** It is thought that persistence of this mediator causes cough — a common side-effect of ACE blockers. As a rule, changing to another ACE blocker alleviates the problem, since patients respond differently to different preparations. Intractable cough on multiple ACE blockers is an indication to try the AT_1 receptor blockers (sartans) instead.

Can't ACE blockers cause angioedema? Yes, though the reported incidence is low. Whether or not persistence of bradykinin plays a role in angioedema, a potentially life-threatening side effect of ACE blockers, is unknown. Any patient who has an episode of angioedema on *any* ACE blocker should not receive any drug in this class. There have also been isolated reports of angioedema resulting from the sartans. The mechanism and actual cause-effect relationships, if any, are unknown.

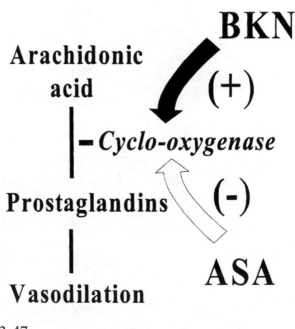

Figure 3-27 — ACE also breaks down bradykinin. The administration of an ACE-blocker will block not only the conversion of angiotensin I to angiotensin II, but the breakdown of bradykinin.

Some experts contend that if a patient has developed angioedema on ACE blockers that both ACE blockers and the sartans are contraindicated;[22] others disagree.[23]

Might elevated bradykinin levels as a result of ACE blockers (inhibitors) be beneficial? Current evidence suggests that increased levels of bradykinin secondary to the inhibition of ACE have significant *beneficial* effects, in addition to a potentially bothersome cough and, perhaps, life-threatening angioedema. Bradykinin stimulates

Figure 3-27A

cyclo-oxygenase (COX), leading to the production of vasodilatory prostaglandins. The resultant vasodilation decreases ventricular preload in CHF and improves cardiac function. **[FIGURE 3-27A]** Experts concur that the potential benefits of ACE inhibition far outweigh the potential drawbacks (i.e., cough and angioedema [rare]).[24]

Do COX inhibitors (e.g., nonsteroidals and aspirin) interfere with the vasodilatory effects of bradykinin? Since both nonsteroidals (NSAIDs) and aspirin (ASA) block COX, they, at least in theory, may inhibit the production of vasodilatory prostaglandins. Studies are limited, but current data suggest that ASA, when used in doses of 80 - 160 mg per day, do not interfere. NSAIDs, on the other hand, are potentially dangerous in patients with a history of CHF, especially those older than sixty years of age. NSAIDs may provoke an acute exacerbation of CHF, or worsen the patient's current status due to loss of vasodilation. This loss may lead to increased ventricular preload, ventricular afterload, or both. Even the newer selective COX-2 inhibitors are considered relatively contraindicated in CHF by many experts.[25]

OBJECTIVE: Describe the molecular mechanisms of action of aldosterone; summarize the most recent data concerning use of spironolactone in chronic congestive heart failure.

The actions of aldosterone. Once secreted via either the AT-II or AT-III pathway, aldosterone binds intracellular receptors, leading to modifications in as yet uncertain regulatory proteins. Aldosterone binds to an intracellular receptor, causing the formation of messenger RNA (mRNA), which fosters the formation of new proteins. These proteins affect both the Na^+ - K^+ exchanger, and Na^+ ion channels in the kidneys, sweat glands, and colon. Aldosterone also increases sodium absorption by intestinal epithelial cells. This causes secondary absorption of chloride ions and water. The effect is most important in the colon, because it allows virtually no loss of sodium chloride in the feces and little water loss.[26] The net effect is Na^+ and water retention, which raises the intravascular volume and blood pressure. **[FIGURE 3-28]**

Adrenal Cortex
↓
Aldosterone
↓
Receptor
↓
Proteins
↓
-Na^+ ion channels
-Na^+ - K^+ exchanger
↓
Na^+ / H_2O Retention

Figure 3-28 — Actions of aldosterone in the kidneys, colon, and sweat glands.

Is this mechanism unique to aldosterone? No, most steroids, as well as thyroid hormones, bind intracellular receptors and initiate production of m-RNA. Binding of the hormone to the intracellular receptor triggers a transformation in the receptor such that a portion of its DNA is exposed. This newly exposed portion (the "DNA-binding domain") binds DNA in the nucleus at what is known as an "enhancer-like element" (essentially a very elegant on-off switch). This binding stimulates transcription of mRNA from the DNA template; mRNA is then translated into proteins by the ribosomes. Each protein produced is specific for a particular reaction. **[FIGURE 3-29]**

Why don't patients with primary hyperaldosteronism (Conn's syndrome) have edema?

Interesting but true — patients with primary aldosteronism *or* those who receive exogenous mineralocorticoids for therapeutic reasons (e.g., orthostatic hypotension) rarely have peripheral edema, even in the presence of expanded intravascular volume and hypertension. In these states, net sodium excretion actually *increases*, reducing the tendency to form peripheral edema. It's been called the **escape phenomenon**.

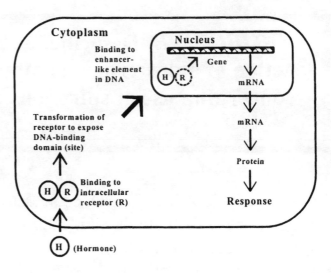

Figure 3-29 — Mechanism of action of steroid and thyroid hormones.

OBJECTIVE: Define the term "escape phenomenon" and explain its role in normal fluid balance, as well as in the pathogenesis of congestive heart failure.

The "great escape." In primary hyperaldosteronism or with exogenous mineralocortocoid administration, the excretion of sodium ions increases, despite an *increase* in extracellular fluid (ECF). Termed the "escape phenomenon," the explanation is twofold:

> **REMEMBER: Natriuretic proteins are essentially endogenous diuretics.**

1. Increased ECF volume increases renal perfusion. This leads to a "volume diuresis" by the kidney.

2.   Increased ECF volume also increases the glomerular filtration pressure, leading to a concomitant "pressure diuresis."

Thus, increased renal perfusion volume and renal perfusion pressure cause the normal kidney to react by excreting sodium and water in the urine (diuresis). The escape phenomenon helps maintain the yin-yang balance of fluid homeostasis

What about atrial natriuretic protein (ANP)? In addition to the above, stretching of the atria by increased plasma volume leads to the production of a protein, atrial natriuretic protein (ANP), by the distended left atrium. When the left atrium distends during ECF expansion, the normal response is release of ANP, which causes increased urinary excretion of sodium (natriuresis) by increasing the glomerular filtration rate (GFR). Four atrial natriuretic proteins has been described (ANP, BNP, CNP, and DNP), but the most is known about ANP.

How does ANP exert its effects? ANP activates guanylyl cyclase via a G-protein. Guanylyl cyclase catalyzes conversion of GTP to cyclic GMP (cGMP). Increased cGMP concentrations in the renal collecting ducts trigger renal excretion of sodium and water. In the vascular smooth muscle, ANP activation of guanylyl cyclase leads to vasodilation.

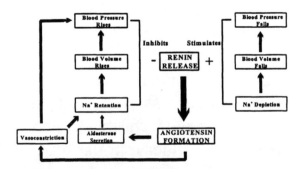

Figure 3-30 — The RAAS is a normal response system designed to maintain plasma volume and normotension.

Remember, CHF is a disease of altered normal response systems. Decreased cardiac output leads to *perceived* hypovolemia. This leads to activation of the RAAS, a normal response system designed to maintain euvolemia. Rather than maintaining normovolemia, activation of the RAAS in patients with CHF *worsens* the situation. Of course, the RAAS "has no idea" that it "fired" inappropriately — its only mission is to detect and try to correct hypovolemia (and hypotension if present). **[FIGURE 3-30]**

At the same time, there is failure of another normal response system, the natriuretic proteins. This failure allows sodium and water retention, already initiated by RAAS activation, to continue. Edema often results.

Why do CHF patients have peripheral edema? As I stated earlier, CHF is a state of decreased renal perfusion (perceived as decreased ECF volume). As such, the "normal" response of volume receptors is to trigger the renin-angiotensin-aldosterone system. In this case, and for as yet unknown reasons, homeostasis fails and edema often results. This makes sense, in light of what is currently known about ANP. The most likely mechanism is down-regulation of the ANP receptor.

What's the problem with ANP in CHF? There are two types of ANPs, with different but related actions — cardiac ANP and brain ATP (BNP). Recent data suggest the existence of at least two other forms, but their specific actions are unknown.[27] Serum elevations of cardiac ANP are predictive of worsened outcome and longer hospitalization in CHF patients.[28] Data suggest that this *normal response* to fluid overload may worsen cardiac function. The reason? Excess ANP *reduces* contraction coupling (interaction of actin and myosin filaments) in the heart.[29] It also appears that there is decreased responsiveness of the distal nephron to brain ANP in CHF, though the exact mechanisms are unclear.[30] Lowered renal response to brain ANP would result in less natriuresis, also worsening fluid retention (and increasing the cardiac preload further). Though not clinically available, synthetic human natriuretic peptides (similar to ANP), administered acutely, improve hemodynamics in severe CHF. When excessive levels of ANP are present, ANP blockers may also be beneficial.[31]

Levels of brain natriuretic protein (BNP) may eventually provide an early diagnostic test for congestive heart failure. Investigators have shown that echocardiographic cardiac dysfunction, *not* evident clinically, correlates with elevated serum BNP levels.[32] Though exciting, the clinical utility of this test remains to be seen.

"Stuff blockers" in CHF. The use of ACE inhibitors in hypertension and chronic CHF is fairly standard treatment. Recent data have suggested a significant synergistic effect of ACE inhibitors and the drug spironolactone (Aldactone®). Used for many years to treat chronic hypertension, often in conjunction with a diuretic (e.g., hydrochlorthiazide), spironolactone blocks aldosterone receptors in the kidneys, sweat glands, and colon. **[FIGURE 3-31]**

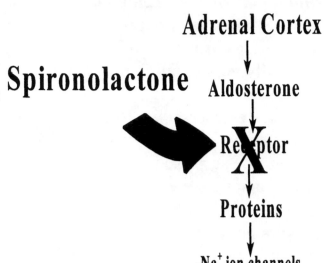

The exciting finding is that the combination of ACE inhibitors and spironolactone in patients with severe chronic CHF led to a significantly decreased two year mortality rate (better than with either agent alone). Researchers were so excited and impressed by the findings that they broke the placebo code, releasing the results to the news media weeks before the final study was published.[33]

Figure 3-31 — Spironolactone blocks aldosterone receptors in the kidneys, the sweat glands, and the colon.

After nearly 30 years of practice, I can remember only a handful of times when a drug effect was *so* pronounced that the "placebo double-blind code" was broken early — this tells me that the findings are *really* important. A fascinating new use for two

PRINCIPLE: A multi-flanked attack works better than just a one-pronged one.

relatively old drugs by combining them. And, all because we're attacking the production of "stuff" or its effects at two different points — a "double whammy" effect, eh?

What about spironolactone in APE? Studies have not been published, as of yet, on this potentially very exciting possibility. Intravenous or sublingual captopril *has* already been shown to be very effective in APE.[34] I wouldn't be surprised if spironolactone were shown to increase the efficacy of ACE blockers both chronically *and* acutely.

Do β-blockers have any role in the treatment of chronic congestive heart failure? At first, it sounds like a silly question — it seems as if β-blockade would only worsen the situation. Not true — chronic stretching of the atria leads to release of massive amounts of catecholamines. When the signal (epinephrine) persists, beta-adrenergic receptors become desensitized ("downregulated"). The result of persistent adrenergic stimulation is activation of a kinase that phosphorylates the receptor, allowing another protein (**beta-arrestin**) to bind the receptor. This binding prevents further interaction between the receptor and the G protein. **[FIGURE 3-32]**

CHF is a disease of neuroendocrine dysfunction and catecholamine excess with hemodynamic manifestions.

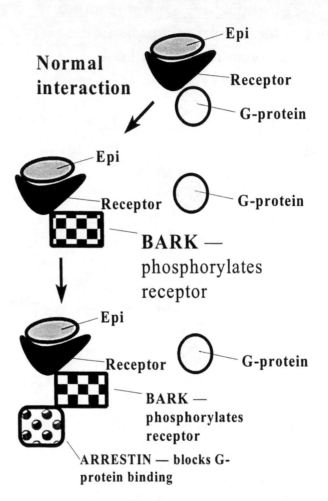

Normal interaction

Epi
Receptor
G-protein

Epi
Receptor
G-protein
BARK — phosphorylates receptor

Epi
Receptor
G-protein
BARK — phosphorylates receptor
ARRESTIN — blocks G-protein binding

Figure 3-32 — Normally, epinephrine binds the surface component of the receptor, while the G-protein binds to the inner part. Excess stimulation leads to displacement of the G-protein and attachment of β-adrenergic receptor kinase (BARK), which phosphorylates the site. Arrestin then attaches to BARK, preventing further attachment of the G-protein. The entire sequence is reversible when the receptor-arrestin complex is absorbed by endocytosis.

CHF is truly a disease of neuroendocrine dysfunction and catecholamine excess with hemodynamic manifestions. Though a double-edged sword, judicious use of β-blockade in chronic CHF usually leads to functional improvement in most patients. Many consider β-blockers standard-of-care therapy in chronic CHF.[35]

A word on treatment strategy in general. The longer I study the science of patient care, the more elegantly straight-forward it seems to be. Military historians have marveled at the ability of great leaders to mount an offensive on several fronts. Scientists have allowed us to fight disease using the same thinking process. The combination of spironolactone and ACE inhibitors discussed above is but one example of a "multi-flanked" approach to disease that is becoming increasingly more common. Of course, the basis behind the approach is an ever-improving understanding of the underlying pathophysiology. Throughout this text, we'll see examples of the "multi-flanked" approach. Already, we've discussed sympathetic stimulation to treat hypoglycemia, via either glucagon or epinephrine, as well as the role of ACE inhibitors combined with spironolactone in CHF.

Myocardial infarction

The most recent recommendations for treatment of acute MI have been published by the American Heart Association and the American College of Cardiology.[36] I encourage the interested reader to pursue these in detail, using the relevant journal references included here. I have limited this discussion to areas that most impact our understanding of the *pathophysiology* of acute myocardial infarction.

> ***OBJECTIVE:* Summarize the newly-discovered interrelationships between inflammation, infection, and rupture of atherosclerotic plaques; describe at least two potential therapeutic implications of these findings, in addition to reperfusion therapy (e.g., bypass, thrombolysis, angioplasty).**

The pendulum swings. Myocardial infarction (MI) is a *great* example of the medical pendulum's constant swinging from one extreme to the other. Some of us are old enough to remember the term "acute coronary thrombosis." It was a popular term for MI in the 1950s and 1960s, though no one could really *prove* that the end pathway in MI was an intracoronary thrombosis. "Believers" even fully anticoagulated MI victims, using warfarin (Coumadin®). Due to the lack of proof, most supporters of this theory were "scoffed at" *despite* the fact that studies repeatedly showed that acute withdrawal of warfarin led to re-infarction (suggesting a rebound hypercoagulable state). And, before investigators could really pursue these data, a new "hot topic" emerged — the role of vasospasm in angina and MI.

It would be years later when investigators in Spokane, Washington *proved* via angiographic studies that the majority of acute Q-wave (transmural) myocardial infarctions (AMIs) *do* occur as a result of "acute coronary thrombosis," and *not* spasm.[37] The same was *not* true, however, for non-Q-wave infarcts (nontransmural).[38] DeWood and colleagues' findings, of course, led to the era of reperfusion therapy, based on the following:

1. The final pathway of more than 85% of acute transmural (Q-wave) myocardial infarctions is total occlusion of an *already narrowed* coronary artery lumen.

2. The pre-existing luminal narrowing is due to atherosclerosis.

3. Total occlusion of the "residual lumen" is *not* usually via an embolism. Rather, thrombosis forms at the site of the narrowing atherosclerotic plaque.

Why does the thrombus occur? Exactly *why* a blood clot had occurred at the plaque site was unclear, though another "trip back in time" will convince you that some had the right idea, even in the old days. You "youngsters" won't remember when obtaining a WBC, ESR (erythrocyte sedimentation rate, or "sed rate"), and CRP (C-reactive protein) were as routine as CPK levels. And, guess what? In most patients, the WBC, ESR, and CRP were all *high*, at least for the first 24 to 48 hours after the acute event.

Aren't all three of these tests (WBC, ESR, CRP) nonspecific measurements of *inflammation*? You bet — my "retrospectoscope" suggests that data supporting *inflammation* as the inciting event in plaque rupture, activation of the clotting cascade, and subsequent "acute coronary thrombosis" have been around since the 1960s. Current data suggest that acute MI patients with increased WBC counts have a higher incidence of in-hospital congestive heart failure.[39] Is it possible that aspirin's anti-inflammatory effect plays a role in reducing the incidence of recurrent MI?

What is the "response to injury" hypothesis of atherosclerosis?
Atherosclerosis is a chronic inflammatory response of the arterial wall initiated by some kind of injury to the endothelium. The **response to injury hypothesis** is the major current pathological theory of atherogenesis in all vessels, not just in the coronary arteries.

The proof's in the mediators. Abundant data support the role of localized plaque inflammation's leading to bleeding as the underlying mechanism of AMI.[40] This explains the fact that factors other than simply the degree of stenosis determine the vulnerability of a lesion to acute occlusion.[41] Markers of inflammation (e.g., CRP levels) correlate with the presence of chronic atherosclerotic disease.[42] (Supportive of these data is the fact that diabetics have earlier and more severe atherosclerosis; insulin has recently been shown to have both an anti-inflammatory and anti-

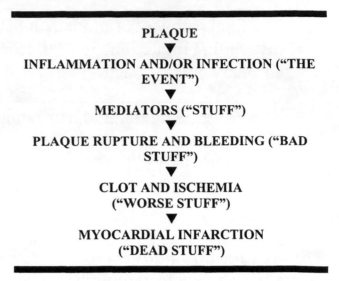

atherosclerotic effect.[43]) The reasons for inflammation in the *first place* are less clear, though some fascinating suggestions have emerged in recent studies.

Is AMI an infectious disease? And before you assume that this question *proves* any doubts left in your mind as to my mental status, let me honestly tell you that the scientific answer is: "At least in some cases, yes." Here's the scoop.

There is an association between elevated levels of antibodies to organisms like Chlamydia (the lung one, not the sexually-transmitted one!) in persons with a history of MI. In addition, persons who were treated with tetracycline or quinolones (e.g., ciprofloxacin) in the three years prior to the index date of the study had a lower risk for MI. Both agents effectively treat Chlamydia. The risk was 30% lower for tetracyclines and 55% less for quinolones. Though this particular study[44] concluded that antibiotics are not indicated at this time for prevention or treatment of acute MI, other authors have been less reserved.[45] The data are very interesting, but far from conclusive. Numerous other data suggest a role of infection, particularly by *Chlamydia pneumonia*, as a major contributor to both chronic and acute arterial occlusion.[46] These include the following:

1. Increased plasma endotoxin levels are associated with a greater prevalence of atherosclerosis.[47]

2. HMG CoA reductase inhibitors ("statins" for hyperlipidemia) modify the inflammatory response of Chlamydia infected cells,[48] and have an anti-atherogenic effect.[49]

3. Elevated plasma levels of interleukin 6 (IL-6) are associated both with Chlamydial infections and increased risk of future myocardial infarctions.[50]

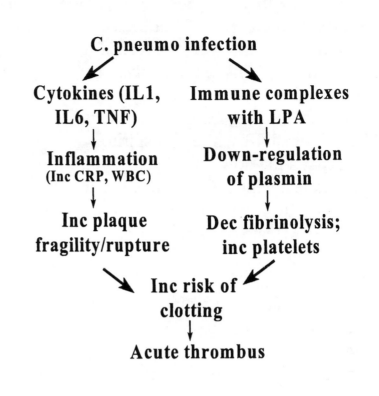

Figure 3-33 — Proposed mechanism to link infection, inflammation, and acute infarction (MI, stroke). The hypothesized chain of events is based on evidence supporting each link separately. No studies to date, however, have proven that the proposed inter-relationships are correct (yet!).

In **Figure 3-33** is a proposed mechanism by which to link Chlamydia pneumonia infection to acute MI (and probably, stroke).

Remember that "multi-flanked" approach? New drugs have amplified a relatively old approach by adding a different "avenue of attack." The target — platelets. We've known for years that platelets form the "net" that is the basis of a blood clot. Plasma clotting proteins then activate fibrinogen and fibrin plugs in the "holes." Newer research has added an interesting wrinkle. The conversion of inactive clotting factors to their active forms takes place on the platelet membrane. Thus, the platelet membranes form the "stage" on which the final clotting reactions take place. **[FIGURE 3-34]**

So, anything that impedes platelet aggregation (e.g., aspirin) would affect not only the "platelet plug," but active fibrin formation as well (to at least some extent). This explains why some people exhibit small, but measurable, increases in either their PT, PTT, or INR while on aspirin. And, that's the down side of antiplatelet agents. Of course, the up side is the ability to decrease recurrent MI, stroke, and transient ischemic attacks (TIAs).

The most recent "anti-platelet" agents affect platelet aggregation via a different mechanism than aspirin's (which inhibits the prostaglandin pathway and the enzyme, cyclooxygenase). These drugs, termed **glycoprotein IIb/IIIa receptor blockers**, interrupt the final common pathway of platelet

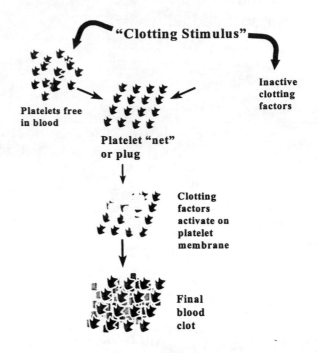

Figure 3-34 — **Mechanism of blood clot formation: Platelets first form a "net." Inactivated plasma clotting factors bind to the platelet membrane and are activated. The final thrombin clot "plugs in" the holes in the net, leading to the completed clot.**

aggregation by binding to (and blocking) the platelet surface receptor.[51] Three are available commercially (abciximab, eptifibatide, tirofiban).

Several studies have suggested an independent mortality-sparing benefit for each of the three currently available drugs (abciximab, eptifibatide, and tirofiban).[52] Though efficacy studies show some differences between each, the common denominator is improved patient outcome, especially in persons with acute coronary ischemic syndromes who are not candidates for reperfusion therapy (e.g., balloon angioplasty or thrombolytics). Studies continue to emerge. Current data suggest that these drugs are, at a minimum, an adjunct to thrombolysis and may be first-line therapy in non-Q-wave MI and in "unstable angina."[53]

Hypertensive emergencies

OBJECTIVE: Describe the role of cerebral autoregulation in the decision whether or not to treat acutely elevated blood pressure levels.

Our biggest challenge in "hypertensive emergencies" is to realize that *true* hypertensive emergencies comprise less than one percent of patients and that the best thing may be to *do nothing*, rather than always succumb to an urge to treat, treat, treat . . . Even *if* the patient qualifies as a "real" hypertensive emergency (markedly elevated BP that will result in death or serious disability, such as MI, stroke, kidney failure, or cerebral

PRINCIPLE: Sometimes the *best* treatment is *no* treatment at all!

hemorrhage, if not lowered within one hour), the proper treatment is *not* an oral agent or a bolus intravenous drug that is out of our control once given. We must use a drug that is easily titratable and can be "turned off" at the first sign of trouble. Read my lips — nitroglycerin or nitroprusside!

Regardless of other available FDA-approved parenteral agents (e.g., diazoxide, labaetolol), none meet the necessary safety criteria outlined above. And oral agents (e.g., nifedipine) are *not* indicated for any hypertensive emergency, though they may be useful in urgencies (BP needs to be lowered within twenty-four hours) *if* carefully monitored.

Still, the most difficult decision is to do nothing. And, this is the appropriate decision in the *majority* of patients with acutely increased blood pressure that we see. Here's why . . .

Cerebral autoregulation maintains normal flow. Through a fairly wide range of mean arterial pressures (MAPs), the various pre- and post-arteriolar sphincters in the cerebral vessels open and close to maintain relatively

3-61

constant cerebral blood flow (CBF). This is a *normal* regulatory mechanism, aptly entitled **cerebral autoregulation**. It's analogous to irrigating farm land. The farmer opens and closes floodgates to each section of crops to keep up the necessary flow, despite varying levels of pressure at the main water source or dam. **[FIGURE 3-35]**

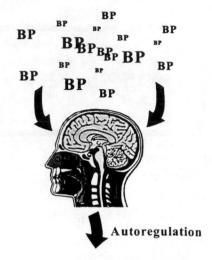

Constant Cerebral Blood Flow

Figure 3-35 — Cerebral autoregulation: within a wide range of mean arterial blood pressures, autoregulation maintains constant cerebral blood flow.

Does autoregulation take place only in the brain? No — autoregulation is a normal response system in many areas of the body. Acute increases in blood pressure will cause an immediate increase in organ and tissue blood flow. This normally persists for less than one minute, though; because of autoregulation, the flow returns back to normal. Two theories have been proposed to explain this normal regulatory process:

1.   The "metabolic theory" states that excessive arterial pressure leads to hyperoxia. Increased oxygen levels result in vasoconstriction with decreased flow, *despite* the presence of increased blood pressure.

2.   The "myogenic theory" suggests that sudden stretch (such as from increased blood pressure), causes smooth muscle in small vessel walls to constrict. The opposite holds true under conditions of low flow — the degree of stretch is less, and the muscle relaxes. The result — decreased vascular resistance and normal flow (at least to a point) despite the presence of *lowered* blood pressure.

The exact mechanisms of autoregulation have not been worked out for each tissue, and likely involve a combination of those outlined above. In addition:

●   The kidneys also regulate blood flow via "tubuloglomerular feedback." The *macula densa* (part of the juxtaglomerular apparatus), located where the tubule abuts the afferent arteriole, monitors fluid volume in the early distal tubule. If too much fluid has filtered across the glomerular filtration membrane, the macula densa sends a signal to the afferent arterioles, causing them to constrict. This reduces renal blood flow and resets the glomerular filtration rate to normal.

- In the brain, local blood flow is also controlled by the concentrations of carbon dioxide and hydrogen. Increases in either rapidly lead to vasodilation, increasing blood flow to rapidly wash out the excess ions.

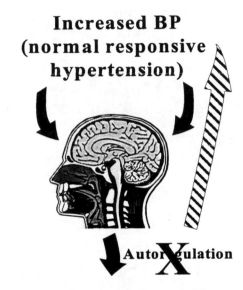

Increased BP (normal responsive hypertension)

Auto **X** **gulation**

Constant Cerebral Blood Flow

Figure 3-36 — When cerebral autoregulation is acutely lost, normal responsive hypertension is the only way to maintain adequate cerebral perfusion.

What happens to cerebral autoregulation in "head problems?"
"Head problems" is my general term for a wide variety of conditions, including stroke (both thrombotic and hemorrhagic) and head trauma, as well as "idiopathic" hypertensive emergencies (formerly termed "crises"). When patients suffer "head problems," they lose cerebral autoregulation. The implication — since the normal "floodgating mechanism" doesn't function, the only way to insure adequate cerebral blood flow is to raise the "main dam" pressure (i.e., the blood pressure).
Similarly, if the floodgates in a farmer's field didn't work, the best way to avoid crop loss is to increase flow from the main dam (which may or may not work!). Thus, the *normal* response to a loss of cerebral autoregulation (an abnormal condition, obviously), is for the mean BP to rise in an attempt to maintain normal cerebral blood flow (CBF). Though it's not medically official, I call this **"normal responsive hypertension."** [FIGURE 3-36]

When, if ever, is "normal responsive hypertension" dangerous for the patient? Make certain you're clear on this: lots of different "head problems" lead to "normal responsive hypertension" due to a loss of autoregulation. This is a *normal* and usually beneficial response. With few exceptions, what would you expect to happen if we came along and lowered this elevated BP, especially *too fast* or *too low*? You guessed it — *worse* cerebral perfusion at a time when the brain is already in trouble.

There is only a *handful* of times when the risks of acutely lowering the BP outweigh the risks of worsening an already compromised cerebral circulation:

1. Ongoing bleeding — remember, *any* head "problem," including bleeding, can lead to loss of cerebral autoregulation and to "normal responsive hypertension." In bleeding, the risks of further damage by bleeding due to elevated blood pressure outweigh those of increasing ischemia by lowering the BP.

2. Cases where the BP continues to increase (systolic > 200 mg Hg) during measurements for sixty minutes or longer — this decision should never be made on a one time measurement, except in the face of bleeding. Depending on patient stability, the upper acceptable blood pressure limit is variable.

3. Cases where the BP continues to increase and the patient appears to be getting worse (again, requiring clinical judgement — a "thinking cook").

Other than in these very limited circumstances, the best thing for the patient (though the most difficult for us) is to "watch and wait." Accept the fact that elevated BP is a normal regulatory response to an *abnormal* condition. With the above exceptions, our intervention may *worsen* an already bad situation.

Now that we "expect" HBP in "head problems," what if it's not present? Hopefully, by this stage you've come to expect "normal responsive hypertension" in "head problems." Its absence should alert you to potential problems, at least in the first 24 to 48 hours of most conditions:

- In many cases of nonhemorrhagic stroke, for example, we *expect* a period of hypertension for the first 12 to 48 hours, due to loss of autoregulation. This response is so common that its *absence* should alert us to look for either concomitant hypovolemia or sepsis from meningitis or endocarditis (the cause of the stroke?).

> **REMEMBER**: "Normal responsive hypertension" is *expected* in most acute "head problems." Its absence is a *red flag*!

- The normal response to head trauma is elevation of the BP, again due to loss of cerebral autoregulation. A *hypotensive* trauma patient, even with head injury, has concomitant hypovolemia (e.g., ruptured spleen, pelvic fracture) until proven otherwise. Only near-terminal isolated head injury causes hypotension.

> **REMEMBER**: There is a huge difference between "baseline" and "normal." Though not normal, "normal responsive hypertension" is the expected *baseline* when a person has lost cerebral autoregulation.

Anaphylaxis

Type I hypersensitivity reactions ("acute anaphylaxis") are a great example of the release of "stuff" and the appropriate use of "stuff blockers." Understanding of the full mechanism of "stuff release" has significant therapeutic implications, some of which are often belittled. Here's why . . .

> **PRINCIPLE**: "Bad stuff" begets more "bad stuff."

> **OBJECTIVE**: Illustrate the pathophysiological basis for an anaphylactic reaction.

The "nuts and bolts" of anaphylaxis. The whole thing starts when we are sensitized at an earlier point to an **antigen**. In response, the body forms **IgE antibodies** that reside on the surface of **mast cells**. Nothing happens unless we are *re-exposed* to the antigen. That's why there is no reaction on a person's first exposure to poison ivy. You have to be lucky enough to stray off the trail *again* to enjoy the weeping of hives and itching! Anaphylaxis is an acute Type I immediate hypersensitivity reaction — regardless of the symptoms present, the underlying mechanism and "stuff" is the same (see the **Table** below for the classification of hypersensitivity reactions).

TABLE — Classification of Hypersensitivity Reactions

TYPE	IMMUNE MECHANISM	EXAMPLE
I — Immediate hypersensitivity	IgE-antigen reaction → release of mediators from basophils and mast cells	Anaphylaxis, asthma (some forms)
II — Cytoxic	Formation of IgG, IgM → bind to antigen on target cell surface → phagocytosis of target cell or lysis by complement	Autoimmune hemolytic anemia, Goodpasture syndrome
III — Immune complex disease	Antigen-antibody complexes → activated complement → neutrophil attraction → release of lysosomal enzymes	Serum sickness, systemic lupus erythematosus, acute glomerulonephritis
IV — Cell-mediated (delayed) hypersensitivity	Sensitized T-lymphocytes → release of lymphokines and T cell-mediated cytotoxicity	Tuberculosis test, contact dermatitis, transplant reaction

What happens the "second time around?" After initial sensitization, repeated exposures to an antigen (Ag) result in binding with the preformed IgE antibody (Ab). This interaction results in degranulation of mast cells with release of numerous vasoactive substances ("stuff"). Initially, histamine is released. Shortly thereafter, additional mediators are also released:

REMEMBER: Many mediators ("stuff") *besides* histamine are released in a Type I allergic reaction (anaphylaxis).

- Slow reacting substance of anaphylaxis.
- Eosinophilic chemotactic factor.
- High molecular weight neutrophilic chemotactic factor (HMW-NCF).
- Prostaglandins.
- Leukotrienes.
- Kinins.
- Bradykinins.

Quite different from the days of simply saying that degranulation of mast cells led to release of "histamine," eh? And *extremely* important in our treatment. Remember that once the "anaphylaxis switch" is pulled, regardless of the extent of a patient's symptoms, the released "stuff" is *not just histamine*! By definition, *any* Type I IgE-mediated allergic reaction is "anaphylaxis," though the severity of symptoms may vary widely from patient to patient, as well as from exposure to exposure in the same patient. **[FIGURE 3-37]**

REMEMBER: By definition, *any* Type I IgE-mediated allergic reaction is "anaphylaxis," though the severity of symptoms may vary widely from patient to patient, as well as from exposure to exposure in the *same* patient.

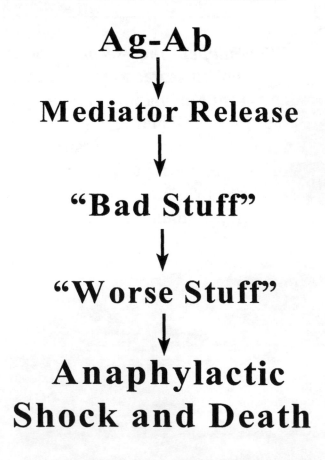

Ag-Ab
↓
Mediator Release
↓
"Bad Stuff"
↓
"Worse Stuff"
↓
Anaphylactic Shock and Death

Figure 3-37 — The pathophysiology of anaphylaxis

Are the signs and symptoms of anaphylaxis always predictable? A difficult question to answer, and the safe answer is "not really." If we remember that the majority of the mast cells in the body "live" in the skin, respiratory tract, and GI tract, then it makes sense that commonly-seen presentations include hives, wheezing, and abdominal pain. When the amount of mediators ("stuff") produced exceeds a certain limit (more metaphorical than measurable), "stuff" spills over into the blood, resulting in vasodilation, hypotension, and eventually, myocardial depression and death. **[FIGURE 3-38]**

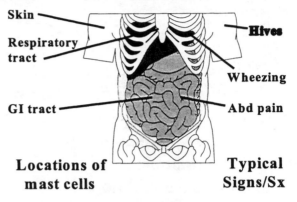
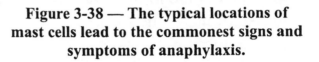

Locations of
mast cells

Typical
Signs/Sx

Figure 3-38 — The typical locations of mast cells lead to the commonest signs and symptoms of anaphylaxis.

When and if this "spillover" will happen is unknown in many patients. Therefore, the most important concept to accept in dealing with Type I allergic reactions is that whenever the "switch" is pulled, at least some mast cells degranulate. "Stuff" is produced and causes clinical effects. There is *always* the potential for this "stuff" (i.e., vasoactive mediators) to cause more problems, including the degranulation of even more mast cells (and release of more "stuff").

Why are antihistamines, by themselves, risky treatment for acute anaphylaxis? This concept usually surprises lots of health care providers — simply because we've gotten away with diphenhydramine (Benadryl®) or cimetidine (Tagamet®) alone in patients with "mild reactions." The most common situation involves progressive urticaria ("hives"). If a patient truly has a Type I IgE-mediated reaction, variable amounts of "stuff" have been released *regardless* of the symptoms. Depending on a number of unpredictable factors, symptoms may range from hives, to wheezing, to shock, myocardial depression, and death. And, *remember* that the "stuff" includes several other compounds besides histamine. True, when we didn't know any better (about the other mediators involved), use of antihistamines alone might have been excusable. Now, this practice reflects ignorance of the pathophysiology of anaphylaxis.

REMEMBER: Progressive hives and anaphylactic shock are opposite ends of the *same* spectrum of "anaphylaxis."

PRINCIPLE: Once "stuff" is released, the patient has a potentially severe problem.

COROLLARY: If you block only some of the "stuff," the patient *still* has a potentially severe problem.

Some health care providers associate the term "anaphylaxis" with *only* "anaphylactic shock." Not true — anaphylaxis is a general term referring to *any* IgE-mediated Type I allergic reaction. "Mild symptoms," such as *progressive hives*, require the same "stuff blockers" as any other anaphylactic reaction. This means epinephrine — a lower dose (0.1 - 0.2 mg SQ) than in more severe symptoms will usually suffice. Adding oral steroids, an oral antihistamine, or even long-acting epinephrine (Susphrine®) usually leads to long-lasting improvement (assuming no further exposure to the "guilty" antigen).

"CYA" really means "Can't you analyze?" I know what some of you are thinking — this is "overkill." Let me (somewhat sarcastically!) suggest that you may be "half-right." Several legal cases I've reviewed involve health care providers who gave *just* antihistamines to persons with progressive hives. By "progressive hives," I mean urticaria that is *actively* continuing to appear or progress, often in our presence. Chronic hives (for our purposes, hives lasting longer than 24 hours without regression) require steroids, antihistamines, and possibly, dermatological consultation.

Back to my story — all of these cases had one thing in common. The health care provider gave only antihistamines (usually 25 - 50 mg of diphenhydramine orally) to persons with progressive hives. Within thirty minutes, patients proceeded to develop more severe symptoms (such as wheezing, airway obstruction, or shock), often *after* leaving the clinic or ED. As a result, patients died before they could receive epinephrine.

> **PRINCIPLE: If you're going to block "stuff," you need to block *all* the stuff.**

Expert testimony in all cases opined (and jurors, as well as Appellate Courts agreed) that *epinephrine* was the initial drug of choice, not antihistamines. Based on the fact that the "stuff" released, even during "just progressive hives," includes more than just histamine, administering epinephrine as a "standard of care" makes sense. There is no reliable way to predict which patients may progress to more severe symptoms.

I thought antihistamines, like diphenhydramine (Benadryl®), were the drug of choice in acute urticaria? And, some authorities agree, depending on the severity of the reaction. Other agents that have been reported to have some success in the management of acute urticaria include H_2 receptor-active antihistamines (cimetidine, famotidine, ranitidine, etc.), newer H_1 antihistamines (doxepin, cyproheptadine, terfenadine, cetirizine, astemizole, loratadine), and subcutaneous epinephrine. All of these agents, plus glucocorticoids, cromolyn, terbutaline, and even nifedipine, are useful in the treatment of *chronic* urticaria.

H_1 antihistamines are competitive inhibitors of histamine at the H_1 receptor. This receptor mediates wheal-and-flare reactions (localized urticaria), bronchial constriction, intestinal smooth muscle contraction, mucous secretion, edema, hypotension, cardiac arrhythmia, and central nervous system depression. Traditional H_1 antihistamines are effective in relieving the pruritus and rash of acute urticaria in at least 70% of patients. Hydroxyzine (Vistaril®) is thought to be superior to diphenhydramine in clinical effect. H_2 antihistamines (e.g., cimetidine [Tagamet®]) compete with histamine at the H_2 receptor, which mediates gastric acid secretion, bronchodilation, mucous secretion, an increase in local cyclic adenosine monophosphate, and cardiac contractility.[54]

The bottom line is simple: the "thinking cook" should always consider both the medical and the legal implications if a patient progresses to more severe symptoms.

Why do some patients in anaphylaxis have a good response to diphenhydramine alone? Part of it is probably sheer luck, since none of us has 100% control over a patients outcome, anyway. The rest has to do with science, receptors, and "stuff." There are actually *three* histamine receptors (H_1, H_2, and H_3). See the **Table** below for complete details.

Because the classic H_1 receptor antagonists are not selective for the H_1 receptor site, they also induce a variety of systemic dopaminergic, serotonergic, and cholinergic responses. This may explain some of the apparent responses of Type I allergic reactions to diphenhydramine (Benadryl®). The second-generation antihistamines were designed for greater specificity at the H_1 receptor. Given their greater selectivity for the H_1 receptor, they cause fewer undesirable central nervous system actions, yet retain similar efficacy to that of the classic antihistamines used in the treatment of allergic rhinitis. The potential cardiotoxic effects of some antihistamines (e.g., torsade de pointes, ventricular tachycardia, ventricular fibrillation) requires caution in prescribing these agents.[55]

Histamine H_3 receptors — H_3 receptors are located in many areas of the body. In the brain, the histamine H_3 receptor combines with G-proteins and controls histamine synthesis and release. H_3 receptors are also present on peripheral neurons of the gastrointestinal and bronchial tract, where they regulate the release of a variety of neurotransmitters. They may decrease histamine release from mast cells, decrease release of proinflammatory kinins (inflammatory "stuff") from unmyelinated nerve in the airways, and also and play a role in modulating inflammatory allergic airway disease. In the cardiovascular system, H_3 receptors innervate the blood vessels and the heart. Their activation leads to the inhibition of noradrenaline release, and consequently, to the reduction of the neurogenic vasopressor and cardiostimulatory responses. In animal models, blockage of H_3 receptors leads to improvement in anaphylaxis.[56] Presynaptic H_3 receptors may also play a role in the pathophysiology of headache and cardiac ischemia.[57]

TABLE — HISTAMINE RECEPTORS

RECEPTOR	H₁ RECEPTOR	H₂ RECEPTOR	H₃ RECEPTOR
Location	Blood vessels, airway and gastrointestinal tract smooth muscle, heart, central nervous system	Gastric mucosa, uterus, heart, central nervous system	Neurons in central nervous system, airways, gastrointestinal tract
Antagonists	Diphenhydramine Loratadine Cetirizine Fexofenadine	Cimetidine Ranitidine Famotidine Nizatidine	Thioperamide Clobenpropit Iodoproxyfan Impentamine
Peripheral effects	Pruritus; pain; vascular permeability; hypotension; flushing; headache; tachycardia; bronchial smooth muscle constriction; activation of airway vagal afferent nerves; stimulation of cough receptors; atrioventricular node conduction time; prostaglandin generation; release of mediators of inflammation; recruitment of inflammatory cells	Gastric acid secretion; vascular permeability; hypotension; flushing; headache; tachycardia; bronchial smooth muscle relaxation; mucus production (airway); chonotropic action (atrium); inotropic action (ventricle); glycoprotein secretion; stimulation of T-suppressor cells; neutrophil and basophil chemotaxis and enzyme release; cytotoxicity and proliferation of lymphocytes; inhibition of natural killer cells	Prevents excessive bronchoconstriction; inhibits gastric acid secretion
CNS Effects	Sleep/wakefulness; food intake; thermal regulation	Neuroendocrine stimulation and hormonal release	Inhibits histamine synthesis; inhibits neurotransmitter release (histamine, dopamine, serotonin, noradrenaline, acetylcholine)

So, how does this all fit together? In the early-phase (initial) response, mast cells are activated when a specific antigen binds membrane bound IgE. This process results in the immediate release by mast cells of stored preformed mediators and to the production of new mediators. In addition, cytokine synthesis and release occurs *consequent* to mast-cell activation (remember: "Stuff begets more stuff!").

Remember: histamine isn't the only "stuff" released. Histamine is one of several molecules that can induce significant symptoms of the immediate allergic response, but it is clearly not the *sole* mediator of allergy (you *already* knew that). The relative contribution of leukotrienes, prostaglandins, and histamines in producing the allergic response depends partly on the end-organ involved.[58]

Once there is "bad stuff," more can be made. During the early-phase allergic response, mediators include LTB4 (leukotriene B4), eosinophil chemotactic factor of anaphylaxis, and neutrophil chemotactic factors. Ultimately, cytokines that up-regulate (i.e., make them work more efficiently) inflammatory cell function and enhance inflammatory cell migration are also produced not only by mast cells but also by eosinophils, basophils, and lymphocytes, which are recruited consequent to mast-cell activation. As we've said before, "damage begets more damage!"

That's why we must block **all** ***the stuff.*** So, the role of histamine in producing early-phase inflammation is end-organ dependent. And, leukotrienes and prostaglandins also play a complementary role. The bottom line — the efficacy of antihistamine therapy is probably dependent on the site of the allergic response and the contribution of histamine to the response in that site. Read my lips — if many types of "stuff" cause the problem, then you must block *all the stuff*, not just some of it.

Is there any role for the "classical antihistamines" in anaphylaxis? We've used diphenhydramine for years to help alleviate acute side effects of epinephrine (a good idea!). The best *therapeutic* benefit of antihistamines is probably for prophylactic treatment, *before* exposure to the allergen, since they are less effective in alleviating symptoms of the immediate allergic response once it is underway. They are most effective when they are occupying the H_1 receptor site before histamine is released.

Are all antihistamines created equal? The answer is clearly "no." The recently-released agent cetirizine (Zyrtec®) has anecdotally helped some patients who previously would have required epinephrine. NOTE: I am not advocating replacing epi with cetirizine — I just wanted to explain what has been the clinical experience of many, including yours truly. In single-dose evaluations, cetirizine is among the most potent of antihistamines. It has been shown to have greater activity than clemastine, hydroxyzine, loratadine, astemizole, mepyramine, and terfenadine.[59] The reason lies in the fact that cetirizine has specific anti-inflammatory ("anti-stuff") effects on both the early and late phases of anaphylaxis — read on . . .

There are two phases of anaphylaxis, early and late. The early phase is the acute reaction we've learned about for years. It usually occurs within thirty minutes of exposure to the antigen. The late phase, on the other hand, may not always occur — only 20% of patients are affected. And, these are the ones who may get into big trouble. The signs and symptoms of the late reaction may be similar to, or more severe than, those of the initial reaction. There are no distinguishing clinical features on initial presentation to identify those at risk for a late reaction. Clinically, we must assume that a patient will have a late reaction, and treat prophylactically.[60]

The late phase reaction depends on the early phase events. In the mid-1970s, several groups of investigators established clearly that the late phase reaction (LPR) is IgE mediated and is dependent on the *initial acute reaction* to antigen. This initial reaction ushers in a complex cascade of inflammatory events that are still the target of intensive investigation. Some of the early "culprits" are the same as the late ones, and some are different, as illustrated in the Table

> ***REMEMBER:*** **The late phase reaction is IgE mediated and directly dependent on the *initial* acute reaction to antigen.**

below.[61] If there were no early reaction, there couldn't be a late one, right?

MEDIATORS AND CELLS IN EARLY AND LATE ANAPHYLAXIS

"Players"	Immediate Response	Late Response
Mediators	Histamine TAME esterase Kinins PGD Leukotrienes C,D,E Leukotriene B Tryptase PAF MBP EDN	Histamine TAME esterase Kinins Eosinophic cationic protein MBD EDN
Cells	Eosinophils	Eosinophils Neutrophils Mononuclear cells Basophils Epithelial cells

EDN: Eosinophil-derived neurotoxin; *MBP:* major basic protein.

Cetirizine modulates the early anaphylactic response. In addition to its effects on H_1 receptors, cetirizine appears to decrease the levels of LTC4 (leukotriene C4) in nasal secretions. It may play other roles in the pathogenesis of acute Type I responses.[62] And, there's more: cetirizine decreases the expression of an inflammatory mediator, intracellular adhesion molecule-1 (ICAM-1), on endothelial cells, thereby inhibiting inflammatory cell migration to the site of allergic inflammation.[63] The best news may be that it doesn't loose efficacy over time (tachyphylaxis).[64]

And, cetirizine also modulates the late response. Cetirizine has significant effects on the late phase response (LPR) of anaphylaxis as well. In fact, it is the *only* antihistamine agent discovered thus far that not only has H_1-blocking antihistamine effects, but affects both the early and late phases of anaphylaxis! This is thought to be due to its ability to inhibit the infiltration of eosinophils, key cells in the pathogenesis of the allergic LPR.[65] It also exhibits independent anti-inflammatory and antiallergic properties through inhibition of the last-phase recruitment of eosinophils, neutrophils, and basophils.[66]

Aren't antihistamines contraindicated in asthma and wheezing? Usually, asthma and wheezing are at least relative contraindications to use of antihistamines. Not so in the case of cetirizine. Research shows that it induces bronchodilation up to 120 minutes after oral administration. In patients with pollen-induced asthma treated during pollen season, relatively high doses of cetirizine decreased beta-agonist and corticosteroid requirements, as well as pulmonary symptoms.[67]

The effect of cetirizine is synergistic to the effect of β2-agonists, such as albuterol, and is also dose dependent.[68] A recent study of patients with both asthma and rhinitis induced by ragweed pollen demonstrated that a 10 mg dose of cetirizine inhibited both rhinitis and asthma symptoms. No adverse effects were noted related to asthma in the cetirizine-treated patients, providing evidence of the safety of cetirizine when administered to patients with concomitant allergic rhinitis and asthma.[69]

If cetirizine is so great, why not use it in place of epinephrine? Understand clearly — cetirizine is probably the best antihistamine agent we currently have available. And, if your patient progresses to life-threatening anaphylactic shock because you failed to give epi, it's an indefensible lawsuit — period! Cetirizine alone works best in urticaria that comes and goes, especially without apparent reason,

PRINCIPLE: As long as the "stuff" that caused the problem in the first place is *still* present, so is the problem.

over a few days. In contrast, an acute progressive bout of hives calls for epi. One could probably make a good argument to use cetirizine in addition to, or maybe even in place of, oral steroids to prevent late phase reactions after an initial response to epinephrine. This hasn't been studied, though, in the direct context of anaphylaxis.

OBJECTIVE: Based on the pathophysiology involved, explain the statement: "Many patients with anaphylaxis should be observed in a medical facility for 4-6 hours, even if they completely respond to initial therapy."

How long should a patient be observed after initial improvement? A good general principle to remember is: *As long as the "stuff" that caused the problem in the first place is still present, so is the problem.* Remember how persons who suffer hypoglycemic reactions from long-acting insulins must be observed, even after initial and complete

---
PRINCIPLE: If the "stuff" outlasts the treatment, there's still a problem.

---

improvement following IV dextrose. And, those who receive intravenous naloxone for narcotic overdose may awaken and sign out against medical advice (AMA), only to have recurrence of life-threatening symptoms. The reason — IV naloxone lasts approximately 1.5 hours; most narcotics persist for 3 to 4 hours. So, another principle: *If the "stuff" outlasts the treatment, there's still a problem.*

In a recent study, biphasic anaphylactic reactions (early, then late, four to six hours later) occurred in 18% of patients. The only predictive factor the investigators were able ascertain was that patients who developed late reactions required higher doses of epinephrine to treat their initial symptoms hours earlier. I find this unhelpful, since we don't know how much epi the "average" patient requires, anyway. And, realistically, keeping a patient in the hospital "under observation" for 4 to 6 hours is difficult these days. Generally, I assume that all patients are at risk for a late phase reaction and administer drug prophylaxis (e.g., steroids, long-acting epinephrine [Susphrine®], cetirizine [Zyrtec®]). Proper patient follow-up instructions are vital as well.

What is Susphrine®? Susphrine® is an oil-based suspension of epinephrine in a 1:1000 concentration. It is long-lasting (6 to 8 hours) and works best as a follow-up medication (prophylaxis against the late phase reaction) after first using aqueous epinephrine to

---

REMEMBER: Susphrine® is a long-acting preparation consisting of epinephrine suspended in sesame seed oil.

"break" the initial attack. The dose is one-half the *total* aqueous epinephrine dose required. So, if a total of 0.4 mg were required to "break" the initial attack, the dose of Susphrine® would be 0.2 mg (or 0.2 cc). The drug should be given SQ, never via the sublingual route (see below). By the way — the oil used is sesame seed oil, so always make certain the patient doesn't have an allergy to this compound.

> *OBJECTIVE:* **Summarize recent evidence regarding the absorption of IM versus SQ epinephrine; formulate a rational approach to treatment based on this information.**

So, how much epinephrine and which route? The general "cookbook recipe" (assuming a thinking cook, of course) is:[70]

- The *dose* (in adults) is 0.1 to 0.5 mg. Depending upon the route, use either the 1:1000 (SQ, IM, sublingual injection) or 1:10,000 dilution (IV). Pre-loaded autoinjectors deliver either 0.3 mg or 0.5 mg, depending on the size of the patient.

- In mild reactions (e.g., progressive urticaria, mild wheezing with no oral involvement), the SQ route is usually adequate.

- Moderate to moderately severe reactions (e.g., more severe wheezing, lip or mouth swelling [without airway obstruction], or mild hypotension) mandate either IM (preferred) or SQ injection. Sublingual injection (see immediately below) is also an option, though this technique is not taught widely in the United States. Use the IV route only in moderately severe to severe patients, and then, only if the IV is already in place. Cutaneous edema makes it difficult to start a new one.

- Severe reactions (e.g., severe wheezing, airway obstruction, shock) requires *immediate* treatment. Use the IV route if an IV is in place already (see above). Otherwise, use either IM or sublingual injection (preferred). SQ administration is inadequate because of decreased subcutaneous tissue perfusion in all but the mildest cases. The SQ route requires approximately 30 minutes to reach an adequate serum level; IM administration results in therapeutic levels within eight minutes.[71]

Sublingual injection — a life-saving technique! Even more rapid than either IM or SQ routes is sublingual injection (SLI); one to two minutes average drug absorption time. Though not widely known or taught, this technique is not new, and it *is* well-documented. Originally, SLI was used in children with status epilepticus, where a spinal needle was utilized to inject succinylcholine into the base of the tongue via a transmental (external inferior midjaw line) approach. Epinephrine, naloxone, succinylcholine, and glucagon have all been administered successfully using SLI.

REMEMBER: Autoinjectors are specifically designed to give an IM injection. DO NOT use them for sublingual injections.

REMEMBER: Don't give Susphrine® via sublingual injection.

Current technique requires a small volume syringe (e.g., TB syringe), so the maximum volume does not exceed 1.0 cc. Limited studies suggest that SLI has similar pharmacodynamics to central vein infusion unless the patient is in complete cardiac arrest.[72] Place the needle in the vascular bed at the inferior base of the tongue; no blood return is necessary.

Many health care providers find SLI aesthetically unpleasant, often out of concern for the patient's comfort. Though I am unaware of any controlled studies on the subject, my anecdotal experience (15 cases) is that patients sick enough to require SLI have enough sublingual edema that the procedure is relatively painless. Typically, they complained more about *arm pain* from multiple fruitless IV start attempts — until I began the routine use of only SLI *unless* there was already a pre-existing IV (rare in the ED). **[Figure 3-39]**

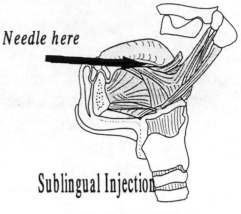

Sublingual Injection

Figure 3-39

A personal opinion. Though I doubt it would stand up in any United States court at this time, I truly believe that if anyone's job description includes administration of epinephrine to anaphylaxis victims, their scope of practice *must also* include the use of sublingual injection!

Summary

Cardiovascular problems comprise a significant percentage of patient care challenges. As always, an understanding of the normal physiology aids us in the treatment of abnormal states. Acute pulmonary edema is a prime example — Starling's law of fluid flux explains the normal mechanism of lung fluid kinetics. A thorough understanding of this over a century old principle continues to form the foundation of modern cardiovascular medicine and classification of acute pulmonary edema as either hydrostatic or hypo-oncotic.

PRINCIPLE: You must appreciate the *normal* to understand the *abnormal.*

PRINCIPLE: Water goes *down*, air goes *up*! This is a fixed law of nature.

Cardiogenic pulmonary edema (APE) secondary to severe coronary artery disease is the most common form of hydrostatic pulmonary edema we deal with. The pathologic changes in both the heart and lungs are nicely reflected, at least sometimes, on the chest x-ray. In addition, by understanding the normal fluid kinetics of the lung, it is easy to appreciate the value of x-ray signs such as Kerley B lines, fluid in the fissures, and pleural effusion. In addition, common treatments including positive pressure breathing, furosemide, nitroglycerine, and morphine all take advantage of Starling's laws.

PRINCIPLE: Patients live/die due to adequacy/failure of Airway, Breathing, and Circulation!

PRINCIPLE: Many diseases result from activation of a *normal response system* under *abnormal* circumstances.

Congestive heart failure (CHF) and APE are excellent examples of the pathophysiologic principle that many diseases occur due to activation of a *normal* regulatory mechanism under *abnormal* circumstances. Activation of the renin-angiotensin-aldosterone (RAAS) system in CHF is a normal response to perceived hypovolemia — with potentially devastating consequences. A thorough understanding of the steps involved in the production of angiotensins I and II and aldosterone offers us a sound pharmacological basis to treat both chronic and acute CHF (APE). Appreciation of the many interrelated steps has led to a "multi-pronged" approach to treatment — a principle that is applicable in many other diseases, as well.

A similar principle applies to acute exacerbation of hypertension. In many cases this simply represents "normal responsive hypertension" due to loss of cerebral autoregulation. Overly aggressive therapy may actually worsen the situation.

Our understanding of myocardial infarction (MI) reflects an interesting "swing of the pendulum," since practitioners in the 1960s and 1970s actually suggested that the final event in MI is thrombotic occlusion of an already-narrowed coronary artery. We now know this to be the case in the majority of transmural (Q-wave) infarcts, leading to the widespread use of and debate concerning the various types of reperfusion therapy. The underlying common pathway to atherosclerotic plaque rupture, with

PRINCIPLE: Sometimes the *best* treatment is *no* treatment at all!

localized bleeding and thrombosis, appears to be inflammation. Again, this concept is not new — witness elevations of CBC, ESR, and CRP levels noted during the 1960s and 1970s eras (when these studies were obtained routinely). Though far from conclusive, evidence suggests that chlamydial infection may be the underlying cause of plaque rupture in acute MI. Finally, better understanding of the role of platelets in formation of the final thrombus has led to new advances in anti-platelet drug therapy.

Anaphylaxis is a classic example of an event (antigen-antibody reaction) that leads to the release of "stuff" (vasoactive substances from mast cells). The concept that far more "stuff" than histamine alone is released directly impacts on the proper treatment with "stuff blockers" — epinephrine. In addition, as long as these mediators ("stuff") persist, the patient still potentially has a problem. Thus, the basis for long-term observation, steroids, and long-acting epinephrine (Susphrine®). A thorough understanding of these principles clarifies why antihistamines, by themselves, are potentially deadly in the treatment of low-grade anaphylactic reactions (e.g., progressive urticaria).

PRINCIPLE: Once "stuff" is released, the patient has a potentially severe problem.

PRINCIPLE: If you're going to block "stuff," you need to block *all* the stuff.

PRINCIPLE: If the "stuff" outlasts the treatment, there's still a problem.

Crossword Puzzle Review

Path Chap 3 -- Cardiovascular

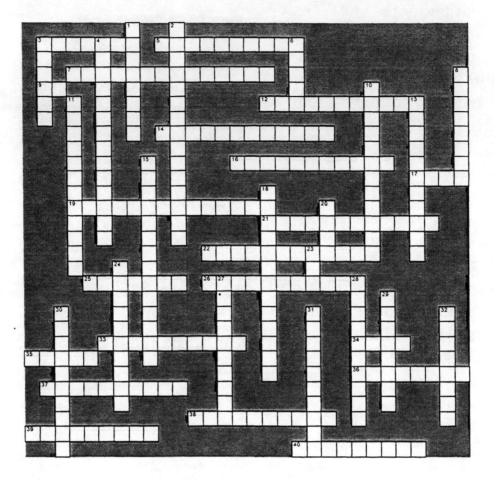

Across

3. Specific blockers of AT-1 receptors.
5. Only common drug for pulmonary edema that increases pulmonary lymphatic efferent flow.
7. Risky therapy, by themselves, for acute and progressive urticaria.
9. General type of receptors bound by angiotensin-II.
12. Any type I IgE-mediated immediate hypersensitivity reaction, regardless of the severity of the symptoms.
14. Cardiac dilation on the chest x-ray in CHF initially reflects a normal _____ mechanism.
16. _____ pressure refers to the "water pressure" either in the tubule or the surrounding tissue.
17. The Starling equation is a mathematical relationship that expresses the net direction of fluid flow into or out of a biologic _____.
19. Specific aldosterone blocker.
21. Pulmonary edema results from leaky vessels (abnormal _____), low oncotic pressure, or increased hydrostatic pressure.
22. Underlying lesion in atherosclerosis, acute and chronic.
25. The amount of blood the heart must pump.
26. Production of _____ proteins by the atria prevents fluid and sodium overload.
33. Stimulation of AT-2 receptors by angiotensin-II leads to _____ of left ventricular hypertrophy.
34. Occurrence of the _____ phase of an anaphylactic reaction depends directly upon the presence of the early phase.
35. Catalyzes the conversion of angiotensinogen to angiotensin-I.
36. You must appreciate the normal to understand the _____.
37. Potentially life-saving route of epinephrine administration in anaphylaxis.
38. Reason for cough in patients on ACE blockers.
39. The workload against which the heart must pump blood.
40. As CHF progresses, the _____ load increases.

Down

1. The underlying lesion in acute pulmonary edema is myocardial _____.
2. Receptors in the macula densa region of _____ apparatus of the kidney monitor intravascular volume and serum sodium concentration.
3. Type of oil contained in Susphrine.
4. Elevated blood pressure is a normal response to loss of cerebral _____.
6. Production of excess fluid in the interstitium or body cavities.
8. The response of the pulmonary circulation to hypoxia is _____ to that of the peripheral vessels.
10. Nitric oxide produces _____.
11. _____ _____ (2 words) are able to dilate and increase their fluid carrying capacity up to fifty times normal.
13. TNF is thought to be released due to _____ stimulation.
15. Beta-blockers are considered a _____ _____ _____ (3 words) in many patients with chronic CHF.
18. _____ of flow on the chest x-ray in CHF is a result of hypoxic vasoconstriction.
20. Side of the lymphatic circulation on which the majority of lymph fluid drains.
23. _____ (abbrev) catalyzes the conversion of AT-I to angiotensin-II.
24. An enlarged cardiac silhouette in late CHF is due to ventricular _____.
27. Life-threatening side effect of ACE blockers.
28. The most common form of hydrostatic pulmonary edema is due to acute loss of left ventricular _____.
29. ARDS is a _____ clinical entity with specific diagnostic criteria.
30. Edema fluid produced by noninflammatory mechanisms is called a _____.
31. By altering the _____ of the renal medulla, fluid is either drawn back into the body from the collecting tubules or allowed to leave as urine.
32. Sildenafil (Viagra) has a potentially life-threatening interaction with _____.

References

1.   Kunis, R, et al. *Coronary revascularization for recurrent pulmonary edema in elderly patients with ischemic heart disease and preserved ventricular function.* N Engl J Med 1985 Nov 7; 313(19):1207-10; Graham, SP, et al. *Comparison of angiographic findings and demographic variables in patients with coronary artery disease presenting with acute pulmonary edema versus those presenting with chest pain.* Am J Cardiol 1991 Dec 15; 68(17):1614-8.

2.   Starling, EH, et al. *The Law of the Heart.* J Physiol 1914; 48:465.

3.   Prabhu, SD, et al. *ß-adrenergic blockade in developing heart failure: effects on myocardial inflammatory cytokines, nitric oxide, and remodeling.* Circulation 2000; 101:2103; Murray, DR, et al. *Chronic ß-adrenergic stimulation induces myocardial proinflammatory cytokine expression.* Circulation 2000; 101:2338.

4.   Herra-Garza, EH. *Tumor necrosis factor-alpha: a mediator of disease progression in the failing human heart.* Chest 1999 Apr; 115(4): 1170-4.

5.   Harada, KK, et al. *Angiotensin II type 1A receptor knockout mice display less left ventricular remodeling and improved survival after myocardial infarction.* Circulation 1999; 100:2093-99.

6.   Chakko, S, et al. *Clinical, radiographic, and hemodynamic correlations in chronic congestive heart failure: conflicting results may lead to inappropriate care.* Am J Med 1991 Mar; 90(3):353-9; Sharma, S, et al. *Can pulmonary venous hypertension be graded by the chest radiograph?* Clin Radiol 1998 Dec; 53(12): 899-902.

7.   Albaum, MN, et al. *Interobserver reliability of the chest radiograph in community-acquired pneumonia.* Chest 1996 Aug; 110(2):343-50.

8.   Parmar, MS and Kanya-Forstner, N. *N-CPAP in the prevention of recurrent intubations and hospitalizations in a patient with refractory congestive heart failure.* Can J Cardiol 1998 Nov; 14(11):1405-8;

Patrick, W, et al. *Noninvasive positive-pressure ventilation in acute respiratory distress without prior chronic respiratory failure.* Am J Respir Crit Care Med 1996 Mar; 153(3):1005-11; Newberry DL, et al. *Noninvasive bilevel positive pressure ventilation in severe acute pulmonary edema.* Am J Emerg Med 1995 Jul; 13(4):479-82.

9.   Mehta, S, et al. *Randomized, prospective trial of bilevel versus continuous positive airway pressure in acute pulmonary edema.* Crit Care Med 1997 Apr; 25(4):620-8.

10.   Yusuf, S, et al. *Effect of intravenous nitrates on mortality in acute myocardial infarction: An overview of the randomised trials.* Lancet 1988; 1:1088-92.

11.   Pickkers, R, et al. *Direct vascular effects of furosemide in humans.* Circulation 1997; 96:1847-52.

12.   Figueras J., and Weil, MH. *Increases in plasma oncotic pressure during acute cardiogenic pulmonary edema.* Circulation 1977 Jan; 55(1):195-9.

13.   Biddle, TL and Yu, PN. *Effect of furosemide on hemodynamics and lung water in acute pulmonary edema secondary to myocardial infarction.* Am J Cardiol 1979 Jan; 43(1):86-90; Ramires, JA, et al. *The effect of intravenous furosemide on the hemodynamic parameters and colloid osmotic pressure in patients with pulmonary edema.* Arq Bras Cardiol 1992 Oct; 59(4):265-8; Demling, RH and Will, JA. *The effect of furosemide on the pulmonary transvascular fluid filtration rate.* Crit Care Med 1978 Sep-Oct; 6(5):317-9; Wickerts, CJ, et al. *Furosemide, when used in combination with positive end-expiratory pressure, facilitates the resorption of extravascular lung water in experimental hydrostatic pulmonary oedema.* Acta Anaesthesiol Scand 1991 Nov; 35(8):776-83.

14.   Opie, LH. Drugs for the Heart, 3rd edition. W.B. Saunders Co., Philadelphia 1991; p. 263; Timmis, AD, et al. *Haemodynamic effects of intravenous morphine in patients with acute myocardial infarction*

complicated by severe left ventricular failure. Br Med J 1980 Apr 5; 280(6219):980-2.

15. Belz, GG. *Irbesartan is a more potent angiotensin II antagonist than valsartan, losartan.* Clin Pharmacol Ther 1999; 66:367-73.

16. Kawano, H.K., et al, *Angiotensin II has multiple profibrotic effects in human cardiac fibroblasts.* Circulation. 2000; 101:1130; Schieffer, BN, et al. *Expression of angiotensin II and interleukin 6 in human coronary atherosclerotic plaques. Potential implications for inflammation and plaque instability.* Circulation 2000; 101:1372.

17. Jorde, U.P., et al. *Maximally recommended doses of angiotensin-converting enzyme (ace) inhibitors do not completely prevent ace-mediated formation of angiotensin II in chronic heart failure.* Circulation 2000; 101:844.

18. Unger, TJ. *Neurohormonal modulation in cardiovascular disease.* Am Heart J 2000; 139:S2-S8.

19. Strawn, WB, et al. *Inhibition of early atherogenesis by losartan in monkeys with diet-induced hypercholesterolemia.* Circulation 2000; 101:1586; Schiffrin, EL, et al. *Correction of arterial structure and endothelial dysfunction in human essential hypertension by the angiotensin receptor antagonist losartan.* Circulation 2000; 101:1653.

20. Devereux, RB. *Therapeutic options in minimizing left ventricular hypertrophy.* Am Heart J 2000; 139:S9.

21. Califf, RM and Cohn, JN. *Cardiac protection: Evolving role of angiotensin receptor blockers.* Am Heart J 2000; 139:S15-S22.

22. Sharma PK, Yium JJ. *Angioedema associated with angiotensin II receptor antagonist losartan. South Med J* 1997; 90: 552-3, 1997; Mimran, A. *Angiotensin receptor blockers: pharmacology and clinical significance.* J Am Soc Nephrol 1999 Apr; 10 Suppl 12: S273-7.

23. Granger, CB. *Randomized trial of candesartan cilexetil in the treatment of patients with congestive heart failure and a history of intolerance to angiotensin-converting enzyme inhibitors.* Am Heart J 2000 Apr; 139(4):609-17.

24. Carson, PE. *Rationale for the use of combination angiotensin-converting enzyme inhibitor/angiotensin II receptor blocker therapy in heart failure.* Am Heart J 2000;140-361-6.

25. Stys, TS, et al. *Does aspirin attenuate the beneficial effects of angiotensin-converting enzyme inhibition in heart failure?* Arch Intern Med 2000; 160:1409-13; Page, J and Henry, D. *Consumption of NSAIDs and the development of congestive heart failure in elderly patients — An underrecognized public health problem.* Arch Intern Med 2000; 160:777-84.

26. Guyton, AC and Hall, JE. Pocket Companion to Textbook of Medical Physiology, Sixth Edition. WB Saunders: Philadelphia, 1999; p. 575.

27. Smith, HJ. *Biochemical diagnosis of ventricular dysfunction in elderly patients in general practice: observational study.* BMJ 2000; 320:906-08.

28. Dickstein, K, et al. *Plasma N-terminal atrial natriuretic peptide predicts hospitalization in patients with heart failure.* Scand Cardiovasc J 1998; 32(6):361-4.

29. De Mello, WC. *Atrial natriuretic factor reduces cell coupling in the failing heart, an effect mediated by cyclic GMP.* J Cardiovasc Pharmacol 1998 Jul;32(1):75-9.

30. Jensen, KT, et al. *Renal effects of brain natriuretic peptide in patients with congestive heart failure.* Clin Sci (Colch) 1999 Jan; 96(1):5-15.

31. Mills, RM, et al. *Sustained hemodynamic effects of an infusion of nesiritide (human b-type natriuretic peptide) in heart failure: a randomized, double-blind, placebo-controlled clinical trial. Natrecor Study Group.* J Am Coll Cardiol 1999 Jul; 34(1):155-62; Kitashiro, S,

et al. *Long-term administration of atrial natriuretic peptide in patients with acute heart failure.* J Cardiovasc Pharmacol 1999 Jun; 33(6):948-52; Northridge, DB, et al. *Comparison of the short-term effects of candoxatril, an orally active neutral endopeptidase inhibitor, and frusemide in the treatment of patients with chronic heart failure.* Am Heart J 1999; 138:1149-57.

32. Murdoch, DR, et al. *Titration of vasodilator therapy in chronic heart failure according to plasma brain natriuretic peptide concentration: randomized comparison of the hemodynamic and neuroendocrine effects of tailored versus empirical therapy.* Am Heart J 1999; 138:1126-32.

33. Pitt, B., et al. *The effect of spironolactone on morbidity and mortality in patients with severe heart failure. Randomized Aldactone Evaluation Study Investigators.* N Engl J Med 1999 Sep 2; 341(10):709-17.

34. Saccheti, AA. *Effect of ED management on ICU use in acute pulmonary edema.* Am J Emerg Med 1999 Oct; 17(6): 571-4.

35. Metra, MC. *A rationale for the use of beta-blockers as standard treatment for heart failure.* Am Heart J 2000; 139:511-21; Hjalmarson, AK, et al. *Effects of controlled-release metoprolol on total mortality, hospitalizations, and well-being in patients with heart failure.* JAMA. 2000; 283:1295-1302.

36. Ryan, TJ, et al. 1999 update: *ACC/AHA guidelines for the management of patients with acute myocardial infarction: executive summary and recommendations: a report of the American College of Cardiology/American Heart Association Task Force on Practice Guidelines (Committee on Management of Acute Myocardial Infarction).* Circulation 1999 Aug 31; 100(9):1016-30; Emergency Cardiac Care Committee, American Heart Association. *Guidelines 2000 for cardiopulmonary resuscitation and emergency cardiovascular care: international consensus on science.* Circulation Aug 22, 2000; 102(8)(entire supplement).

37.	DeWood, MA, et al. *Prevalence of total coronary occlusion during the early hours of transmural myocardial infarction.* N Engl J Med 1980 Oct 16; 303(16):897-902; DeWood MA, et al. *Coronary arteriographic findings in acute transmural myocardial infarction.* Circulation 1983 Aug; 68(2 Pt 2):I39-49.

38.	DeWood, MA, et al. *Coronary arteriographic findings soon after non-Q-wave myocardial infarction.* N Engl J Med 1986 Aug 14; 315(7):417-23.

39.	Kyne LL. *Neutrophilia and congestive heart failure after acute myocardial infarction.* Am Heart J 2000; 139:94-100.

40.	See, for example: Kamijikkoku S, et al. *Acute myocardial infarction and increased soluble intercellular adhesion molecule-1: a marker of vascular inflammation and a risk of early restenosis?* Am Heart J 1998 Aug; 136(2): 231-6.

41.	Shaw, P.K. *Plaque disruption and thrombosis. Potential role of inflammation and infection.* Cardiol Clin 1999 May; 17(2): 271-81.

42.	Abdelmouttaleb, I, et al. *C-Reactive protein and coronary artery disease: additional evidence of the implication of an inflammatory process in acute coronary syndromes.* Am Heart J 1999 Feb; 137(2): 346-51.

43.	Dandona, PL, et al. *Insulin may have anti-inflammatory and anti-atherosclerotic effects.* J Clin Endocrinol Metab 2000; 85:2572-5.

44.	Meier, CR, et al. *Antibiotics and risk of subsequent first-time acute myocardial infarction.* JAMA. 1999; 281:427-31.

45.	Danesh, J, et al. *Helicobacter pylori infection and early onset myocardial infarction: case-control and sibling pairs study.* BMJ 1999 Oct 30; 319(7218):1157-62; Valtonen, VV. *Role of infections in atherosclerosis.* Am Heart J 1999 Nov; 138(5 Pt 2):431-3.

46. Roivainen, MM,et al. *Infections, inflammation, and the risk of coronary heart disease.* Circulation 2000; 101:252.

47. Wiedermann, CJ, et al. *Endotoxin may cause atherosclerosis in patients with certain bacterial infections.* J Am Coll Cardiol 1999; 34:1975-84.

48. Kothe, H.J, et al. *Hydroxymethylglutaryl coenzyme A reductase inhibitors modify the inflammatory response of human macrophages and endothelial cells infected with chlamydia pneumoniae.* Circulation 2000; 101:1760.

49. LaRosa, JC, et al. *Effect of Statins on Risk of Coronary Disease. A Meta-analysis of Randomized Controlled Trials.* JAMA. 1999; 282:2340-6.

50. Ridker, PM, et al. *Plasma Concentration of Interleukin-6 and the Risk of Future Myocardial Infarction Among Apparently Healthy Men.* Circulation 2000; 101:1767.

51. Lefkovits, J, et al. *Platelet glycoprotein IIb/IIIa receptors in cardiovascular medicine.* N Engl J Med 1995; 332:1553-9.

52. Kong, DF, et al. *Clinical outcomes of therapeutic agents that block the platelet glycoprotein IIb/IIIa integrin in ischemic heart disease.* Circulation 1998; 98: 2829-35; *Randomised placebo-controlled trial of abciximab before and during coronary intervention in refractory unstable angina: the CAPTURE Study.* Lancet 1997; 349: 1429-35; The PURSUIT Investigators. *Inhibition of platelet glycoprotein IIb/IIIa with eptifibatide in patients with acute coronary syndromes: the PURSUIT Trial investigators, Platelet glycoprotein IIb/IIIa in unstable angina: receptor suppression using integrilin therapy.* N Engl J Med 1998; 339: 436-43.

53. The Platelet Receptor Inhibition in Ischemic Syndrome Management (PRISM) Study Investigators. *A comparison of aspirin plus tirofiban with aspirin plus heparin for unstable angina.* N Engl J Med 1998; 338: 1498-505; The Platelet Receptor Inhibition in Ischemic Syndrome Management (PRISM) Study Investigators. *Inhibition of the platelet*

glycoprotein IIb/IIIa receptor with tirofiban in unstable angina and non-Q-wave myocardial infarction. N Engl Jour Med 1998; 338: 1489-97; The PURSUIT Trial Investigators, *Inhibition of platelet glycoprotein Iib/IIIa with eptifibatide in patients with acute coronary syndromes.* N Engl Jour Med 1998; 339: 436-43; Gibler, WB, et al. *Prospective use of glycoprotein IIb/IIIa receptors in the emergency department.* Ann Emerg Dec 1998; 32: 712-22; Coller, BS, et al. *Abolition of in vivo platelet thrombus formation in primates with monoclonal antibodies to the platelet GPIIb/IIIa receptor: correlation with bleeding time, platelet aggregation, and blockade of GPIIb/IIIa receptors.* Circulation 1989; 80: 1766-74.

54.   Pollack, CV, Jr. *Outpatient management of acute urticaria: the role of prednisone.* Ann Emerg Med 1995 Nov; 26(5): 547-51.

55.   DuBuske, M. *Clinical comparison of histamine H_1-receptor antagonist drugs.* J Allergy Clin Immunol 1996; 98:S307-18.

56.   Chrusch, C, et al. *Histamine H_3 receptor blockade improves cardiac function in canine anaphylaxis.* Am. J. Respir. Crit. Care Med. October 1999; 160: 1142-9.

57.   Malinowska, B, et al. *Histamine H_3 receptors--general characterization and their function in the cardiovascular system.* J Physiol Pharmacol 1998 Jun; 49(2): 191-211.

58.   Simons, EF and Simons, KJ. *The pharmacology and use of H_3-receptor-antagonist drugs.* N Engl J Med 1994; 330:1663-9.

59.   De Vos, C, et al. *Inhibition of histamine and allergen skin wheal by cetirizine in four animal species.* Ann Allergy 1987; 59:278-82.

60.   MacNamara, BE. *"Not so immediate" hypersensitivity -- the danger of biphasic anaphylactic reactions.* J Accid Emerg Med 1998 Jul; 15(4):252-3.

61.   Charlesworth, EN. *Late-phase inflammation: influence on morbidity.* J Allergy Clin Immunol 1996 Dec; 98(6 Pt 3): S291-7.

62. Naclerio, RM, et al. *The effect of cetirizine on early allergic response.* Laryngoscope 1989; 99:596-9.

63. Canonica GW, et al. *Adhesional molecules: a review of their clinical roles in allergic inflammation.* ACI News 1993; 5:80-4.

64. Simons, FR, et al. *A double-blind, single-dose crossover comparison of cetirizine, terfenadine, loratadine, astemizole, and chlorpheniramine versus placebo, suppression effects on histamine-induced wheals and flares during 24 hours in normal subjects.* Ann Allergy and Immunology 1990; 86:540-7.

65. DeVos, M, et al. *Cetirizine effects on the cutaneous allergic reaction in humans.* Ann Allergy 1990; 65:512-6.

66. Ciprandi, G, et al. *Ceterizine reduces inflammatory cell recruitment and ICAM-1 (or CD54) expression on conjunctival epithelium in both early- and late-phase reactions after allergen-specific challenge.* J Allergy Clin Immunol 1995; 95:612-21.

67. Buttmann, G, et al. *Protective effect of cetirizine in patients suffering from pollen asthma.* Ann Allergy 1990; 64:224-8.

68. Spector SL, et al. *Comparison of the bronchodilatory effects of cetirizine, albuterol, and both together versus placebo in patients with mild to moderate asthma.* Journal Allergy Clin Immunol 1995; 96:174-81.

69. Grant JA, et al. *Ceterizine in patients with seasonal rhinitis and concomitant asthma: prospective, randomized, placebo-controlled trial.* J Allergy Clin Immunol 1995; 95:923-32.

70. Joint Task Force on Practice Parameters, American Academy of Allergy, Asthma and Immunology, American College of Allergy, Asthma and Immunology, and the Joint Council of Allergy, Asthma and Immunology. *The diagnosis and management of anaphylaxis.* J Allergy Clin Immunol 1998 Aug; 102(2):264; Bochner, BS and Lichtenstein, DS. *Anaphylaxis*, New Engl Jour Med 1991; 324: 1785-

90; Hollingsworth, HM, et. al., *Anaphylaxis*, J Intensive Care Med 1991; 6:55-70.

71.   Simons, FE, et al. *Epinephrine absorption in children with a history of anaphylaxis*. J Allergy Clin Immunol 1998 Jan;101(1 Pt 1):33-37; Hughes, G and Fitzharris, P. *Managing acute anaphylaxis. New guidelines emphasise importance of intramuscular adrenaline* [editorial]. BMJ 1999 Jul 3; 319(7201):1-2.

72.   Heniff, MS, et al. *Comparison of routes of flumazenil administration to reverse midazolam- induced respiratory depression in a canine model*. Acad Emerg Med 1997 Dec; 4(12):1115-8; Rothrock, SG, et al. *Successful resuscitation from cardiac arrest using sublingual injection for medication delivery*. Ann Emerg Med 1993 Apr; 22(4):751-3.

CHAPTER 4
RESPIRATORY PROBLEMS

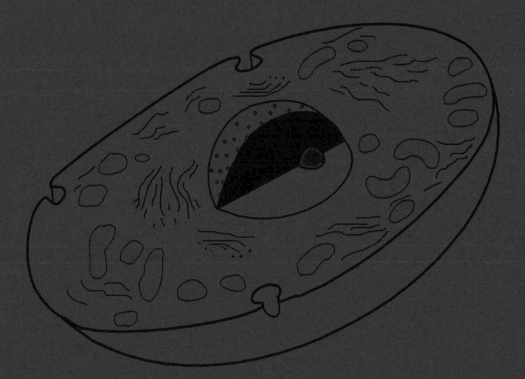

CHAPTER 4 — RESPIRATORY PROBLEMS

Contents

Objectives

After reading this chapter, you'll be able to:

- Summarize recent developments regarding the role of inflammation in asthma.
- Explain and defend the role of steroids and leukotriene inhibitors in the therapy of chronic asthma.
- List and explain at least two reasons why the incidence of asthma deaths is increasing in the United States.
- Defend the use of parasympatholytic agents (e.g., atropine, ipratroprium bromide) in the treatment of asthma and COPD.
- Summarize potential problems with COPD, chronic CO_2 retention, and oxygen therapy; formulate a reasonable clinical approach based on your understanding of these concepts.

- Formulate and summarize a simple, but effective, approach to rapidly identify the primary process (respiratory or metabolic, acidosis or alkalosis) in any set of arterial blood gases.
- List the basic principles of: respiratory compensation for metabolic acidosis or alkalosis; metabolic compensation for respiratory acidosis or alkalosis.
- Defend the statement: "All hyperventilating patients have something seriously wrong until proven otherwise."
- List and explain at least three situations where the use of "brown paper bag" treatment for hyperventilation may result in serious harm or death to the patient.

Introduction

Respiratory problems comprise a large portion of both emergency and nonemergency primary care. Our understanding of pathophysiology has increased significantly, though patient outcome (especially in asthma) does not necessarily reflect it. Nonetheless, our challenge remains — by understanding the normal, we may better appreciate and apply our treatment to what happens in disease states. First, we'll discuss obstructive lung diseases (COPD and asthma), then see how easy arterial blood gases can really be! We then turn to hyperventilation and shortness of breath — an area where slipshod thinking may be rapidly fatal for the patient. This section concludes with a review of the oxyhemoglobin dissociation curve and pulmonary function tests — and how to use them clinically.

Asthma

Our understanding of asthma in recent years has led to significant changes in the treatment approach. Despite our improved insight, the death rate from asthma continues to rise, internationally, as well as in the United States. As we'll see, failure of another normal "warning system" may be responsible. The challenge to researchers is clear. Note that one recent study (definitely a minority "view") suggested that the death rate from asthma has been stable since 1988, primarily due to better health care provider compliance with recommended national guidelines.[1]

What's old? I won't insult you by detailing what we've known for years about asthma. At the same time, the "new stuff" just fills in some unknown "blanks" in our "old" knowledge. Seems it's that way in a lot of things. In fact, I think it's time for another principle: *To understand what's new, you must first be comfortable with what's old.* In a nutshell, we've known the following about asthma for quite a while:

> ***PRINCIPLE:*** **To understand what's new, you must first be comfortable with what's old.**

- During attacks, patients suffer bronchospasm with variable degrees of air trapping. Typically, bronchospasm reverses totally or near-totally with appropriate treatment, except in patients with severe disease.

- The airways are plugged with mucus and other secretions during the attack; these clear when the attack improves.

Notice, I did not use the "standard" definition of "reversible bronchospasm, mucus plugging, and airway obstruction." The reason — the bulleted points above are still considered correct. As far as "totally reversible" or "normal between attacks," our thinking has changed radically.

What's new? Besides bronchospasm, air trapping, and mucus plugging, the majority of patients, even in the absence of clinical symptoms, have pathological evidence of chronic airway inflammation. Bronchoalveolar lavage reveals inflammatory cell infiltrate and other evidence of airway inflammation between attacks. Acute attacks involve not only bronchospasm, but desquamative bronchitis with eosinhophilia, mediator release (leukotrienes, neuropeptides)[2], and the production of free radicals.[3] And the production of this "stuff" does not appear to abate completely between attacks, even if the patient is asymptomatic. Inflammation is common to *all* asthmatics, including those with cough-variant asthma. These patients still benefit from anti-inflammatory therapy.[4] **[FIGURE 4-1]**

Airway cross-section

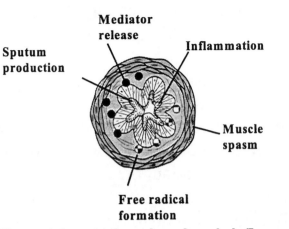

Figure 4-1 — Asthma is a chronic inflammatory condition accompanied by cell infiltrates, mediator release, and free radical activation.

The steroid switch. Our understanding of the chronic inflammatory nature of asthma led to a switch from inhaled adrenergic agents (e.g., albuterol) as primary ongoing therapy to inhaled corticosteroids (e.g., beclamethasone). Inhaled sympathomimetic drugs were relegated to an "as needed" (PRN) only basis, except for the newly released agent, salmeterol (Serevent®). Recent data support this trend, suggesting that chronic use of inhaled sympathomimetics may worsen the underlying inflammatory state.[5]

Important note. Salmeterol is *only* indicated for chronic therapy, usually no more than twice per 24-hour period, despite the fact that it is a β-sympathomimetic drug. It has a very long half life and may take up to 45 minutes to reach full effect. Thus, it has virtually no use as a "rescue inhaler" in an acute attack. Use of this agent more frequently than twice daily, especially in combination with other β-stimulant agents (e.g., albuterol, isoethrane) may *cause* deadly cardiac dysrhythmias.[6] When used properly, the drug is safe and may allow patients to reduce their steroid dose.[7] One study; however, suggested that long-acting beta-agonists, such as salmeterol, should not be used as monotherapy in patients with persistent asthma. The investigator's data showed that this practice could delay awareness of an acute asthma exacerbation.[8]

Now, back to inhaled steroids. The use of oral corticosteroids in all but the most severe asthmatics has always been frowned upon because drug side effects outweighed potential benefits. With the advent of inhaled preparations, at just about the same time that the pivotal role of airway inflammation was discovered, our treatment approach was altered forever. Inhaled steroids on an ongoing, *not* a PRN basis, became the primary form of treatment for most asthmatics, as well as for many COPDers.

Enter the double edge sword. Initially, researchers felt that inhaled steroids did not have the same side effect risk as did their oral counterparts. And, this is *still correct*, with qualifications. Most of the major side effects from oral steroids (cataracts, adrenal suppression, osteoporosis) have also been reported in patients taking only inhaled steroids. The incidence with inhaled steroids is lower, but *not* negligible. The chances of

PRINCIPLE: There's usually more than one side to any story!

having side effects increase with increasing doses, including steroids taken both nasally (for local allergies) and inhaled. The common denominator is the total dose (as measured in beclamethasone equivalents). Based on the type of steroid and the total daily dose, experts have proposed a level of risk stratification:[9]

1. Low risk — inhaled corticosteroid dosage of 800 µg of beclomethasone dipropionate (BDP) per day, or its equivalent in other corticosteroid preparations, in adults or 400 µg BDP or equivalent in children.

2. Moderate risk — inhaled BDP >800 μg in adults or >400 μg in children.

3. High risk — systemic corticosteroid therapy four times a year or daily or alternate-day systemic corticosteroid therapy.

Dosages of nasal corticosteroid probably should be added to the oral or inhaled corticosteroid dose for total burden of inhaled corticosteroid.

Is the sword really "triple-edged?" Maybe the sword contains even another edge — despite all of our research findings, the death rate from asthma continues to rise. Most experts feel this is due to insufficient suppression of chronic inflammation (read my lips — *not enough* steroids), rather than "overdose" of β-adrenergic agents (including salmeterol). So, we feel the need to further suppress chronic inflammation, while at the same time recognize more potential side effects from inhaled steroids than first believed. Steroids are effective, and relatively nonspecific, "stuff blockers." Recent data suggest that their use, alone, may reduce the death rate from asthma by more than 20 percent.[10] Current research and treatment advances focus on inhibition of specific mediators, such as leukotrienes.

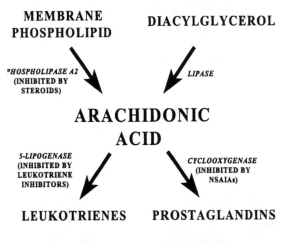

Figure 4-2 — Leukotrienes are produced from arachidonic acid via the 5-lipogenase pathway.

The role of leukotrienes. Leukotrienes are produced from arachidonic acid, as are prostaglandins, but via a different pathway. They are one of several inflammatory mediators ("stuff") that play a role in asthma, particularly in the ongoing inflammation proven to be present between attacks. It has also been established that the leukotrienes exert their pro-inflammatory effect by binding a specific receptor. Whether G-proteins and second messengers are then involved is currently unknown. **[FIGURE 4-2]**

Steroids suppress one of the major pathways that lead to formation of arachadonic acid; another biosynthetic pathway remains, allowing for continued production of leukotrienes, despite maximum doses of steroids. The synthesis and initial actions of leukotrienes allow us to utilize the "multi-pronged" attack concept to treat asthma. The final enzyme in this second branch of the arachidonic acid pathway is 5-lipogenase, which catalyzes the final formation of the various leukotrienes.

REMEMBER:

- **Arachidonic acid may be metabolized to either prostaglandins or to leukotrienes.**
- **Leukotrienes exert their final pro-inflammatory effect by binding a receptor.**
- **The mechanisms by which leukotriene-receptor binding aggravates inflammation are as yet unknown.**

Of course, the next step is to ask, "If 'stuff' causes the problem, then shouldn't blocking that 'stuff' be helpful?" And, the answer is "yes." Three anti-leukotriene drugs are commercially available in the United States for the treatment of chronic asthma. Two, zafirlukast (Accolate®) and montelukast (Singulair®), block the cysteinyl leukotriene receptor. The other, zileuton (Zyflo®), inhibits 5-lipogenase. These agents may help reduce airway inflammation and possibly decrease the need for steroids. Most studies have shown each, used individually, as safe and effective in *chronic* asthma. They are *not* indicated as "rescue" medications during an acute attack[11] but may decrease the inhaled steroid dose requirement.[12] Recent data show that zafirlukast

PRINCIPLE: A multi-flanked attack is more effective than a one-pronged one.

reduces the risk of acute exacerbations by nearly 50 percent.[13] Of course, as with any drug, not everyone responds. This makes sense, since leukotrienes are only one of *several* mediators released in asthma.

The only significant side effect is emergence of Churg-Strauss vasculitis (primarily involving the abdominal viscera) in a few patients. Though a direct causative effect is possible, an equally plausible alternative explanation is that withdrawal of steroids (facilitated by leukotriene blockers) led to clinical presentation of a disease that was already present, but suppressed by steroids.

Another use of the two-pronged approach, parasympathetic blockade. We've all known for years that whatever sympathetic nervous system stimulation causes, stimulation of the *parasympathetic nervous system* will result in an opposite effect, right? The principle holds true for asthma, as well as numerous other conditions. Other than "stuff blockers," many of our treatment modalities (old and new) involve β-adrenergic (sympathetic) stimulation, which leads to bronchodilation (e.g., epinephrine, inhaled sympathomimetics). Theophylline preparations *also* cause sympathetic stimulation, though via a different mechanism (i.e., increased levels of cyclic AMP [cAMP]).

Research over the past twenty years has established, and it makes sense, that parasympathetic stimulation leads to the opposite effect — bronchoconstriction. The mediator is thought to be cyclic GMP (cGMP). In addition, cholinergic (parasympathetic) stimulation leads to the formation of arachidonic acid (and hence, leukotrienes) via the diacylglycerol (DAG) pathway. Thus, blocking the parasympathetic nervous system, such as with atropine, should offer a "two-pronged" attack on bronchospasm.

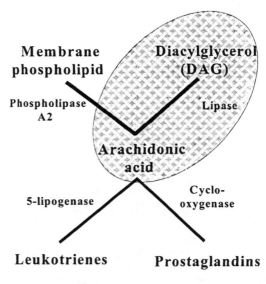

The DAG Pathway

Use of inhaled atropine and, more recently, ipratropium bromide (an atropine-like agent with fewer side effects) is effective in many patients, both acutely and in chronic therapy in asthmatics, as well as COPDers. Current data are not definitive as to the benefit of routinely adding inhaled ipratropium to inhaled sympathomimetics, though no studies have demonstrated a worsened outcome.[14] Since the "battle of the data" continues, the most helpful angle to take here is that this drug combination represents a reasoned physiologically-based attempt to "attack" disease on "multiple fronts."

If allergy (IgE) plays a role in asthma, would an IgE antibody help? The answer is a somewhat qualified "yes." Many asthmatics (70%) have an allergic component to their disease. Limited data suggest that administration of monoclonal antibodies against Ig-E are effective in reducing the frequency of allergic asthma, as well as the steroid dose.[15]

Where do theophylline preparations fit into the treatment protocol? There is still widespread debate regarding the efficacy and role of both oral and intravenous aminophylline (theophylline) derivative in both asthma and COPD. On balance, the literature indicates that there are patients who will benefit, though it is difficult to identify them prospectively. These drugs remain an *option* for clinicians.

How do theophylline preparations work? Traditionally, theophylline was thought to work primarily by inhibiting phosphodiesterases that metabolize cyclic adenosine monophosphate (cAMP). Phosphodiesterase inhibition would increase intracellular cAMP, causing bronchodilation. However, several lines of evidence suggest that this mechanism may not be of primary importance:

1. Drug concentrations needed to elevate cAMP in vitro may exceed therapeutic levels in vivo.

Possible mechanisms of methylxanthines (e.g., theophylline):

- **Inhibition of phosphodiesterase.**
- **Sympathetic stimulation.**
- **Adenosne inhibition.**
- **Anti-inflammatory.**

---

2.   Other phosphodiesterase inhibitors are not effective in asthma.

3.   Theophylline-induced relaxation of airway smooth muscle in vitro can occur without changes in intracellular cAMP levels.

Other mechanisms demonstrable in laboratory preparations, including antagonism of adenosine and stimulation of endogenous catecholamine release, also are of questionable importance to the clinical actions of theophylline. Recent evidence supports an anti-inflammatory role for theophylline in asthma. Methylxanthines, such as theophylline, reduce the activity of many of the inflammatory cells implicated in the pathogenesis of asthma and increase the activity and numbers of suppressor T cells, which may play an important role in airway inflammation.[16]

Does angiotensin II play a role in asthma? Glad you asked. Exciting new data proves a role of angiotensin II (AT-II) in pulmonary fibrosis. AT-II induces fibroblast proliferation via activation of the AT_1 receptor and also involves an interaction with **transforming growth factor**.[17] Both human and animal data have shown that AT-II promotes antigen-induced airway hyperresponsiveness and eosinophil accumulation by the same mechanism (i.e., activation of the AT_1 receptor).[18] Limited data also suggest a potential therapeutic role for the AT_1 receptor blocking agents (sartans; ARBs) in bronchospasm.[19]

The death rate is still ***rising, despite our progress.*** Sad, and true: I've already mentioned that part of the reason involves *undermedication* with anti-inflammatory agents. A second is that severe asthmatics don't realize they are in trouble until it is too late. In other words, they lack the "early warning system" and don't sense dyspnea until they are quite ill. **[FIGURE 4-3]** Failure to sense dyspnea early enough

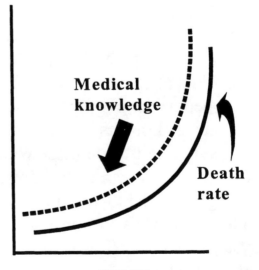

Figure 4-3 — The curves representing our increasing knowledge of asthma and the asthma death rate are nearly superimposable.

in an attack is a common underlying pattern in patients who have had near-fatal asthma attacks, as well as those who actually succumb. Once the components of the "early warning system" are identified, we can take steps to restore them, as I suggested using coffee in hypoglycemia (see **Chapter 2**). A patient profile of "high risk" patients has been identified:

1.   Females between 20 and 40 years of age.

2.   Long-standing history of asthma.

3.   History of previous episodes where care was obtained (for whatever the reason) in an untimely fashion (i.e., *later* than it should have been!).[20]

What is known about loss of the "early warning system" in fatal asthma?
One possible explanation for loss of the "early warning system" in asthma is a blunted perception of increased airflow resistance that occurs during an acute asthma attack. This reduces the patient's ability to estimate the severity of an attack. Blunted perception to resistive loads has been shown both in adults and in children with a history of near-fatal asthma. When asked to inspire against resistance, control patients easily perceived differences in airway resistance, while those with a history of near-fatal asthma did not. The severity of asthma does not account for this difference. Certain of these individuals may be identifiable with chromosomal studies.[21] Other researchers believe that histamine challenge, rather than resistive loading tests, better identify persons with decreased stretch receptor sensitivity.[22] Teenage asthmatics with prolonged wheezing do not perceive the severity of their symptoms as do those with sudden acute worsening.[23] These findings suggest that there may be "down-regulation" of pulmonary stretch receptors during prolonged wheezing, leading to loss of the "early warning system" when airflow obstruction becomes critical.

If there is an intrinsic sensing defect in patients with near-fatal asthma, it would be challenging to correct

REMEMBER: Early detection of exacerbations and near-fatal asthma episodes may be easier by frequent monitoring of peak expiratory flow and perhaps, sputum eosinophil counts.

directly. Experts suggest that the best approach may be to identify prospectively patients with poor perception of airflow limitation. Once identified, these patients would be ideal candidates for close monitoring of lung function, using a device like the Airwatch™, a hand-held device that can download lung function (PEF and FEV_1 values) for several weeks over standard telephone lines. At the first sign of decreasing lung function, intensification of therapy should occur.[24] Telemonitoring using the Internet has been shown to be easily learned and appears to work effectively.[25] Another potential method involves monitoring of the sputum eosinophil count. This has been shown to increase two to three days *prior* to clinical symptoms.[26] Recently, experts have recommended routine screening for allergic aspergillosis (a fungal infection common in allergic asthma) in all patients with allergic asthma.[27] Whether or not aspergillosis screening will impact mortality is unclear.

COPD

Obstructive lung disease. Many experts now group asthma and COPD together under the "umbrella" of **obstructive lung disease**. [FIGURE 4-4] There is good reason for this, as the underlying pathophysiology and the treatments are more similar than they are different. Inflammation has also been shown to play a major role in COPD, leading to increased used of inhaled corticosteroids, as in asthma.[28] Current data suggest that release of tumor necrosis factor (TNF) may be a prime instigator during an acute exacerbation.[29] Many of the pharmacologic approaches to asthma are also applicable, at least to an extent, in COPD. The most serious problem in our therapeutic approach remains an unfortunately too common *misunderstanding* of a patient's need for the drug, oxygen.

What about α-1 antitrypsin deficiency (AAT) and emphysema? α-1 antitrypsin (AAT) is part of the "yin-yang" balance between proteases (elastase) and anti-proteases (AAT, elastase inhibitor) theat takes place in the lung (and also in the liver). In normal lung, the alveoli are chronically exposed to low levels of neutrophil elastase released from activated and degenerating neutrophils. This proteolytic activity can destroy the elastin in alveolar walls, if unopposed by the inhibitory action of AAT. Because lung tissue cannot regenerate, destruction of the connective tissue of alveolar walls leads to emphysema. Under normal conditions, elastase and AAT balance out each other's effects.

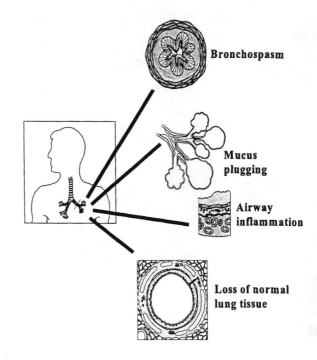

Figure 4-4 — Obstructive lung disease is a group of inter-related conditions (asthma, COPD) with similar pathogenesis (inflammation) and treatment (anti-inflammatory drugs).

Any imbalance in normal homeostasis is problematic. Excess functioning of elastase results from cigarette smoking. Decreased function of elastase inhibitor results from a deficiency of AAT. So, persons with AAT deficiency have an increases risk for developing liver disease and lung disease. Smoking increases the risk of COPD (particularly emphysema) even more. Weekly IV administration of AAT reverse the deficiency of elastase inhibitor.

Why we breathe. We have two stimuli to breath, the carbon dioxide drive (CO_2 drive) and the hypoxic drive (O_2 drive). Normally, the CO_2 drive is the primary breathing stimulus. The hypoxic drive only functions in a "backup" capacity in normal individuals. A small percentage (less than 20%) of COPDers are chronic CO_2 retainers — in other words, they have lost their CO_2 drive and retain large amounts of

---

Why we breathe:

1. **Hybercarbic drive (CO_2).**
2. **Hypoxic drive (O_2).**

CO_2 in their blood. Over time, the kidneys compensate for increased CO_2 levels by retaining bicarbonate, so that the net pH is normal. The only remaining breathing stimulus for these few individuals is the hypoxic drive. Thus, they often run lower than normal pO_2 levels (e.g., 50 to 55 mm Hg), which serve to drive breathing. Though patients may benefit from chronic low-flow oxygen,[30] many COPD patients appear relatively intact mentally even without it. Despite this appearance, neuropsychological testing demonstrates intellectual defects of varying degrees in nearly all chronic CO_2 retainers.[31]

Many of us learned the "nonphysiological approach." Many of us are taught *incorrectly* that by giving oxygen to *any* patient with COPD, we will cause them to stop breathing due to suppression of the hypoxic drive. ***PLEASE*** — don't be bullied into believing this. The generally accepted recommendation around the world is "Give 'em what they need!" Let me elaborate.

Here are the facts:[32]

1.   Only a small number of COPD patients are chronic CO_2 retainers.

2.   Even in CO_2 retainers, administration of oxygen has been shown to have a negligible effect on *minute ventilation* (the rate at which new air reaches the lungs), even if the pCO_2 level does *rise*. In other words, despite laboratory changes (increased pCO_2), net oxygen exchange remains relatively unchanged. When and if it occurs, increased pCO_2 is thought to be due to an increase in pulmonary dead space, rather than suppression of the ventilatory drive.[33]

> **REMEMBER**: The risk that oxygen administration will lead to respiratory arrest in a COPD patient is more theoretical than real. The risk of hypoxemia from inadequate O_2 therapy is far more real!

3.   Hypoxia, especially in the face of acute disease, is likely to be *more* dangerous than a theoretical risk of apnea due to oxygen administration.

4.   There is no guarantee that a CO_2 retainer given oxygen will stop breathing; in fact, odds are probably *better* that an acutely ill and hypoxic patient, whether a CO_2 retainer or not, *will* get worse *without* oxygen. Try explaining that one to the jury, gang!

5.   Even *if* patients did stop breathing, isn't it possible that if hypoxia (worse than the patient's "baseline") were already present, they were on the brink of respiratory failure anyway?

Now, I'm not advocating giving high concentrations of oxygen to every patient with COPD. And, I wouldn't do it in any other patient, either, unless there were a darn good reason. On the other hand,

> **PRINCIPLE**: The *best* treatment for a hypoxic patient is *oxygen*!

withholding potentially lifesaving oxygen from a hypoxic patient is worse. And, I don't mean "chronically hypoxic." As mentioned earlier, I mean worse than their usual baseline. To be fair, data also suggest that even when we decide to give oxygen to known CO_2 retainers, we don't need to strive for as high an oxygen saturation (> 90%) as normal — 85% to 88% will suffice. This recommendation is based on the fact that patients with acute respiratory failure complicating COPD, when treated with controlled oxygen administration with only partial correction of hypoxia and continued respiratory acidosis, will continue to have a high respiratory drive.[34] Think I'm done — well, not quite yet.

The ventilator argument. The typical "finger-pointing" scenario in a COPD patient goes something like this: (feel free to fill in the names and titles of either Actor A or Actor B; I'll play myself, thank you). "Them" refers to a patient or patients, regardless of sex.

- Actor A: "You gave them too much oxygen and made them stop breathing."

- Actor B: "They weren't doing well anyway and needed oxygen."

  PRINCIPLE: There is a *big* difference between *baseline* and *normal.*

- Actor A (looking enraged): "Now by making them stop breathing, you had to intubate them."

- Actor B (looking relatively calm and collected): "Apneic patients tend to oxygenate better with endotracheal intubation than bag valve mask."

- Actor A (face red, nearly in tears): "How will I ever get them off the ventilator?"

- Rothenberg (enters to clear up the misunderstanding): "The major reason it's difficult to get COPD patients 'off the ventilator' is because we try to ventilate them to *normal blood gases*, rather than to their *baseline*. They haven't been 'normal' for years, else we wouldn't have the problem in the first place. Learn about permissive hypercapnea or consult with someone who already knows."

Note that the same arguments summarized above have been made for severe asthma attacks. One recent study showed slight increases in the pCO_2 following administration of 100% oxygen in acute asthmatics, but there was no significant impact on patient outcome.[35]

***COROLLARY*: Trying to achieve normal blood gas levels in chronically compensated patients, rather than just returning them to their usual baseline, is often dangerous!**

Arterial blood gases made simple (REALLY!)

More health care professionals lose sleep over arterial blood gases (ABGs) than just about any other lab test we get. I just can't believe how complex this straightforward test is made to appear. *PLEASE* — try it my way; thousands of our colleagues who had near panic attacks in the past are now very comfortable with ABGs.

REMEMBER: ABGs *are* easy and straight-forward. Unfortunately, few of us were lucky enough to learn these facts the first time around!

You only need to look at four items — and *one* of them is the patient's name. The other three are: pH, pCO_2, and pO_2. Just about everything else on an ABG report represents calculated parameters that are *not needed* to identify the primary underlying acid-base disorder in most patients. Try it — I guarantee results ☺ . . .

NORMAL ABG VALUES (SEA LEVEL)

pH	7.35-7.45
pCO_2	35-45 mm Hg (torr)
pO_2	> 80 mm Hg (torr)

NOTE: torr is another unit of pressure that is sometimes used interchangeably with mm Hg

Why we get confused reading ABGs. There are three main reasons we have trouble with ABGs:

1. *Trying to figure out all the extraneous material on the report* — thus, my suggestion is to look at only the four most important items — the patient's name, pH, pCO_2, and pO_2.

2. *Trying to make pH, pCO_2, and pO_2 interrelate predictably.* It just doesn't happen that way (remember why the apple fell on Newton's head — don't try to rock the boat and rewrite the laws of physics!). True, there is a solid "marriage" between pH and pCO_2, which we'll talk about shortly. However, the relationship between pCO_2 and pO_2 is far less predictable. One day, they get along; the next, you find yourself in the middle of an ugly "domestic" situation. Get the hint? **[FIGURE 4-5]**

3. *Always trying to find a logical correlation between the pH and pCO_2 on the ABG and the serum bicarbonate level on the electrolyte panel.* Remember when I said that findings on the bicarbonate level were *independent* of the pH and pCO_2? At least for now, assume that the pH, pCO_2, and pO_2 are *independent* of the serum bicarbonate level on the electrolyte panel.

PRINCIPLE: **An apple fell from the tree, hitting Sir Isaac Newton because of *gravity*. Like all laws of Nature, we're not about to change this fact any time soon.**

CORROLARY: **The main reason we don't understand concepts is that we try to rewrite the Laws of Nature...**

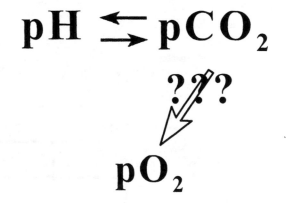

Figure 4-5 — The pH and pCO_2 are predictably related; there is no predictable relationship between the pCO_2 and the pO_2.

With the above *caveats* in mind, let's make sure we understand what each of the three measured parameters really means . . .

Separate and only sometimes-related physiological processes. The arterial pH, pCO_2, and pO_2 represent separate physiological processes. Sometimes, they are closely related; other times not:

- **pH** — represents acid-base balance; the sum of all respiratory and metabolic acid-base processes.

- **pCO_2** — chemically, the partial pressure of CO_2 dissolved in the blood. It is a respiratory acid, and is controlled by the lungs. The process of CO_2 exchange is known as **ventilation**. Changes in the pCO_2 result in near-instantaneous changes in the pH (unlike changes in the serum bicarbonate, which may take hours to days to occur, if at all).

- **pO_2** — chemically, the partial pressure of O_2 dissolved in the blood. The process of O_2 exchange is known as **oxygenation**.

What causes cyanosis? Cyanosis is not related directly to the pO_2. It appears whenever the arterial blood contains more than five grams of deoxygenated hemoglobin per 100 milliliters of blood. Anemic patients rarely show significant cyanosis because they don't have enough hemoglobin for five grams of it to be deoxygenated in the arterial blood. On the other hand, patients with polycythemia have excess available hemoglobin and may appear cyanotic, even under otherwise normal conditions.

The "happy marriage." Oxygenation and ventilation are not always directly related. On the other hand, ventilation (pCO_2) and acid-base balance (pH) *are* predictably related ("happily married forever"). Remember that respiratory changes occur rapidly through the lungs, versus metabolic ones, which take hours to days via the kidneys:

- pCO_2 represents *respiratory acid*. **Increased** blood levels of pCO_2 means *increased* acid, therefore *decreased* pH.

- Since pCO_2 represents respiratory acid, **decreases** in the blood pCO_2 level mean a *decrease* in acid, therefore *increased* pH.

Do you notice a pattern? Sure hope so. With a *decrease* in the pCO_2 there is an *increase* in the pH, and vice versa. This "marriage" is so stable because of this predictable inverse relationship: *when the pCO_2 moves one way, the pH always moves in the* opposite *direction*. In fact, we can quantitate this relationship as follows: *for every 10 mg Hg increase or decrease in pCO_2, the pH moves 0.1 units in the* opposite *direction*. Make certain you are comfortable why this has to be true. Increased pCO_2 levels add acid (more acidotic), lowering the pH; decreased pCO_2 levels take away acid (more alkalotic), leading to an

> *REMEMBER*: When the pCO_2 moves one way, the pH always moves in the *opposite* direction.

> *REMEMBER*: For every 10 mg Hg increase or decrease in pCO_2, the pH moves 0.1 units in the *opposite* direction.

increase in the pH. The 10 to 0.1 ratio merely represents empiric findings — use it to your favor.

Now, let's put it all together using a simple, yet elegant, "three question approach."

I have only three questions — To properly identify the primary underlying abnormality (respiratory/metabolic, acidosis/alkalosis) follow these rules:

1.   Look at the pO_2. **Is it low?** If it's low, *fix it!* Otherwise, move on to the next step. I'm not trying to minimize the importance of hypoxia; once you've identified it, the presence contributes nothing more to the test interpretation. Give oxygen and look at the pH.

2.   Look at the pH. Assuming it's not normal, is it too high or too low? If it's normal, maybe the test shouldn't have been done in the first place — or there is a compensatory process present. Patients *rarely* completely compensate, at least acutely, and *never* overcompensate. For the sake of understanding, let's just learn the system with either a high pH (alkalotic) or a low pH (acidotic). Note that the suffix "tic" refers to the net pH, while "sis" refers to a *process*. There may be more than one process contributing to the net pH. Our system helps identify the *primary* culprit — yes, there is always an "instigator," regardless of what else might be going on. So, look at what the pH did — **which way did it go, up (too high; alkalotic) or down (too low; acidotic)?**

3.   Look at the pCO_2. Only one question left: **"Did the pCO_2 move in the *opposite* direction as the pH?"** If so, the primary underlying process is *respiratory*. If not, the primary underlying process is *metabolic*. Trust me on this one, and please understand why these statements are correct; don't just memorize (though the "cookbook approach" *is* correct as well as helpful). Note, I didn't ask the alternative two questions (did the pCO_2 move in the *same* direction as the pH or not

change at all?). Why ask two questions when one will do?
Think about it — if the pCO_2 and pH move in opposite directions, the primary process *must* be respiratory, based on the 10 to 0.1 ratio discussed above. Otherwise, the primary process *must* be metabolic, and the pCO_2 remains unchanged or moves in the *same* direction as the pH.

Combining the pH and pCO_2 information as above, it's simple to classify the primary process as either alkalosis or acidosis (depending on whether the pH is too high or too low), and either respiratory or metabolic (depending on whether the pCO_2 moves in the *opposite* direction of the pH). Don't try to make the process more complicated than it really is. If you follow this system, you're going to get it right most of the time!

Let's try some examples to be sure. For our purposes here (and to make my math easy), let's assume that the normal pH is 7.40, the pCO_2 is 40 mm Hg, and the pO_2 is greater than 80 mm Hg.

Example 1 — 21-year-old male with acute narcotic intoxication. His respiratory rate is 4/min.

Parameter	Patient	Normal
pH	7.20	**7.35-7.45**
pCO2	60	**35-45 mm Hg (torr)**
pO2	45	**> 80 mm Hg (torr)**

Now, ask the "three questions":

1. Look at the pO_2. Is it low?. It's *too low*; the patient is hypoxic, so please fix it. Now, move on to the next question.

2. Look at the pH. Assuming it's not normal, is it too high or too low? It's *too low*; thus, the patient is acidotic — the pH went *down*. Only one question left . . .

3. Look at the pCO_2. Did it move opposite from the pH? The pH went *down*, so we are really asking if the pCO_2 went *up*. Well, did it? You bet. Since the pH and pCO_2 moved in *opposite* directions, the primary underlying problem is *respiratory*.

Putting everything together, the patient has a *respiratory acidosis* with concomitant hypoxia. Of course, in light of the clinical history, it shouldn't surprise us that the pO_2 would be low, unless the patient overdoses in a hyperbaric chamber!

Now, lets *prove* that we're right, rather than memorizing. Here, let's simply ask what would the effect on pCO_2 *have* to be if, via a primary respiratory process, he (the overdosed male) retained 20 "units" of pCO_2? Based on our 10 to 0.1 "opposite" ratio above, an increase of 20 mm Hg in the pCO_2 should *decrease* the pH by 0.2 units — which is exactly what happened. Thus, we've proven that the system works so far. Let's try another case . . .

Example 2 — 35-year-old female with pleuritic chest pain; her respiratory rate is 35/min.

Parameter	Patient	Normal
pH	7.60	7.35-7.45
pCO2	20	35-45 mm Hg (torr)
pO2	55	> 80 mm Hg (torr)

Now, ask the "three questions":

1. Look at the pO_2. Is it low?. It's *too low*; the patient is hypoxic, so please fix it. Now, move on to the next question.

2.   Look at the pH. Assuming it's not normal, is it too high or too low? It's *too high;* thus, the patient is alkalotic — the pH went *up.* Only one question left . . .

3.   Look at the pCO_2. Did it move opposite from the pH? The pH went *up,* so we are really asking if the pCO_2 went *down.* Well, did it? You bet. Since the pH and pCO_2 moved in *opposite* directions, the primary underlying problem is *respiratory.*

Putting everything together, the patient has a *respiratory alkalosis* with concomitant hypoxia. The low pO_2 points out why we should always *assume* that even the most "obvious" anxiety-hyperventilator has something seriously wrong until proven otherwise.

Again, lets *prove* that we're right, rather than memorizing. Here, let's ask what would the effect on pCO_2 *have* to be if, via a primary respiratory process, we "blew off" 20 "units" of pCO_2? Based on our 10 to 0.1 "opposite" ratio above, a decrease of 20 mm Hg in the pCO_2 should *increase* the pH by 0.2 units — which is exactly what happened. Thus, we've proven that the system works, again. Here's your next patient:

Example 3 — 60-year-old male in acute renal failure following an intravenous pyelogram.

Parameter	Patient	Normal
pH	7.25	**7.35-7.45**
pCO2	40	**35-45 mm Hg (torr)**
pO2	70	**> 80 mm Hg (torr)**

Now, ask the "three questions":

1.   Look at the pO_2. Is it low?. It's *too low;* the patient is hypoxic, so please fix it. Now, move on to the next question.

2. Look at the pH. Assuming it's not normal, is it too high or too low? It's *too low*; thus, the patient is acidotic — the pH went *down*. Only one question left . . .

3. Look at the pCO_2. Did it move opposite from the pH? The pH went *down*, so we are really asking if the pCO_2 went *up*. Well, did it? No. Since the pH and pCO_2 did *not* move in *opposite* directions, the primary underlying problem is *metabolic*.

   NOTE: The only question you really need to ask is whether the pCO_2 moved* opposite *from the pH. The remaining two options are that it did not change, or that it moved in the same direction. Either way, since it did not move in the* opposite *direction, the primary problem is metabolic. Why ask two questions when just one will do?

Putting everything together, the patient has a *metabolic acidosis* with mild concomitant hypoxia. Now, lets *prove* that we're right, rather than memorizing. Here, we'll use the mathematical technique of proof by "assuming the opposite" and discovering we were right the first time.

What if we're wrong and the primary problem is *really* respiratory? Well, what would the effect on the pCO_2 be in a primary respiratory situation if the pH were *decreased* by 0.15 units? The pCO_2 should *increase* by 15 mm Hg. Obviously, this is *not* the case, proving that we were correct in the first place. Let's try one more example before discussing compensation . . .

Example 4 — 45-year-old woman who has received NG suction X 36 h and inappropriate fluid-replacement.

Parameter	Patient	Normal
pH	7.56	**7.35-7.45**
pCO2	35	**35-45 mm Hg (torr)**
pO2	80	**> 80 mm Hg (torr)**

Now, ask the "three questions":

1. Look at the pO$_2$. Is it low?. Seems *OK* to me; be happy and move on to the next question.

2. Look at the pH. Assuming it's not normal, is it too high or too low? It's *too high*; thus, the patient is alkalotic— the pH went *up*. Only one question left . . .

3. Look at the pCO$_2$. Did it move opposite from the pH? The pH went *up,* so we are really asking if the pCO$_2$ went *down*. Well, did it? No way. Since the pH and pCO$_2$ did *not* move in *opposite* directions, the primary underlying problem is *metabolic*.

Putting everything together, the patient has a *metabolic alkalosis* with no significant hypoxia. Now, lets *prove* that we're right, rather than memorizing. Again, let's use the same mathematical technique. What if we're wrong and the primary problem is *really* respiratory. Well, what would the effect on the pCO$_2$ be in a primary respiratory situation if the pH were *increased* by 0.16 units? The pCO$_2$ should *decrease* by 16 mm Hg. Obviously, this is *not* the case, proving that we were correct originally. Now, let's consider compensation.

GOOD NEWS! **That's the *entire* ABGs system; if you're waiting for it to get more complex, please take a "chill pill" now. Compensation involves the *same* rules and asks the *same* three questions.**

Compensation. Rather than present lots of complicated tables to memorize, let's review the rules of compensation, then try a case:

- Respiratory compensation via the lungs for a primary metabolic process is quick (minutes to hours).

- Metabolic compensation via the kidneys for a respiratory process is slower (hours to days).

- Complete compensation is unusual; overcompensation is rare.

Example 5 — 35-year-old female with a known history of diabetes. She complains of nausea and vomiting for two days. The serum pregnancy test is negative. Her respiratory rate is 25/min.

Parameter	Patient	**Normal**
pH	7.25	**7.35-7.45**
pCO2	20	**35-45 mm Hg (torr)**
pO2	110	**> 80 mm Hg (torr)**

Now, ask the "three questions":

1. Look at the pO_2. Is it low?. It's *normal;* not a problem here, so let's move on.

2. Look at the pH. Assuming it's not normal, is it too high or too low? It's *too low*; thus, the patient is acidotic — the pH went *down*. Only one question left . . .

3. Look at the pCO_2. Did it move opposite from the pH? The pH went *down*, so we are really asking if the pCO_2 went *up*. Well, did it? No. Since the pH and pCO_2 did *not* move in *opposite* directions, the primary underlying problem is *metabolic*.

Putting everything together, the patient has a *metabolic acidosis* with no significant hypoxia. Now, lets *prove* that we're right, rather than memorizing. Again, let's use the mathematical technique of proof by "assuming the opposite." What if we're wrong and the primary problem is *really* respiratory? Well, what would the effect on the pCO_2 be in a primary respiratory situation if the pH were *decreased* by 0.15 units? The pCO_2 should *increase* by 15 mm Hg. Obviously, this is *not* the case, proving that we were correct originally.

REMEMBER: There *is* a method to my madness — repetition works wonders!

But, wait, there's more . . . look at the pCO_2. It's low, indicating that in addition to the primary underlying metabolic acidosis, the patient has a *compensatory* respiratory alkalosis. Think about it — if you've got a metabolic acidosis and want to compensate, what would you do? "Blow off" *respiratory* acid. It's really the only acute alternative, since the kidneys won't get rid of the abnormal metabolic acid for a while, right? And, deep sighing ventilations (Kussmaul's respirations) are a common clinical finding in patients with metabolic acidosis from any of a number of causes. These indicate *respiratory* compensation (respiratory alkalosis) for a *metabolic* problem.

REMEMBER: Respiratory compensation for metabolic acidosis via hyperventilation occurs quickly. Acidotic patients often demonstrate rapid, sighing ventilations, representing a compensatory respiratory alkalosis.

If you're up to it, I have a compensation question:

Assuming that we could actually identify the exact moment at which the above patient began her respiratory compensation (which is, in reality, nearly impossible), what was her pH *prior* to the onset of respiratory compensation? Give it some thought, then look at the hints below (commercial break!).

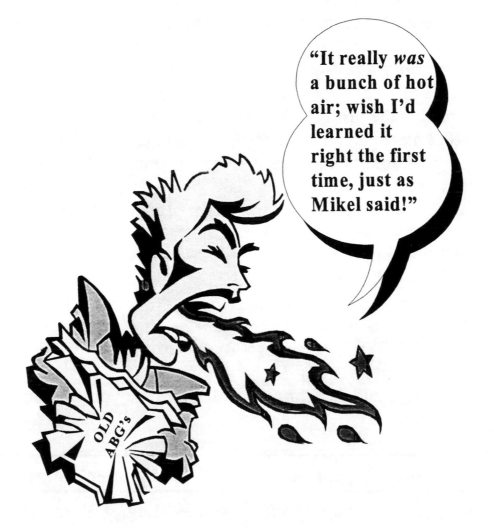

"It really *was* a bunch of hot air; wish I'd learned it right the first time, just as Mikel said!"

A commercial message from the author.

If we assume that the pCO_2 was normal (40 mm Hg) prior to the onset of compensation, the question really becomes "what is the effect on the pH of *lowering* the pCO_2 by 20 mm Hg?" The answer, (based on the "happy marriage", is that it should *increase* by 0.2 units. If the pH, with compensation, is now 7.20, we assume it's 0.2 units *higher* than before compensation occurred. Do the math — 7.25 minus 0.20 equals 7.05, the approximate starting pH prior to the onset of respiratory compensation. Since pH is a logarithmic scale (remember, $pH = - Log [H^+]$), a change in pH of 0.2 units translates to a significant decrease in acid content of the patient's blood.

A trip down logarithm row (optional). If the patient in the above example started with a pH of 7.05, she hyperventilated away ("blew off") 20 mm Hg of her pCO_2, raising the pH to 7.25. The question is: by raising the pH from 7.05 to 7.25 (0.2 pH units), how much did the acid level ($[H^+]$) in her blood change? First of all, intuition tells us that the $[H^+]$ must have *decreased*, else the pH wouldn't have increased — agreed? The easiest way to answer the question is using the mathematical formula for pH and to solve for the $[H^+]$:

$$pH = - Log_{10} [H^+]$$

Remember the definition of a logarithm:

$$If\ Log_A (B) = X,\ then\ A^X = B$$

So, for each pH (7.05 and 7.25), we can solve for the hydrogen ion concentration, $[H^+]$:

pH = 7.05 (before compensation)	pH = 7.25 (after compensation)
$7.05 = - Log_{10} [H^+]$ *(multiply both sides by -1)*	$7.25 = - Log_{10} [H^+]$ *(multiply both sides by -1)*
$10^{-7.05} = [H^+]$	$10^{-7.25} = [H^+]$
$8.9 \times 10^{-8} = [H^+]$	$5.6 \times 10^{-8} = [H^+]$

Now, compare the [H⁺] before and after compensation. After respiratory compensation, the [H⁺] level *decreased*, leading to an *increase* in the pH. So, the acid level *decreased* by (8.9 - 5.6)/8.9 = .37 or 37% (remember, the exponents cancel out). **Small *changes in pH reflect relatively* large *changes in [H⁺] levels due to the logarithmic scale.***

And, in summary . . . That's all there really is to it. Whether or not a compensatory process is present, you should always use the "three questions" to identify the primary process. Once you've got that issue settled, look for respiratory compensation if the primary process is metabolic. If the primary process is respiratory, look now at the serum electrolytes and the bicarbonate level to determine if a compensatory metabolic process is present.

ASK ONLY THREE QUESTIONS:

1. **Look at the pO_2. Is it low?**

2. **Look at the pH. Which way did it go, up (too high) or down (too low)?**

3. **Look at the pCO_2. Did the pCO_2 move in the *opposite* direction of the pH?**

Hyperventilation and shortness of breath

A trip down memory lane. Recall the last ABG case above — the patient had a metabolic acidosis with a *compensatory respiratory alkalosis*. She was hyperventilating to "blow off" respiratory acid in an attempt to compensate for accumulated metabolic acid. OK so far?

Well, consider what the effect of breathing in and out of a paper bag would have on this patient's pCO_2. Logic dictates that rebreathing would increase the pCO_2. Now, what would this do to the patients "acid load?" There's already metabolic acid on board and now she would have even more, this time in the form of rebreathed CO_2 (respiratory acid).

What's *wrong* with this picture? None of us would *deliberately* try to increase the pCO_2 in a patient with metabolic acidosis who is trying to compensate by hyperventilating. But how about doing so inadvertently (read my lips: *without thinking and understanding the pathophysiology of respiratory compensation*)? Isn't that *exactly* what we do by having apparent "anxiety hyperventilators" rebreathe

---

PRINCIPLE: Hyperventilation is a normal respiratory compensatory mechanism for metabolic acidosis. Having the patient rebreathe CO_2 through a "brown paper bag" does little to improve the pH!

---

from a brown paper bag? What if a patient turns out to be hyperventilating as a normal response ("normal response system") to a metabolic acidosis? We just made the situation worse. And, there's more . . .

A "brown paper bag" is not an oxygen tent. Besides the risk of rebreathing carbon dioxide and worsening a metabolic acidosis (by increasing *respiratory acid*), there is also a significant risk of worsening pre-existing hypoxia. Studies have shown that after only 30 seconds the FIO_2 in a "brown paper bag" or the medical equivalent, a mask with the tubing tied or ports occluded (or both), is 0.1.[36] As I recall, room air, *before we ever get involved*, is 0.21 (21% oxygen).

Remember, people "hyperventilate" for a number of reasons, including:

- Myocardial infarction.
- Pulmonary embolism.
- Metabolic acidosis.
- Pneumothorax.

And there are lots more conditions, all of which mandate administration of oxygen (ABCs). Think of the potential effect if we assume first that the patient is just hyperventilating due to anxiety, rather than assume the *worst* first. This is a guaranteed way to hurt someone, and the legal "defense" is called "settle out of court as soon as possible." Give the patient the benefit of the doubt — administer appropriate concentrations of oxygen, and avoid any possibility of rebreathing carbon dioxide and *worsening* a metabolic acidosis.

PRINCIPLE: The proper treatment of hypoxia is oxygen, not worsening the situation by a "brown paper bag."

PRINCIPLE: Apparent "anxiety hyperventilators" have something *seriously wrong* until proven otherwise!

COROLLARY: Give the patient the benefit of the doubt and administer oxygen first!

The oxygen-hemoglobin dissociation curve

Often simply called the "oxyhemoglobin saturation curve," the oxygen-hemoglobin dissociation curve shows the percent saturation of hemoglobin plotted as a function of pO_2. [FIGURE 4-6] This curve shows

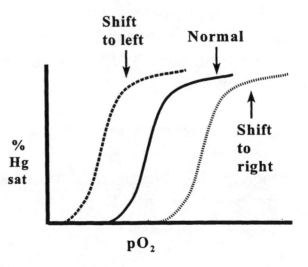

Figure 4-6 — The Oxyhemoglobin Dissociation Curve

a progressive rise in the percentage of hemoglobin (Hg) that is bound to oxygen as the pO_2 rises. This is commonly referred to as the **percentage saturation of hemoglobin**.

Why the sigmoid shape to the curve? The sigmoid shape of the curve is due to stronger binding of oxygen to hemoglobin as more oxygen molecules become bound. Hg is capable of binding four molecules of oxygen. After one oxygen molecule binds, the affinity of Hg for the second oxygen molecule increases, and so on. As you'd suspect, the affinity for the fourth oxygen molecule is greatest. This is sometimes referred to as the **Haldane effect**. Regardless of the name, increased affinity for subsequent oxygen molecules causes the sigmoid shape to the curve. The steep rise means that hemoglobin will be highly saturated at relatively low pO_2 levels.

What is the significance of the curve's shifting to the left or to the right? Right-left shifts in the oxyhemoglobin saturation curve indicate changes in the affinity of Hg for oxygen. When the curve shifts to the right, the affinity of Hg for oxygen *decreases*; the result is an *increase* in tissue oxygen delivery (oxygen "falls off" hemoglobin more easily). The opposite occurs when the curve shifts to the left — tissue oxygen delivery *decreases* due to an *increase* in the affinity of Hg for oxygen (i.e., it "holds on" more tightly).

What factors cause right or left shifts of the curve? The curve shifts to the right in metabolically active tissues. The result is increased tissue oxygen delivery. Chronic hypoxemia increases the synthesis of 2,3-diphosphoglycerate (2,3-DPG), which binds hemoglobin, also increasing tissue oxygen delivery. So, the factors shifting the curve to the right are:

- Increased temperature.
- Increased pCO_2 levels.
- Increased hydrogen concentrations (acidosis, or low pH).
- Increased 2,3-DPG levels.

Opposing factors shift the curve to the left, resulting in increased affinity of Hg for oxygen. As a result, tissue oxygen delivery is decreased. These factors are:

- Decreased temperature.
- Decreased pCO_2 levels.
- Decreased hydrogen concentrations (alkalosis, or high pH).
- Decreased 2,3-DPG levels.

The binding of H^+ and CO_2 to hemoglobin is inversely related to the binding of oxygen. At tissue pH (low pH, high CO_2 concentration), the affinity of hemoglobin for oxygen decreases as H^+ and CO_2 are bound, resulting in oxygen release to the tissues. The reverse occurs in the lungs — CO_2 is excreted, leading to a rise in the blood pH. The affinity of hemoglobin for oxygen increases, and more oxygen binds. This is sometimes called the **Bohr effect**. Chemically, this principle is illustrated in the equation below:

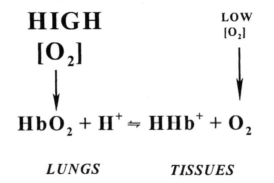

$$HbO_2 + H^+ \rightleftharpoons HHb^+ + O_2$$

LUNGS   *TISSUES*

Both O_2 and H^+ are bound by hemoglobin, but with inverse affinity. When the oxygen concentration is high, as in the lungs, hemoglobin binds O_2 and releases protons (H^+). When the oxygen concentration is low, as in the peripheral tissues, H^+ is bound to hemoglobin and O_2 is released to the tissues.

Changes in the affinity of hemoglobin for oxygen explain several empirical observations:

- Fever (increased temperature) increases tissue oxygenation.
- Acidosis (decreased pH) increases tissue oxygenation while alkalosis *decreases* it.
- Hypermetabolic states (requiring more oxygen) lead to increased production of 2,3 DPG.

Pulmonary function tests — a brief guide

Pulmonary function tests (PFTs) are used commonly in diagnosing and monitoring treatment of many respiratory diseases. Detailed discussion of all available techniques is beyond the scope of this text. On the other hand, there are some basics we should all be familiar with.

What is a spirometer? A spirometer is a device that measures respiratory excursions and air movement. Various devices are available, each generating different graphic patterns. We'll limit our discussion here to what is present on the "standard spirogram." **[FIGURE 4-7]** This device consists of a drum inverted in water with a tube extending from the air space in the drum to the patient's mouth. As the person breathes, the drum moves up and down, recording respiratory excursions. Parameters that may be determined from standard spirometry include lung volumes, lung capacities, and flow rates.

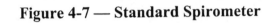

Figure 4-7 — Standard Spirometer

Inspiratory reserve volume				
Tidal volume	Inspiratory capacity	Vital capacity	Total lung capacity	
Expiratory reserve volume	Functional residual capacity			
Residual volume				

Figure 4-8 — Standard spirometry curve and values. Calculation of residual volume requires measurement of functional residual capacity by other means (body plethysmography, nitrogen washout).

There are four **pulmonary volumes**, all of which, added together, equal the maximum volume to which the lungs can be expanded: **[FIGURE 4-8]**

- **Tidal volume** (V_t) — the volume of air inspired or expired with each normal breath.
- **Inspiratory reserve volume** (IRV) — the extra volume that can be inspired above and beyond the normal tidal volume.
- **Expiratory reserve volume** (ERV) — the additional amount of air that can be expired by forceful expiration after the end of a normal tidal expiration.
- **Residual volume** (RV) — the volume of air remaining in the lungs after a maximum forced expiration.

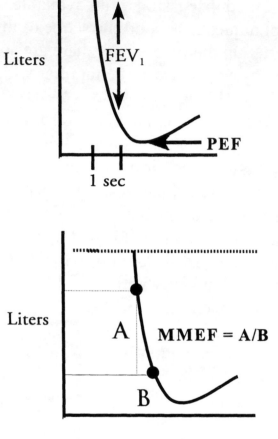

There are four **pulmonary capacities**, which are combinations of two or more lung volumes:

Figure 4-9 — Flow Rates

- **Inspiratory capacity** (IC) — the maximum amount of air a person can inhale at a normal expiratory level; $IC = V_t + IRV$.

- **Functional residual capacity** (FRC) — the amount of air remaining in the lungs at the end of normal expiration; $FRC = ERV + RV$.

- **Vital capacity** (VC) — the maximum amount of air a person can expel from the lungs after a maximum inspiration followed by maximum expiration; $VC = IRV + V_t + ERV$.

- **Total lung capacity** (TLC) — maximum volume to which the lungs can be expanded with maximum inspiratory effort; $TLC = VC + RV$.

During a forced expiration (as fast as possible), the shape of the spirometric curve changes. Based on the rate of change, certain flow rates have been defined: **[FIGURE 4-9]**

- **Forced expiratory volume in one second** (FEV_1) — the amount of air that can be expired in one second during a forced exhalation.

- **Mid-maximal expiratory flow** (MMEF) — the slope of the midportion of the expiratory flow curve during a maximal forced exhalation.

- **Peak expiratory flow** (PEF) — the fastest measured rate of air expulsion during a maximum forced exhalation.

In addition to the above volumes, capacities, and flow rates, several other terms are used commonly regarding pulmonary function:

- **Minute volume** — the total amount of new air that is moved into the respiratory passages each minute. Minute volume = tidal volume X respiratory rate (breaths per minute).

- **Alveolar ventilation** (sometimes called minute ventilation) — the rate at which new air reaches the gas exchange areas of the lungs. Understanding of alveolar ventilation requires us to discuss the concept of *dead space* . . . Then, I'll come back to the formulas we use.

What is dead space? Dead space air is air that fills the respiratory passages but never reaches the gas exchange areas. There are three types of dead space air:

- **Anatomic dead space** — air in the conducting airways (e.g., trachea, mainstem bronchi) that does not take part in gas exchange. This volume averages 150 ml in adults.

- **Alveolar dead space** — air in the gas exchange portions of the lung that cannot take part in gas exchange. In normal persons, the amount of alveolar dead space is negligible.

- **Physiological dead space** — the sum of anatomic and alveolar dead space (i.e., the total dead space air volume). As stated above, physiological dead space in normal individuals should be nearly the same as the anatomical dead space.

Now, back to alveolar ventilation. Remember that alveolar ventilation measures the amount of *new air* that enters the alveoli, it equals the respiratory rate times the amount of new air that enters the alveoli during each breath:

$$V_a = RR \times [V_T - V_D]$$

where V_a is the alveolar ventilation per minute, RR is the respiratory rate, V_T the tidal volume, and V_D the physiological dead space volume.

How do we use PFTs clinically? The most common use of PFTs is to differentiate obstructive from restrictive lung disease:

- Obstructive lung disease — any of a number of diseases whose net effect is obstruction to expiratory air flow. Common examples include asthma and COPD.

- Restrictive lung disease — any of a number of diseases that limit the ability of the lungs to expand, but expiratory flow is usually unaffected. Common examples include interstitial fibrosis of the lungs, severe spinal deformities, and neurologic lesions that impair the efficacy of the muscles of respiration.

The most commonly used diagnostic parameters are the vital capacity (VC) and forced expiratory volume in one second (FEV_1). Normals vary, depending upon sex and age and the results are often expressed as a percentage of predicted, as well as "raw scores." Sometimes, the ratio of FEV_1 to VC (FEV_1/VC ratio) is helpful. It should normally be greater than 75%.

Obstructive lung disease is characterized by increased resistance to air flow and high lung volumes. Greater radial traction on the airways at higher lung volumes due to loss of elastic recoil tend to increase their caliber and decrease resistance to airflow. In obstructive disease, the VC is often increased, but expiratory flow markedly depressed. So the expected findings are:

Obstructive Disease:

- **Increased VC.**
- **Decreased FEV_1.**
- **FEV_1/VC ratio less than 75%%.**

- Increased VC.
- Decreased FEV_1.
- FEV_1/VC ratio less than 75%.

Many laboratories also calculate the MMEF, derived from the midportion of the FEV_1 curve.

PRINCIPLE: **A normal test *doesn't* mean a normal patient!**

Decreases in the MMEF are far more sensitive to early obstructive lung disease than changes in the FEV_1.

In restrictive disease, flow rates are usually normal, but the lungs are unable to expand fully. And, it's easier for these patients to breath at low lung volumes, since they have difficulty expanding the lungs. We'd expect to find:

- Relatively normal FEV_1.
- Decreased VC.
- FEV_1/VC ratio greater than 75% of normal.

Some diseases exhibit both restrictive *and* obstructive components. We should never make a diagnosis based on a test alone.

Restrictive Disease:

- **Relatively normal FEV_1.**
- **Decreased VC.**
- **FEV_1/VC ratio greater than 75% of normal.**

Summary

Asthma is now known to be a chronic inflammatory condition with periodic exacerbations. Release and persistence of inflammatory mediators plays a pivotal role in the pathophysiology, as well as in our multi-pronged treatment approach. To date, steroids (both inhaled and oral), as well as leukotriene antagonists, have proven helpful. Recent data concerning the possible role of angiotensin II and AT_1 receptor blockers (sartans) in asthma appears promising.

PRINCIPLE: If "stuff" causes the problem, as long as the "stuff's" still around, there's still a problem!

PRINCIPLE: A multi-flanked attack is more effective than a one-pronged one.

Despite our incredible advances in understanding, the death rate from acute asthma continues to rise. The major reasons are *undermedication*, particularly with anti-inflammatory drugs (e.g., steroids), and *loss of the "early warning system" for dyspnea*. Many severe asthmatics are just not aware of how sick they really are until it's too late. Current research centers on identifying controllable factors in this "normal response system" as we attempt to reverse this deadly trend.

PRINCIPLE: Many diseases arise from *loss* of a normal response system (NRS) or *normal activation* of a NRS under *abnormal* circumstances, with untoward results.

Many of the newer therapeutic approaches to asthma also work in COPD. Unfortunately, there is still an occassional misunderstanding regarding the proper role for oxygen in patients with COPD. The bottom line is clear: "give patients the

PRINCIPLE: The *best* treatment for a hypoxic patient is *oxygen*!

amount of oxygen they need under the circumstances." Fears of giving "too much oxygen" and causing COPDer's to stop breathing are misguided. Even in CO_2 retainers, administration of oxygen has been shown to have a negligible effect on *minute ventilation*, even if the pCO_2 level does *rise*.

Arterial blood gases (ABGs) are very straightforward if you realize that they measure three separate, and only sometimes related, physiological processes:

1. **pH** — acid-base balance in the body.

2. **pCO$_2$** — measures ventilation; chemically, the partial pressure of CO_2 dissolved in the blood.

3. **pO2** — measures oxygenation; chemically, the partial pressure of O_2 dissolved in the blood.

By remembering a couple of basic principles, and asking only three questions, it's easy to identify the *major* underlying acid-base disorder, regardless of whether compensation or other processes are also present.

REMEMBER: For every 10 mg Hg increase or decrease in pCO$_2$, the pH moves 0.1 units in the *opposite* direction.

ASK ONLY THREE QUESTIONS:

1. Look at the pO$_2$. Is it low?

2. Look at the pH. Which way did it go; up (too high) or down (too low)?

3. Look at the pCO$_2$. Did the pCO$_2$ move in the *opposite* direction of the pH?

Crossword Puzzle Review

Path Chap 4 -- Respiratory

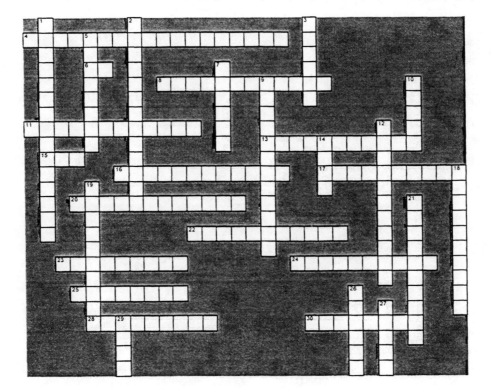

<table>
</table>

Across

4. Primary normal breathing stimulus.
6. Sum of all potentially competing and compensatory respiratory and metabolic acid-base processes.
8. _____ are produced from arachidonic acid, as are prostaglandins, but via a different pathway.
11. Blocks bronchoconstriction induced by cGMP.
13. During attacks, asthma patients suffer bronchospasm with variable degrees of _____ _____ (2 words).
15. Potential mediator during acute exacerbation of COPD.
16. Total amount of new air moved into the respiratory passages each minute.
17. Inhaled beta-sympathomimetic agents indicated only for chronic therapy.
20. Cyanosis appears when the amount of _____ hemoglobin is > 5 gm per 100 ml of blood.

22. Increase in sputum 2-3 days prior to an acute exacerbation.
23. Hyperventilation is a normal respiratory compensatory mechanism for _____ acidosis.
24. FEV1 is the amount of air that can be expired in one second during a forced _____.
25. Shifts of the oxyhemoglobin dissociation curve to the left _____ the affinity of hemoglobin for oxygen.
28. Peak expiratory flow is the fastest measured rate of air _____ during a maximum forced exhalation.
30. There is a big difference between _____ and normal.

Down

1. _____ (cholinergic) stimulation leads to the formation of arachidonic acid.
2. Maximum amount of air a person can expel from the lungs after a maximum inspiration followed by maximum expiration.

3. The best treatment for a hypoxic patient.
5. The pH and the pCO2 move in _____ directions.
7. In restrictive disease, flow rates are usually _____, but the lungs are unable to expand fully.
9. Underlying chronic state in obstructive lung disease.
10. Apparent "anxiety hyperventilators" have something _____ until proven otherwise.
12. Lower risk with inhaled steroids, but still present.
14. Despite advances, the death rate from asthma continues to _____.
18. Enzyme that produces leukotrienes from arachidonic acid.
19. Persons with near fatal asthma appear to have blunted perception of increased airflow _____.

19. Obstructive lung disease is characterized by increased _____ to air flow and high lung volumes.
21. Device that measures respiratory excursions and air movement.
26. Tidal volume is the volume of air inspired or expired with each normal _____.
27. Oxygen delivery to the tissues increases when the oxyhemoglobin dissociation curve shifts to the _____.
29. Respiratory acid level in the blood.

References

1.   Sly, RM, et al. *Asthma deaths falling in the United States*. Ann Allergy Asthma Immunol 2000; 85:121-7.

2.   Bousquet, J, et. al. *Eosinophilic inflammation in asthma*. NEJM, 1990; 323:1033-9.

3.   Kanazawa, H, et. al., *The role of free radicals in airway obstruction in asthmatic patients*. Chest 199; 100:1319-22.

4.   Niimi, AA, et al. *Airway remodeling seen in cough-variant asthma*. Lancet 2000; 356:564-5.

5.   Town, IG, et al. *Regular beta-agonists may not be helpful in asthma therapy*. Am J Respir Crit Care Med 2000; 161:1459-64.

6.   D'Alonzo, GE and Tolep, K. *Salmeterol: a long-acting beta 2-agonist*. J Am Osteopath Assoc 1998 Apr; 98(4):216-8, 221-31.

7.   Shrewsbury, SS, et al. *Salmeterol addition more effective than corticosteroid increase in asthma therapy*. BMJ 2000; 320:1368-73.

8.   McIvor RA, et al. *Potential masking effects of salmeterol on airway inflammation in asthma*. Am J Respir Crit Care Med 1998; 158:924-30.

9.   Ledford, D. *Osteoporosis in the corticosteroid-treated patient with asthma*. J Allergy Clin Immunol 1998; 102:353-62.

10.   Suissa, SS, et al. *Low-dose inhaled corticosteroids and the prevention of death from asthma*. N Engl J Med 2000; 343:332-6.

11.   Drazen, J. *Clinical pharmacology of leukotriene receptor antagonists and 5-lipoxygenase inhibitors*. Am J Respir Crit Care Med 1998 Jun; 157(6 Pt 2):S233-7.

12.   Löfdahl, CG, et al. *Randomised, placebo controlled trial of effect of a leukotriene receptor antagonist, montelukast, on tapering inhaled*

corticosteroids in asthmatic patients. BMJ 1999; 319:87-90.

13. Barnes, NJ, et al. *Zafirlukast reduces risk of asthma exacerbations.* Thorax 2000; 55:478-83.

14. Rodrigo, G, et al. *A meta-analysis of the effects of ipratropium bromide in adults with acute asthma.* Am J Med 1999 Oct; 107(4):363-70.

15. Milgrom, HA, et al. *Treatment of Allergic Asthma with Monoclonal Anti-IgE Antibody.* N Engl J Med 1999; 341:1966-73.

16. Warner, DO. *Asthma — Current Pathophysiology and Treatment.* Anesthes Clin N Am 1998; 16:1-60.

17. Marshall, RP, et al. *Angiotensin II is mitogenic for human lung fibroblasts via activation of the type 1 receptor.* Am J Respir Crit Care Med 2000; 161:1999-2004.

18. Myou, S, et al. *Type 1 angiotensin II receptor antagonism reduces antigen-induced airway reactions.* Am J Respir Crit Care Med 2000; 162:45-9.

19. Myou, S, et al. *Effect of lorsartan, a type 1 angiotensin II receptor antagonist, on bronchial hyperresponsiveness to mechacholine in patients with bronchial asthma.* Am J Respir Crit Care Med 2000; 162:40-4.

20. Spitzer, WO. *The use of β-agonists and the risk of death and near death from asthma.* N Engl J Med 1992; 326:501-6; Molfino, NA, et. al.. *The fatality-prone asthmatic patient: Follow-up study after near-fatal attacks.* Chest 1992; 101:621-3; Kikuchi, Y, et al. *Chemosensitivity and perception of dyspnea in patients with a history of near-fatal asthma.* N Engl J Med 1994; 330:1329-34.

21. Kifle, Y, et al. *Magnitude estimation of inspiratory resistive loads in children with life-threatening asthma.* Am J Respir Crit Care Med 1997; 156:1530-5.

22. Bijl-Hofland, ID. *Perception of respiratory sensation assessed by means of histamine challenge and threshold loading tests.* Chest 2000 Apr; 117(4): 954-9.

23. Rietveld, SS, et al. *Perceptions of asthma by adolescents at home.* Chest. 2000; 117:434-9.

24. Martin, RJ. *Assessment of the AirWatch lung function monitoring system.Asthma Clinical Research Network (ACRN).* J Allergy Clin Immunol 1999 Mar; 103(3 Pt 1): 535-6.

25. Finkelstein, JJ, et al. *Internet-based home asthma telemonitoring. Can patients handle the technology?* Chest. 2000; 117:148-155.

26. Ajatakanon, AA, et al. *Changes in sputum eosinophils predict loss of asthma control.* Am. J. Respir. Crit. Care Med. 2000; 161:64-72.

27. Eaton, TT, et al. *Routine aspergillosis screening worthwhile in asthmatics.* Chest 2000; 118:7-8, 66-72.

28. Balzano, G, et al. *Eosinophilic Inflammation in Stable Chronic Obstructive Pulmonary Disease Relationship with Neutrophils and Airway Function.* Am. J. Respir. Crit. Care Med. 1999; 160:1486-92; Barnes, PJ. *Novel approaches and targets for treatment of chronic obstructive pulmonary disease.* Am. J. Respir. Crit. Care Med. 1999; 160:S72-7.

29. Takabatake, NT, et al. *The relationship between chronic hypoxemia and activation of the tumor necrosis factor-system in patients with chronic obstructive pulmonary disease.* Am. J. Respir. Crit. Care Med. 2000; 161:1179-84.

30. Petty, TL. *Supportive therapy in COPD.* Chest 1998 Apr; 113(4 Suppl):256S-262S.

31. Hjalmarsen, A, et al. *Effect of long-term oxygen therapy on cognitive and neurological dysfunction in chronic obstructive pulmonary disease.* Eur Neurol 1999 Jul; 42(1):27-35; Stuss, DT, et al. *Chronic obstructive*

pulmonary disease: effects of hypoxia on neurological and neuropsychological measures. J Clin Exp Neuropsychol 1997 Aug; 19(4):515-24.

32. Crossley, DJ, et al. *Influence of inspired oxygen concentration on deadspace, respiratory drive, and PaCO₂ in intubated patients with chronic obstructive pulmonary disease.* Crit Care Med 1997 Sep; 25(9):1522-6.

33. Hanson, CW III, et al. *Causes of hypercarbia with oxygen therapy in patients with chronic obstructive pulmonary disease.* Crit Care Med 1996 Jan; 24(1):23-8; Similowski, T and Derenne, JP. *Relationship between hypercapnia and hypoxemia in chronic obstructive respiratory insufficiency.* Rev Mal Respir 1988; 5(4):373-80.

34. Erbland, ML, et al. *Interaction of hypoxia and hypercapnia on respiratory drive in patients with COPD.* Chest 1990 Jun; 97(6):1289-94.

35. Chien, JW, et al. *Uncontrolled oxygen administration and respiratory failure in acute asthma.* Chest. 2000; 117:728-33.

36. Callaham, M. *Hypoxic hazards of traditional paper bag rebreathing in hyperventilating patients.* Ann Emerg Med 1989 Jun; 18(6):622-8.

CHAPTER 5
NEUROLOGICAL PROBLEMS

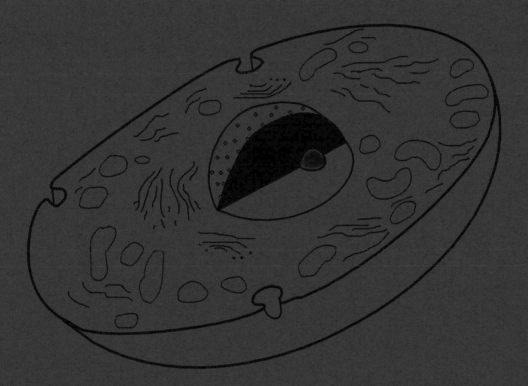

CHAPTER 5 — NEUROLOGICAL PROBLEMS

Contents

Objectives

After reading this chapter, you'll be able to:

- Defend the statement: "Seizures are the electrophysiologic equivalent of 'VF' of the brain." Include pharmacologic evidence to support your argument(s).
- Describe the mechanism by which benzodiazepines exert their effects during seizures.
- Explain and defend the statement: "Λ stroke is a brain attack; a TIA (transient ischemic attack) is 'unstable angina' of the brain."
- Describe the current and future role of thrombolytic therapy in stroke.
- Describe the "ischemic penumbra" in stroke.
- Summarize potential methods of "neuroprotection" after a stroke.

Introduction

From early in my training, I was always mystified and confused by the workings of the nervous system. Seemed as if neurophysiology was something for neurologists and neurosurgeons, not internists and emergency physicians. It finally hit me that I was wrong. Most of us are *very* comfortable with cardiovascular physiology (at least, when compared to neuro stuff). Once I realized that the two are extremely similar in many ways, neuro became significantly less threatening and

PRINCIPLES: There are far more *similarities* than *differences* among the body's cells and organs.

even became fun! I urge you to try and utilize this way of thinking also.

Two of the most common neurologic conditions facing the primary care provider are seizures and stroke. Both nicely illustrate "generic" principles of pathophysiology. Altered level of consciousness or "coma" may result from a variety of different situations. As such, it is really a symptom rather than a separate disease. For this reason, I have chosen not to discuss it as a separate section here.

Before we launch into specific conditions, let's review the basis for my suggestion that the underlying neuro and cardiac processes are similar. I presented the "heart-lung-brain" triad in Chapter 1 (p. 1-70). **[FIGURE 5-1]** Clinically, when one organ is affected, the others suffer as well. The same is true on a pathophysiological level; other than some name changes, the anatomic and molecular events in many cardiac and neurologic events (e.g., seizures, dysrhythmias, stroke, infarction) are similar.

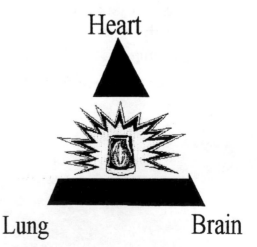

Figure 5-1 — The Heart-Lung-Brain Triad

Seizures

Seizures are sudden, paroxysmal episodes of exaggerated motor activity or abnormal behavior caused by excessive electrical discharge of cerebral neurons. Seizures recurring spontaneously over a span of years are termed **epilepsy.** Up to 5.9% of the population will experience at least one non-febrile seizure at some stage of life. Seventy-five percent of patients with epilepsy have their first seizure before 20 years of age.[1]

Pathophysiology of a generalized seizure: For the purposes of this discussion, we'll limit ourselves to generalized ("grand mal") seizures. The steps leading to a generalized seizure are: **[FIGURE 5-2]**

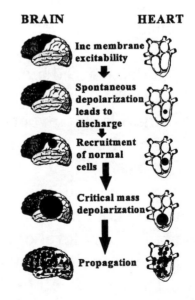

1. Increased cell membrane excitability (for any of a number of reasons) results in hypersensitive neurons.

2. Hypersensitive neurons spontaneously depolarize, leading to neuronal discharge.

3. Surrounding normal neurons are "recruited" until a "critical mass" of brain tissue has depolarized.

4. The seizure discharge then propagates throughout the brain, resulting in a generalized tonic-clonic motor seizure.

REMEMBER: Great minds and hearts fibrillate alike!

Seizures may terminate for a variety of natural causes including exhaustion of neuronal energy sources, depletion of excitatory transmitters, release of inhibitor substances, or failure of oxidative metabolism.

Doesn't this all sound familiar?
Sure does, because the above description of the pathophysiology of a generalized seizure in the brain is nearly identical to that of ventricular fibrillation (VF) of the heart. The only differences are name changes to protect the "innocent." In fact, the "critical mass" of depolarized brain tissue is identical to the concept of a "critical mass of fibrillating myocardium" required for the propagation of VF.

Once I realized that generalized seizures are nothing more than "VF of the brain," my level of comfort with neurophysiology got a lot better. Though I won't explore it in detail, it turns out that the molecular events (e.g., ion channel activity) are also very similar.[2]

PATHOPHYSIOLOGY OF VF:

- **Increased membrane excitability results in hypersensitive cardiac cells (myocytes).**

- **Hypersensitive myocytes spontaneously depolarize.**

- **Surrounding normal myocytes are "recruited" until a "critical mass" of myocardium has depolarized.**

- **The discharge then propagates throughout the heart, resulting in VF.**

SEIZURES

DEFINITION	COMMON CAUSES	HISTORY (SYMPTOMS)	PHYSICAL (SIGNS)	"TESTS"	TREATMENT
Sudden, paroxysmal episode of exaggerated motor activity caused by excessive electrical discharge of cerebral neurons	*NON-CNS ORIGIN:* metabolic, drug/alcohol withdrawal/OD organ related (liver/kidney failure); *CNS ORIGIN:* infection, fever, epilepsy, trauma, stroke, tumor	"Seizure FACTS": Focus, Activity, Color, Time; Secondary information (what was patient doing before, aura, incontinence, bite mouth or tongue, hit head, previous history, etc.); COCAINE??	Post-ictal state; loss of urine/feces, skin signs, spinal tenderness, neurological examination; Complete return to normal preictal cerebral function can take up to two hours	ABGs, CBC, electrolytes, glucose, renal function tests, Ca++, Mg ++, toxicology screen, anticonvulsant blood levels	"Four fixes"; benzodiazepine, phenytoin or derivatives, phenobarbital, lidocaine, general anesthesia

How do benzodiazepines stop seizures?

The benzodiazepine (BD) drugs (e.g., diazepam [Valium®]) all have a common mechanism of action. They bind a receptor in the brain that is near grouped cells (the GABA nucleus) that produce gamma aminobutyric acid (GABA), an inhibitory neurotransmitter. BDs stimulate the release of GABA by the GABA nucleus, providing a generalized CNS depressant effect. GABA has no intrinsic anti-seizure (membrane-stabilizing) activity. [**FIGURE 5-3**]

Though the role of GABA in seizure inhibition, as well as in other disease states (e.g., delirium tremens) is well-established, "designer" versions of GABA stimulants have been abused as "date rape" drugs and intoxicants. For this reason, commercial preparations are unlikely to become available anytime soon.

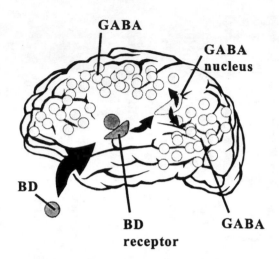

Figure 5-3 — BDs bind their brain receptor; this causes release of GABA from the GABA nucleus. GABA acts as a nonspecific inhibitory neurotransmitter and suppresses the seizure.

Why don't BD's always work in status epilepticus?

BDs often suppress ongoing seizure activity. Depending on the half-life of the drug, they may effectively prevent seizure recurrence over the next few hours as well. BDs are not always effective, by themselves, particularly in status epilepticus.

The mechanisms that determine progression of a single seizure to status epilepticus are uncertain. However, two general concepts of the

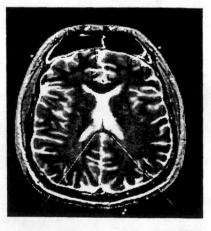

Figure 5-4 — White lines indicate vicinity of the hippocampus.

pathophysiology of status epilepticus are known and seem to provide potential answers to our question:

1.   The hippocampus (an elevation of the floor of the lateral ventricle) **[FIGURE 5-4]** is consistently activated during status epilepticus.

2.   Loss of GABA-mediated inhibitory synaptic transmission ("GABAnergic receptor inhibition") in the hippocampus is critical for emergence of status epilepticus.

If *reduction* in GABAnergic receptor inhibition leads to development of status epilepticus, *enhancement* of GABAnergic inhibition would be expected to interrupt status epilepticus, agreed? Both benzodiazepines and barbiturates bind the "BD" receptor, leading to release of GABA from the "GABA nucleus." The result — enhancement of GABAnergic inhibition. However, patients often become refractory to benzodiazepines when seizures are prolonged. Then, barbiturates are used.

> *PRINCIPLE*: **If lack of "stuff" contributes to the problem, give 'em back the necessary "stuff" to improve things!**

Recent evidence suggests the presence of multiple BD receptor subtypes ("isoforms") in the hippocampus with *different* sensitivity to benzodiazepines but *similar* sensitivity to barbiturates. This exciting finding explains why the two drug classes might have different clinical effects.

It's all plastic to me! In addition, rapid functional **plasticity** (the ability to alter its functional properties "on the fly") of BD receptors has been demonstrated to occur during status epilepticus in animal studies. The animals lost substantial sensitivity to diazepam during status epilepticus. An alteration in the functional properties of hippocampal BD accompanied the sensitivity loss. Receptors develop *reduced*

> *REMEMBER*: **Neuronal plasticity is the ability of a cell to alter its functional properties "on the fly."**

sensitivity to diazepam but retain *normal* sensitivity to pentobarbital. Therefore, the prolonged seizures of status epilepticus rapidly alter the functional properties of hippocampal BD receptors, possibly explaining why benzodiazepines and barbiturates may not be equally effective during treatment of the prolonged seizures of status epilepticus.[3]

Reasons for receptor plasticity during status epilepticus are unknown. Some data suggest that the receptor transiently loses its normal inhibition by zinc.[4] Glutamate is also believed to play a role, and the therapeutic value of glutamate receptor antagonists is being actively investigated.[5] Animal data suggests that at least some of these changes may be permanent, perhaps due to the production of an abnormal protein (serum response factor).[6] This finding may explain the clinical tendency of patients to be *more* likely to have status epilepticus in the future after their first episode. **[FIGURE 5-5]** Glutamate is also believed to play a role in post-stroke ischemic neuronal damage.

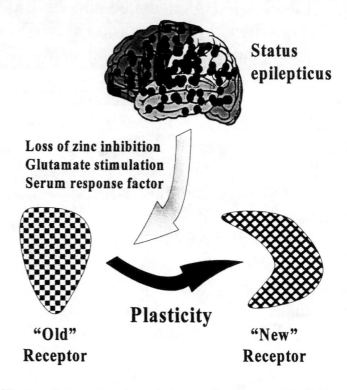

Figure 5-5 — During status epilepticus, plasticity causes functional changes in the BD receptor that affect the ability of BD's, but not barbiturates, to bind.

[**Note:** *The use of the term "BD receptors" is somewhat creative on my part. These are actually called GABA(A) receptors and are physically linked to the "GABA nucleus." I think it's easier to understand the drugs' mechanism of action by taking "poetic license" with the term. The concept is far more important here than neuroanatomical terms. The concept that benzodiazepines or barbiturates bind a receptor that causes release of GABA is correct.*]

What about "true" anti-seizure medications? Since the BDs have no intrinsic long-term anti-seizure activity, other drugs are necessary in the prevention of further seizures or to stop status epilepticus. Over the years, the two most popular agents have been phenytoin (Dilantin®) and phenobarbital. Recently, intravenous phenytoin has been supplanted by fosphenytoin (Cerebyx®) in many areas. Lidocaine, though potentially epileptogenic by itself, has also proven helpful in status epilepticus.[7] **[FIGURE 5-6]**

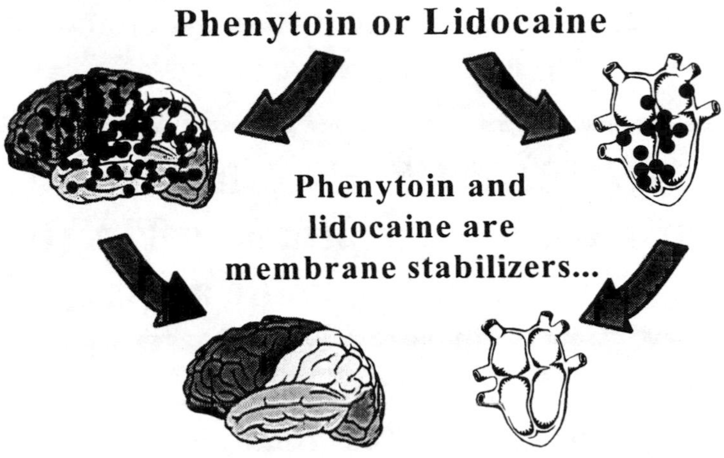

Phenytoin or Lidocaine

Phenytoin and lidocaine are membrane stabilizers...

Figure 5-6 — Both lidocaine and phenytoin are membrane stabilizing agents.

The most interesting fact about phenytoin and lidocaine is that they are also cardiac anti-dysrhythmics. They have membrane-stabilizing actions — since the underlying pathophysiology of "VF of the brain" and "VF of the heart" is similar, it makes sense that they should work for both. In fact, I suspect that newer cardiac agents such as amiodarone[8] may also find their way into the treatment of status epilepticus, based on the same logic.

Stroke

Stroke is a cerebral ischemic syndrome resulting from disruption of the cerebral circulation with a subsequent loss of neurologic function. Eighty-five percent are of vascular origin; of these, 85% are occlusive (2/3 thrombotic, 1/3 embolic) and 15% hemorrhagic. Nonvascular causes of stroke include seizures, tumors, demyelination syndromes, and psychogenic causes.

OBJECTIVE: **Explain and defend the statement: "A stroke is a brain attack; a TIA (transient ischemic attack) is 'unstable angina' of the brain."**

The "heart analogy" continues. Similarity makes learning easier, and there is not only a metaphorical likeness between "heart attack" and "brain attack," but a scientific one as well:

1. The "final event" in both stroke and MI involves, in many cases, total occlusion of an already-narrowed atherosclerotic artery by a blood clot. There is increasing evidence that atherosclerosis is a chronic inflammatory disorder resulting from a combination of processes, and that acute exacerbations of this inflammation are associated with the acute coronary syndromes such as myocardial infarction and unstable angina. Studies have shown that higher serum acute phase protein levels, such as C-reactive protein and serum amyloid A protein, are associated with increased risk of myocardial infarction (MI), stroke, or peripheral vascular disease, and predict risk of infarction and death among high-risk patients.[9]

PRINCIPLE: **By concentrating on** *similarities* **rather than** *differences*, **you only need to learn the underlying "principles" once. The rest involves** *applying* **the principle** *with understanding* **to various diseases.**

2. Whether or not plaque inflammation plays as pivotal a role in stroke as in MI is unknown.[10] Current data, however, are compatible with an inflammatory etiology. Inflammatory mediators are released following stroke, and levels are higher in persons with a history of stroke.[11]

> **REMEMBER: The underlying pathophysiology of thrombotic stroke and myocardial infarction is very similar.**

3. Embolic stroke is far more common than is embolic myocardial infarction. In stroke, the blood clot is less likely to represent an *in situ* thrombus than in MI.

4. Regardless of the origin (embolic or thrombotic), dissolution of the clot will likely improve cerebral flow (or myocardial flow in MI).

The bottom line. So, it is reasonable to state: "A stroke is a brain attack; a transient ischemic attack (TIA) is 'unstable angina' of the brain." These statements hold true both in treatment (e.g., thrombolytic therapy, anti-platelet agents) and in prioritization of patient care — persons with "unstable angina" (or unstable myocardial ischemic syndrome, as the new name goes)

> **REMEMBER: A stroke is a brain attack; a transient ischemic attack (TIA) is 'unstable angina' of the brain.**

are at a risk for development of MI and life-threatening dysrhythmias. Similarly, persons with TIAs are at risk for a full-blown stroke.

OBJECTIVE: Describe the current and future role of thrombolytic therapy in stroke.

Thrombolytic therapy in stroke — Various intra-arterial and intravenous agents, especially tissue plasminogen activator (tPA), have been used to treat acute thrombotic stroke in selected patients for several years. The basis for clot dissolution is the same as in acute MI — improve brain oxygenation as soon as possible. Unfortunately, the data in stroke look less promising than in MI. Only a very small percentage of persons with thrombotic stroke receive thrombolytic therapy:[12]

1. The time frame from symptom onset to recommended tPA administration is shorterthan in myocardial infarction; the *maximum* in most institutions is three hours. Clinical trials using new MRI techniques to screen patients may be able to identify a subset of acute stroke patients who are ideal candidates for thrombolytic therapy even beyond three hours after stroke onset.[13]

2. Current data suggest that tPA administered from three to five hours following the onset of stroke has no significant effect on clinical outcome at 90 days, and increases the risk of intracranial hemorrhage significantly.[14]

> **REMEMBER: Even under ideal circumstances, many persons with thrombotic stroke won't receive reperfusion therapy.**

3. The majority of potentially-qualifying patients (thrombotic stroke) present too late (mean time = 5.7 hours after onset of symptoms) to benefit from tPA.[15]

4. Even of the 20% of stroke patients who reach the hospital *within* that three-hour window, few ultimately receive tPA. Reasons for this are unclear, but include patients' preconceived attitudes and lack of sufficient health care provider education.[16]

Of those stroke victims who *do* receive thrombolytic therapy, most see significant improvement in their outcome, provided the time-frame criteria are met.[17] One recent study, however, suggested that tPA offered no significant benefit, even when administered within the appropriate time frame. In addition, the drug led to a marked increase in intracranial hemorrhage.[18]

Intra-arterial administration of a newer, experimental agent, prourokinase, may extend the stroke treatment window to six hours. A recent study showed significantly improved clinical outcome at 90 days, in spite of an increased frequency of symptomatic intracranial hemorrhage.[19]

Late presentation occurs *notwithstanding* widespread educational efforts, both to the public and to health care professionals (e.g., "Code Stroke" programs). Though frustrating, delayed patient awareness of symptoms is likely when we consider the "natural history" of thrombotic stroke:

- Patients go to sleep feeling fine.

- They wake up with completed or nearly-completed stroke in the morning.

> **REMEMBER**: The natural history of thrombotic stroke is that the patient goes to sleep and wakes up in the morning with a neurological deficit. The time of onset of the stroke *must* be assumed to be bedtime.

- If the patient awakens with the deficit, the clinician *must* assume the time of onset to be the last time the patient was awake and normal. Similarly, if the patient is aphasic or otherwise unable to report the time of onset, and there are no witnesses, the patient should not be treated.[20]

Unless newer thrombolytic agents with an extended window of safety are discovered, or we invent some type of "nocturnal stroke detector," I don't see that the use of thrombolytics in acute stroke will become as widespread as in acute MI. Does this mean that all our "early identification" efforts are wasted? I think not.

Why we still ***need early identification of stroke victims.*** Even if only a small percentage of stroke patients will qualify for thrombolytics, efforts at earlier identification still hold great promise. The reason — production of "stuff" by ischemic brain tissue.

Remember when cerebral resuscitation studies in cardiac arrest were the "talk of the town?" We knew that it was far easier to get back a perfusing cardiac rhythm than a functioning brain. Though few clinically practical techniques evolved, scientific study revealed:

REMEMBER: In MI, "time is muscle." Similarly, in stroke, "time is brain."

- Even after restoration of normal cardiac flow, the brain suffers damage.

- The degree of damage suffered reflects the total "global" ischemic time (since cardiac arrest).

- During the period of total cerebral ischemia, as well as following reperfusion, a set of chemical reactions takes place leading to the formation of free radicals, leukotrienes, and other mediators ("stuff"). Calcium is also involved in the cascade.

Unfortunately, attempts to block free radicals or calcium led to little clinical success in terms of improved post-resuscitation neurological function. Other than occasionally trying head or total body hypothermia during

---

***PRINCIPLE*: If "stuff" (e.g., free radicals) causes the problem, the longer it's around, the worse the problem!**

---

resuscitation, most research *and* clinical efforts refocused on early defibrillation and the principle that "You can't save the brain if you don't save the heart first!"

The ischemic penumbra — As in acute MI, a peri-stroke (peri-infarct) zone of severely hypoperfused, nonfunctional, but still viable cortex surrounds the irreversibly damaged ischemic core. This has been referred to as the **ischemic**

REMEMBER: Our mission is to "save the penumbra!"

penumbra (though the concept is *far* more important than the name). With elapsing time, more penumbra becomes irreversibly damaged and gets "added" into the ischemic core. Tissue reperfusion may halt this deleterious process until a certain point in time. **[FIGURE 5-7]**

The existence of the penumbra has been known in experimental animals for a long time. Recent positron emission tomography (PET) studies performed in humans 5 to 18 hours after stroke onset have documented the existence of penumbra tissue in about one third of the cases. Potentially viable penumbral tissue has been detected as late as 16 hours after symptom onset in occasional patients, suggesting the therapeutic window may be

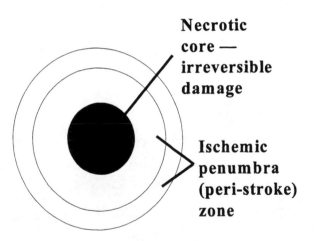

Necrotic core — irreversible damage

Ischemic penumbra (peri-stroke) zone

Figure 5-7 — The Ischemic Penumbra

longer than thought. Long-term neurological recovery is proportional to the volume of penumbra that eventually escapes infarction. The penumbral region is potentially salvageable, and is therefore the *ultimate* target of therapy for acute stroke. Thus, many of our current efforts are directed toward saving the penumbra.[21]

What factors determine the extent of the penumbra (peri-stroke) zone? The ischemic cascade starts within seconds to minutes of loss of perfusion. As we've said, obstruction of a blood vessel creates a central area of irreversible infarction ("ischemic core") and a surrounding area of potentially reversible ischemic penumbra ("peri-stroke zone"). During the hours to days after a stroke, the ischemic territory activates specific

---

PRINCIPLE: "Bad stuff" begets more "bad stuff."

---

genes. These cause the formation of cytokines and cell adhesion molecules that stimulate local inflammation and may further impair blood flow in the microcirculation. Finally, apoptotic gene ("self-destruct" genes) activation promotes programmed cell death in the population of surviving neurons. Without timely intervention, the entire ischemic penumbra eventually succumbs to these progressive insults and becomes part of the infarct core. **[FIGURE 5-8]**

Apoptosis may be a major mechanism of neuronal loss during stroke.[22] Experimental work currently centers on drugs that inhibit the release of caspases, self-destruct enzymes released during apoptotic cell death.[23]

In human beings, the presence of an ischemic penumbra may be detected through the use of positron emission tomography and the magnetic resonance techniques of diffusion- and perfusion-weighted imaging.[24] These techniques demonstrate that in most cases the penumbra merges with the infarct core within several hours of the onset of stroke.[25]

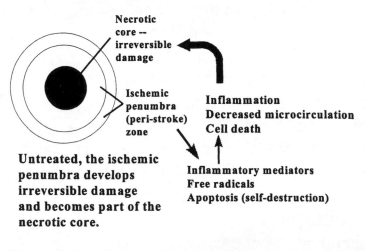

Figure 5-8 — Factors that determine the size of the ischemic penumbra.

On the basis of current understanding of the ischemic cascade and the evolving penumbra, it appears that acute intervention must occur very early for a substantial portion of brain tissue to be preserved. The time window, if any, in which to alter the course of the ischemic cascade remains less well defined than that for thrombolytic therapy, but it is also presumed to be relatively brief.[26]

> ## OBJECTIVE: Summarize potential methods of "neuroprotection" after a stroke.

The concept of neuroprotection in stroke. Along with increased interest in reperfusion therapy in stroke came the awareness than many patients would never qualify — whether due to time frame limitations or because they had had a hemorrhagic stroke. Researchers again turned to alternative therapeutic approaches,

PRINCIPLE: If "stuff" leads to problems, give "anti-stuff" to stop the formation of "stuff," block its action, or both...

based on some of the older post-cardiac arrest work noted above. As it turns out, a similar cascade of events takes place during stroke (see *The Ischemic Penumbra*, above). "Stuff" is produced, including free radicals and inflammatory mediators. Prior to these revealing studies, brain tissue was not believed to produce cytokines and other inflammatory mediators.

More on the inflammatory cascade after acute stroke. It is now well established that brain cells can produce cytokines and chemokines, and can express adhesion molecules that enable a localized inflammatory reaction. The accumulation of neutrophils early after brain injury is also believed to contribute to brain tissue loss.[27] Clinically, simple measurements of inflammation, such as the ESR (erythrocyte

REMEMBER: Inflammation and mediator production is present in acute stroke, as well as in chronic atherosclerosis of cerebral (and all other) blood vessels.

sedimentation rate), have been shown to provide meaningful prognostic information.[28] As with any other "bad stuff," the longer it persists, the more damage it can cause. Therefore, administration of either "stuff blockers" or "anti-stuff" as soon as possible makes sense, yes? So, even in persons who are not thrombolytic therapy candidates, earlier identification would lead to earlier treatment with "stuff blockers" — *if* they were available!

So, what "stuff blockers" are available for stroke patients? At this point, there are *no* commercially-available neuroprotective agents. Current research centers around:[29]

Drug	Proposed Mechanism of Neuroprotection	Time Window
Nimodipine	Calcium channel blocker	<12 hours
Lubeluzole	Inhibitor of glutamate release and glutamate toxicity	<6-8 hours
Cerestat	Glutamate (NMDA) receptor antagonist	<6 hours
Cervene	Opiate antagonist, indirect glutamate antagonist	<6 hours
Fosphenytoin	Ion channel blocker, indirect glutamate antagonist	<6 hours
Tirilazad	Free-radical scavenger	<6 hours
Enlimomab	Inhibitor of cellular adhesion molecules	<6 hours
Citicoline	Free-radical scavenger, membrane stabilization	<24 hours

Investigators have also evaluated gangliosides[30] (components of the neural membrane) and aminophylline.[31] On balance, neither currently appears promising. Promising animal work includes:

- Limited data suggest a neuroprotective role of both caffeine and pentoxifylline during experimental cerebral ischemia.[32]

- Animal studies have demonstrated that hypothermia improves the post-stroke outcome.[33]

- Propofol (Diprovan®) increases excitatory amino acid uptake in astrocytes in vitro. This may decrease formation of glutamate, a substance thought critical to further cerebral damage.[34] Similar results have been noted for the inhalational anesthetic isoflurane.[35]

- Blockade of central angiotensin II receptors (AT_1 receptors) — the selective AT_1 receptor antagonist irbesartan was infused intracerebroventricularly over a 5-day period before the induction of ischemia, at a dose that inhibited brain but not vascular AT_1 receptors. There was a significant effect on animal outcome.[36]

- Several lines of evidence indicate that estrogen therapy may be of neuroprotective benefit in animals, but this has not yet been studied in humans.[37] Progesterone also appears to be of benefit in rat models.[38]

  NOTE: Several currently available drugs (e.g., estrogen) have shown excellent results in animal neuroprotection studies. Off-label use in humans may not be far away.

- The antihypertensive agent diazoxide opens potassium channels in mitochondria and has been used successfully as a neuroprotectant in pig models of stroke.[39]

Despite wide discrepancies between these animal models and human stroke, the most promising aspect is that most of these agents are currently available commercially for other purposes. Thus, off-label use (using a drug without an "official" FDA indication), which is relatively common with many drugs, may lead to early human studies if the animal work pans out.

What do the latest human data show? Human data suggest that sublingual administration of glycine (an inhibitory neurotransmitter precursor) led to short-term clinical improvement.[40] On the other hand, administration of the calcium channel blocker nimodipine seems to offer no significant benefit when given after human stroke.[41]

In randomized trials of middle-aged patients with coronary artery disease, the cholesterol-lowering statins reduced the incidence of stroke. Statins also reduced the size of cerebral infarction in a murine stroke model, suggesting a neuroprotective effect. Pravastatin reduces the risk of stroke in patients with coronary artery disease and average cholesterol levels; simvastatin reduces the risk of the combined endpoint of stroke and transient ischemic attack in hypercholesterolemic patients with coronary artery disease.[42] Human data have also shown that aspirin, 160 to 300 mg per day for four weeks after stroke, markedly decreases the incidence of in-hospital relapse or extension.[43] Many experts urge early use of aspirin in nonhemorrhagic stroke, especially in persons who do not receive thrombolytic therapy. This is not, however, considered a standard of care at this time.

The **TABLES** below summarize other aspects of cerebral ischemic syndromes:

THROMBOTIC CEREBRAL ISCHEMIC SYNDROMES — 1

TRANSIENT ISCHEMIC ATTACK (TIA)	REVERSIBLE ISCHEMIC NEUROLOGIC DEFICIT (RIND)
Episode of neurologic impairment, attributed to focal cerebral ischemia, that resolves completely within 24 h. Patients with TIAs face an annual risk of permanent stroke damage or death of approximately 10%; > 50% of the strokes that follow a TIA occur within the first year, and more than 20% occur within the first month. TIAs lasting over 1 to 2 hours also place that subset of patients at higher risk of stroke.	Focal cerebral ischemic event lasting longer than 24 hours. Complete resolution usually requires 1 to 3 days and always occurs before 3 to 4 weeks; initially clinically indistinguishable from a completed stroke, but the prognosis and underlying structural lesions have been shown to resemble more closely the TIA. Can be caused by both thrombotic and embolic events.

THROMBOTIC CEREBRAL ISCHEMIC SYNDROMES — 2

PROGRESSING THROMBOTIC STROKE	COMPLETED THROMBOTIC STROKE
Focal neurologic impairment attributed to thrombosis in an artery serving the brain, and exhibiting a stepwise worsening of the neurologic deficit over minutes, hours, or days following presentation. Up to 40% of patients with thrombotic stroke may exhibit such progression. The deficit persists, by definition, greater than 3 weeks.	Stable (for at least 24 h) focal neurologic impairment attributed to thrombosis in an artery serving the brain. The deficit persists, by definition, greater than 3 weeks.

OTHER CEREBRAL ISCHEMIC SYNDROMES

CARDIOGENIC BRAIN EMBOLUS	HEMORRHAGIC SYNDROMES
Focal neurologic deficit attributed to an embolism originating from the heart. The deficit persists, by definition, greater than 3 weeks.	15% of strokes; intracerebral hemorrhage, intracerebellar hemorrhage, subarachnoid hemorrhage, subdural/epidural hemorrhage.

CAUSES OF CEREBRAL ISCHEMIC SYNDROMES

OCCLUSIVE	HEMORRHAGIC
Thrombosis = 2/3 of events (atherosclerosis, hypertension, or both); emboli = 1/3 of events (atrial fibrillation, mural thrombus, carotid artery); about 1 stroke in 6 is cardioembolic in nature.	Hypertension, aneurysm or vascular malformation rupture, trauma (46% of post-traumatic bleeds present more than 24 hours after the inciting event); oral anticoagulants and amphetamines (vasculitis) can also cause; alcohol/cigarettes markedly increase the risk, especially in previously hypertensive individuals.

Summary

Understanding various neurological problems, especially seizure and stroke, is far easier when we realize the striking similarities to the heart. The molecular pathophysiology of a generalized seizure is nearly *identical* to that of the heart during ventricular fibrillation. And, excluding electrical therapy, so is much of the treatment (e.g., membrane stabilizing drugs such as phenytoin or lidocaine). This knowledge will likely lead to even more cross-research between anti-arrhythmic and anti-seizure drugs, such as amiodarone.

PRINCIPLES: There are far more *similarities* than *differences* among the body's cells and organs.

Under the same principles, a stroke is really just a "heart attack of the brain," or a "brain attack." And, a transient ischemic attack carries the same implications for the nervous system (and the patient's life) as does any unstable myocardial ischemic syndrome for the heart (e.g., "unstable angina"). The similarity continues with regard to thrombolytic therapy, though with current thrombolytic agents, few stroke patients qualify. However, our understanding of reperfusion injury should soon lead to clinically available neuroprotective drugs, lending support to our ongoing educational efforts to improve stroke awareness.

PRINCIPLE: If "stuff" leads to problems, give "anti-stuff" to stop the formation of "stuff," block its action, or both.

Crossword Puzzle Review

Path Chap 5 -- Neuro

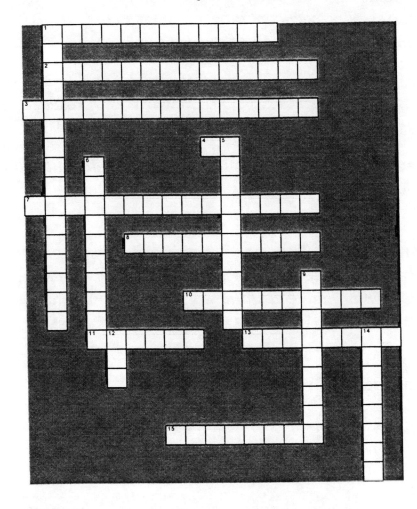

Across

1. Underlying lesion in cerebrovascular disease.
2. Neurophysiology is very similar to that of the _____ system.
3. Stop seizures by causing release of GABA.
4. The pathophysiology of a seizure in the brain is nearly identical to that of _____ (abbrev) of the heart.
7. Why we still need early identification of stroke victims.
8. GABA is an _____ neurotransmitter.
10. Reason patients with seizures become refractory to benzodiazepines.
11. Cerebral ischemic syndrome resulting from disruption of the cerebral circulation.
13. Seizures recurring spontaneously over a span of years.
15. Both lidocaine and phenytoin have _____-stabilizing actions.

Down

1. The "peri-stroke" zone.
5. Neuronal plasticity is the ability of a cell to alter its _____ properties "on the fly."
6. Usual upper limit "window of opportunity" for thrombolytic therapy in stroke.
9. The majority of vascular strokes are _____ in nature.
12. "Unstable angina of the brain" (abbrev).
14. sudden, paroxysmal episodes caused by excessive electrical discharge of cerebral neurons.

References

1. Hopkins, A, et al. *The first seizure in adult life. Value of clinical features, electroencephalography, and computerised tomographic scanning in prediction of seizure recurrence.* Lancet 1988 Apr 2; 1(8588):721-6.

2. Delgado-Escueta, AV, et al. *New waves of research in the epilepsies: crossing into the third millennium.* Adv Neurol 1999; 79:3-58.

3. Macdonald, RL and Kapur, J. *Acute cellular alterations in the hippocampus after status epilepticus.* Epilepsia 1999; 40 Suppl 1:S9-20.

4. Banerjee, PK, et al. *Zinc inhibition of gamma-aminobutyric acid(A) receptor function is decreased in the cerebral cortex during pilocarpine-induced status epilepticus.* J Pharmacol Exp Ther 1999 Oct; 291(1):361-6.

5. Sahai, S. *Glutamate in the mammalian CNS.* Eur Arch Psychiatry Clin Neurosci 1990; 240(2):121-33.

6. Morris, TA, et al. *Persistent increased DNA-binding and expression of serum response factor occur with epilepsy-associated long-term plasticity changes.* J Neurosci 1999 Oct 1; 19(19):8234-43.

7. Walker, IA and Slovis, CM. *Lidocaine in the treatment of status epilepticus.* Acad Emerg Med 1997 Sep; 4(9):918-22.

8. Kudenchuk, PJ, et al. *Amiodarone for resuscitation after out-of-hospital cardiac arrest due to ventricular fibrillation.* N Engl J Med 1999; 341:871-8.

9. Whicher, J, et al. *Inflammation, the acute phase response and atherosclerosis.* Clin Chem Lab Med 1999 May; 37(5):495-503.

10. Glader, CA, et al. *Chlamydia pneumoniae antibodies and high lipoprotein(a) levels do not predict ischemic cerebral infarctions.* Stroke 1999; 30:2033-37.

11. Hallenbeck JM. *Cytokines, macrophages, and leukocytes in brain ischemia.* Neurology 1997; 49(suppl 4):S5-9; Clark, WM. *Cytokines and reperfusion injury.* Neurology 1997; 49(suppl 4):S10-14.

12. Casetta, I, et al. *Temporal trend and factors associated with delayed hospital admission of stroke patients.* Neuroepidemiology 1999; 18(5):255-64.

13. Albers, GW. *Expanding the window for thrombolytic therapy in acute stroke : the potential role of acute mri for patient selection.* Stroke 1999 Oct; 30(10):2230-37.

14. Clark, WM, et al. *Recombinant tissue-type plasminogen activator (alteplase) for ischemic stroke 3 to 5 hours after symptom onset. The ATLANTIS study: a randomized controlled trial.* JAMA. 1999; 282:2019-26.

15. O'Connor, RE, et al. *Thrombolytic therapy for acute ischemic stroke: why the majority of patients remain ineligible for treatment.* Ann Emerg Med 1999 Jan; 33(1):9-14; Kothari, R, et al. *Acute stroke: delays to presentation and emergency department evaluation.* Ann Emerg Med 1999 Jan; 33(1):3-8; Hacke, W, et al. *Thrombolysis in acute ischemic stroke: controlled trials and clinical experience.* Neurology 1999; 53(7 Suppl 4):S3-14.

16. Furlan, AJ. *Acute ischemic stroke: new strategies for management and prevention.* Geriatrics 1999 Aug; 54(8):47-52.

17. Osborn, TM, et al. *Intravenous thrombolytic therapy for stroke: a review of recent studies and controversies.* Ann Emerg Med 1999 Aug; 34(2):244-55; Albers, GW, et al. *Intravenous tissue-type plasminogen activator for treatment of acute stroke. The standard treatment with*

alteplase to reverse stroke (STARS) study. JAMA 2000; 283:1145-1150.

18. Katzan, IL, et al. *Use of tissue-type plasminogen activator for acute ischemic stroke. The Cleveland area experience.* JAMA. 2000; 283:1151-58.

19. Furlan, A, et al. *Intra-arterial prourokinase for acute ischemic stroke. The PROACT II study: a randomized controlled trial.* JAMA. 1999; 282:2003-2011.

20. Kasner, SE. *Emergency identification and treatment of acute ischemic stroke.* Ann Emerg Med 1997 Nov; 30(5): 642-53.

21. Baron, J. *Mapping the ischaemic penumbra with PET: implications for acute stroke treatment.* Cerebrovasc Dis 1999 Jul-Aug; 9(4):193-201.

22. Cohen GM. *Caspases: The executioners of apoptosis.* Biochem J 1997; 1:326.

23. Robertson, GS. *Neuroprotection by the inhibition of apoptosis.* Brain Pathol 2000 Apr; 10(2): 283-92; Fink, KB. *Reduction of post-traumatic brain injury and free radical production by inhibition of the caspase-1 cascade.* Neuroscience 1999; 94(4):1213-8.

24. Read, SJ. *Identifying hypoxic tissue after acute ischemic stroke using PET and 18F-fluoromisonidazole.* Neurology 1998 Dec; 51(6):1617-21.

25. Marks, MP. *Evaluation of early reperfusion and i.v. tPA therapy using diffusion- and perfusion-weighted MRI.* Neurology 1999 Jun 10; 52(9): 1792-8.

26. Hossman, KA. *Viability thresholds and the penumbra of focal ischemia.* Ann Neurol 1994; 36: 557-65; Fisher M and Garcia JH. *Evolving stroke and the ischemic penumbra.* Neurology 1996; 47:884-8; Heiss WD, et al. *Assessment of pathophysiology of stroke by positron emission tomography.* Eur J Nucl Med 1994; 21:455-65; Marchal G, et

al. *Prolonged persistence of substantial volumes of potentially viable brain tissue after stroke: a correlative PET-CT study with voxel-based data analysis.* Stroke 1996; 27:599-606.

27. Barone, FC and Feuerstein, GZ. *Inflammatory mediators and stroke: new opportunities for novel therapeutics.* J Cereb Blood Flow Metab 1999 Aug; 19(8):819-34.

28. Vila, N, et al. *Cytokine-induced inflammation and long-term stroke functional outcome.* J Neurol Sci 1999 Jan 15; 162(2):185-8.

29. Tortella, FC, et al. *Neuroprotection (focal ischemia) and neurotoxicity (electroencephalographic) studies in rats with AHN649, a 3-amino analog of dextromethorphan and low-affinity N-methyl-D-aspartate antagonist.* J Pharmacol Exp Ther 1999 Oct; 291(1):399-408; Chabrier, PE, et al. *BN 80933, a dual inhibitor of neuronal nitric oxide synthase and lipid peroxidation: a promising neuroprotective strategy.* Proc Natl Acad Sci USA 1999 Sep 14; 96(19):10824-9.

30. Mohiuddin AA, Bath FJ, Bath PMW. Theophylline, aminophylline, caffeine and analogues for acute ischaemic stroke (Cochrane Review). In: *The Cochrane Library,* Issue 4, 1999. Oxford: Update Software.

31. Candelise, L and Ciccone, A. Gangliosides for acute ischaemic stroke (Cochrane Review). In: *The Cochrane Library,* Issue 4, 1999. Oxford: Update Software.

32. Evans, SM, et al. *Neuroprotection by caffeine and pentoxifylline during experimental cerebral ischaemia.* West Indian Med J 1999 Mar; 48(1):23-5.

33. Sick, TJ, et al. *Mild hypothermia improves recovery of cortical extracellular potassium ion activity and excitability after middle cerebral artery occlusion in the rat.* Stroke 1999; 30:2385-91.

34. Sitar, SM. *Propofol prevents peroxide-induced inhibition of glutamate transport in cultured astrocytes.* Anesthesiology 1999 May; 90(5): 1446-53.

35.   Kawaguchi, MM. *Isoflurane delays but does not prevent cerebral infarction in rats subjected to focal ischemia.* Anesthesiology 2000 May; 92(5): 1335-42.

36.   Wen-Jie, D, et al. *Blockade of central angiotensin AT1 receptors improves neurological outcome and reduces expression of AP-1 transcription factors after focal brain ischemia in rats.* Stroke 1999; 30:2391-99.

37.   Hurn, PD. *Estrogen as a neuroprotectant in stroke.* J Cereb Blood Flow Metab 2000 Apr; 20(4): 631-52; Yang, SH, et al. *Estradiol exerts neuroprotective effects when administered after ischemic insult.* Stroke 2000; 31:745.

38.   Chen, JJ. *Neuroprotective effects of progesterone after transient middle cerebral artery occlusion in rat.* J Neurol Sci 1999 Dec 1; 171(1): 24-30.

39.   Domoki, FV, et al. *Mitochondrial potassium channel opener diazoxide preserves neuronal-vascular function after cerebral ischemia in newborn pigs.* Stroke 1999; 30:2713.

40.   Gusev, EI.*Neuroprotective effects of glycine for therapy of acute ischaemic stroke.* Cerebrovasc Dis 2000 Jan-Feb; 10(1): 49-60.

41.   Ahmed, NN. *Effect of intravenous nimodipine on blood pressure and outcome after acute stroke.* Stroke 2000 Jun; 31(6): 1250.

42.   Hess, DC. *HMG-CoA reductase inhibitors (statins): a promising approach to stroke prevention.* Neurology 2000 Feb 22; 54(4): 760-6.

43.   Chen, ZM, et al. *Aspirin after acute stroke may decrease risk of nosocomial relapse.* Stroke 2000; 31:1240-49.

CHAPTER 6
SHOCK

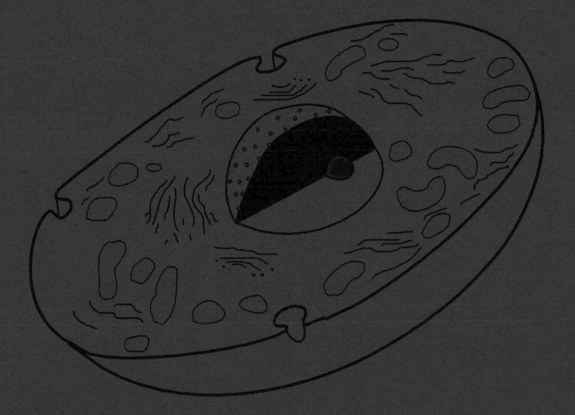

CHAPTER 6 — SHOCK

Contents

Objectives

After reading this chapter, you'll be able to:

- State a pathophysiological definition of shock.
- Describe the Weil-Shubin classification of shock.
- Define and describe the systemic inflammatory response syndrome (SIRS).
- Draw a summary diagram for the generic model of shock.

- Defend the following statements:
    "Shock does not necessarily equal hypotension."
    "Raising the blood pressure in shock may worsen bleeding."
    "We really don't know how best to monitor a patient in shock."
    "There are no compelling data to change fluid therapy at this time."
- Summarize the evidence favoring and the physiologic basis for the following treatments of shock: steroids, immune therapy, anti-opiates, pentoxyfilline.

NOTE: Due to the large amount of information covered in this chapter, there are detailed outlines prior to certain sections to guide the reader in meeting his or her learning goals.

Introduction

Our current understanding of shock reflects the beginning, *and* the future of "what's new in pathophysiology." It was in understanding shock that I first realized the importance of "stuff." Debates involving fluid therapy and use of the MAST suit in shock are interesting, but as in CHF, these treatments attack the hemodynamic *effects* of shock rather than the *cause*. We'll spend most of our time in this chapter learning the proper physiological classification of shock, based on the mechanism, and then apply the model of "stuff," as was done originally by investigators nearly thirty years ago.

NOTE: Shock is one of the hottest topics in medical research today. As such, I have included much detailed information on study results. It is not absolutely necessary to read and understand every word of the research if you are clear on the essence of each section. To help you, I've put experimental data that I consider "not essential reading" in a smaller font.

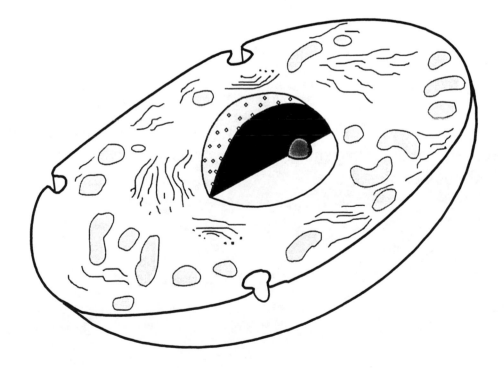

Definition

OBJECTIVE: State a pathophysiological definition of "shock."

Shock is a clinical syndrome involving widespread cellular dysfunction due to inadequate delivery and use of oxygen at the cellular level. Cell dysfunction leads to release of mediators. Shock may occur with normal, increased, or most frequently, decreased cardiac output. Low-flow states are also characterized by excess CO_2 in venous blood, in organs, and in tissues.[1]

REMEMBER: Shock involves widespread cellular dysfunction due to inadequate delivery and use of oxygen at the cellular level.

Diagnosing shock

How do we diagnose shock? One of the most important questions I've come across is, "How do we diagnose shock?" Most of us are aware of the "standard" findings (**Table**, p. 6-5).

Table — "Standard" Findings in Shock

Test	Normal	Mild Shock	Moderate Shock	Severe Shock
Sensorium	Oriented	Slightly anxious but oriented	Anxious, confused	Lethargic, confused, incoherent
Pulse	60-100	100-120	120-150	> 140; rapid, thready
Pupils	Equal, 2-4 mm	Normal	Normal	May be dilated, slow to react
Blood pressure	120/80	110/80	70-90/50-60	< 50-60 systolic
Pulse pressure	40	30	20-30	10-20
Capillary blanch	Normal	Normal	Slow	Very slow
Respiratory rate	12-16	14-20	20-30	> 35
Urine output cc/H	40-50	30-35	15-30	Negligible
Skin	Dry	Slightly moist	Sweaty	Cool, clammy

Even assuming that "hypotension is not necessary to diagnose shock,"[2] the reliability of other parameters, such as tachycardia, has been questioned for years.

Is tachycardia always a reliable indicator of shock? Unfortunately, the answer is "no." Tachycardia is not a reliable sign of hypovolemic shock in penetrating abdominal injuries.[3] Nearly 50% of hypotensive patients are not tachycardic. Proposed mechanisms for this unexpected finding may involve a parasympathetic reflex, resulting in relative bradycardia despite the presence of hypotension. Bradycardia in response to trauma has been noted

> ***PRINCIPLE*: If the patient looks *sick* and the test looks good, the patient is still *sick*!**

in other studies, both animal and human. Tissue damage may attenuate the expected heart rate response to hemorrhage. World War II data showed that the pulse rate had little value as an index of severe traumatic shock. In shock cases seen shortly after injury, finding a low pulse rate was common.[4]

The concept that tachycardia is a reliable indicator of shock has also been challenged in patients with hemoperitoneum due to ruptured ectopic pregnancy. In one study, 55% of hypotensive patients were not tachycardic. The quantity of hemoperitoneum varied widely in each group and did not correlate with the hemodynamic response. These results support the proposed theory that hemoperitoneum may trigger a parasympathetic reflex, resulting in a pulse rate inappropriate for the degree of hypotension. A vasovagal reflex may play a role in those patients without significant hemoperitoneum. The diagnosis of hypovolemic shock must be considered even without tachycardia.[5]

PRINCIPLE: **Tachycardia is not always a reliable indicator of shock.**

What's the bottom line, then? If "classic" findings are present, they corroborate your impression of shock. Their absence, however, does *not* rule out shock. Remember, if the finding is present, it helps you. If not, it doesn't matter, meaning a negative test does *not* mean a normal patient. Shock is a prime example of this principle.

PRINCIPLE: **A normal test does not necessarily mean a normal patient!**

Classification

OBJECTIVE: Describe the Weil-Shubin classification of shock.

Mechanistically, shock is divided into four types: hypovolemic, cardiogenic, obstructive, and distributive.[6] When identifying the underlying cause, first determine whether shock is central or peripheral in origin. **[FIGURE 6-1]**

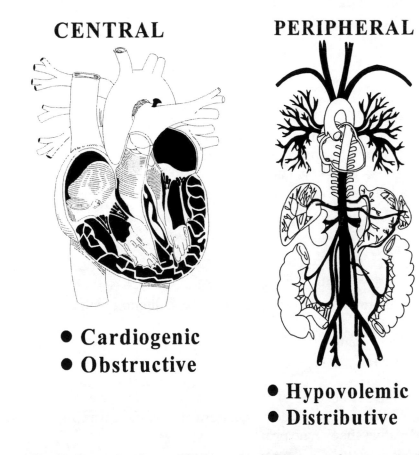

CENTRAL

PERIPHERAL

- Cardiogenic
- Obstructive

- Hypovolemic
- Distributive

Weil-Shubin Classification of Shock

Figure 6-1 — The Weil-Shubin classification of shock

CAUSES OF SHOCK

CENTRAL

Cardiogenic Shock
- Myocardial infarction
- Acute mitral insufficiency
- Ventricular septal defect
- Heart failure
- Hemodynamically significant dysrhythmias

Obstructive Shock
- Vena cava — compression
- Pericardium — tamponade
- Cardiac chambers — ball-valve thrombus, tumor
- Pulmonary circuit — pulmonary embolism
- Aorta — dissecting aneurysm

PERIPHERAL

Hypovolemic Shock

Exogenous Causes
- Hemorrhage
- Plasma loss — burns, inflammation
- Electrolyte loss — diarrhea, dehydration

Endogenous Causes — extravasation due to:
- Inflammation
- Trauma
- Anaphylaxis
- Envenomation

Distributive Shock

Low resistance — normal or high cardiac output; vasodilation with arteriovenous shunting
- Cervical spine transection
- Inflammation
- Peritonitis
- Gram-negative shock (early)

High or normal resistance — cardiac output normal/low; increased venous capacitance
- Gram-negative shock (late phase)
- Barbiturate intoxication
- Ganglionic blockade

Central shock — Central shock occurs when the central circulation (heart and great vessels) is unable to pump sufficient blood to maintain tissue oxygen needs. This results from direct (cardiogenic) or indirect (obstructive) impairment in cardiac emptying. There are two types of central shock:

1. **Cardiogenic** — The cardiac pump cannot adequately circulate the available volume. The most common cause is myocardial infarction; cardiogenic shock complicates myocardial infarction (MI) in five to ten percent of patients. Fifty percent of the patients who develop this syndrome do so within 24 hours following their MI.[7]

   Anterior infarcts lead to cardiogenic shock more commonly than do inferior ones. If over 40% of the left ventricular muscle is lost, shock will result. Without appropriate treatment, mortality is 55 to 85% within 24 hours. Patients with a cardiac index (cardiac output/body surface area) less than 2.0 $L/min/m^2$ (normal = 3.2-5.2 $L/min/m^2$) and a pulmonary artery wedge pressure (a measure of left ventricular filling) greater than 15 mm Hg (normal = 7-10 mm Hg) have a very high mortality.[8]

   Other potential cardiogenic causes include dysrhythmias, ventricular septal defects, or congestive heart failure. Ventricular fibrillation may be viewed as the "ultimate" form of cardiogenic shock. [**Figure 6-2**].

CENTRAL

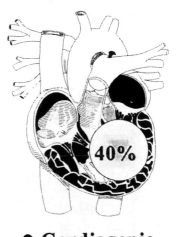

- **Cardiogenic**
- Obstructive

Figure 6-2 — Cardiogenic shock usually occurs when over 40% of the left ventricular myocardium is nonfunctional.

2. **Obstructive** — The pumping action of the heart is normal, but a physical obstruction to blood flow is present in the heart or great vessels. Possibilities include blockage in the vena cava (vena caval syndromes), pericardium (tamponade), cardiac chambers (ball-valve thrombus, tumor), pulmonary circuit (pulmonary embolus), or aorta (dissecting aneurysm). As a result, insufficient blood leaves the central circulation to oxygenate the tissues adequately. **[FIGURE 6-3]**

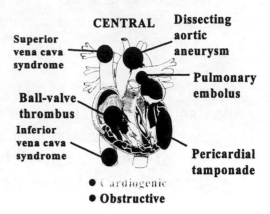
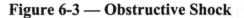

Figure 6-3 — Obstructive Shock

Peripheral shock — Peripheral shock occurs at the level of the peripheral vascular bed. There are two major types:

1. **Hypovolemic** — The intravascular compartment is filled inadequately for proper tissue perfusion. Sources of fluid loss may be *exogenous* (e.g., hemorrhage, diarrhea, dehydration) or *endogenous* (e.g., internal bleeding, "third-spacing" [inflammation, trauma, envenomation]).

2. **Distributive** — The name may be new to you, but the concept isn't. Remember the terms "pooling," "capacitance vessels," "warm shock," or "vasodilation?" Same concept. Distributive shock results from a normal total blood volume but too many "open vessels." This maldistribution is due to a defect in arterial resistance, venous capacitance, or both, with loss of vascular tone. As the vessels expand, the quantity of fluid in them becomes insufficient to meet metabolic demands. Despite appearing well perfused, the patient's metabolic demand exceeds the oxygen supply. The most common causes are sepsis, drug overdose, anaphylaxis, and spinal cord injury. Ganglionic blockade or barbiturate poisoning also result in distributive shock. **[FIGURE 6-4]**

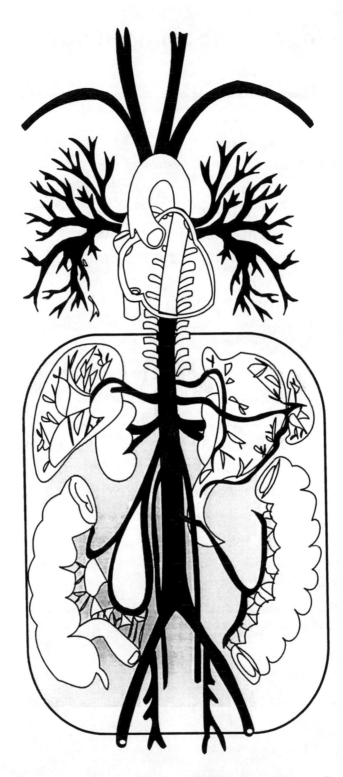

**Figure 6-4 — Distributive shock involves loss of
vascular tone that leads to pooling, particularly
in the viscera and lower extremities.**

Pathophysiology — the common link

Human Hypovolemic Shock
- The compensated stage
- Decompensation
- Energy failure occurs
- Progressive cardiac failure follows
- Other organ systems are affected as well
- Coagulation abnormalities and disseminated intravascular coagulation (DIC)
- The important role of protein C
- The crucial point

Human Septic Shock
- Human septic shock compared to hypovolemic shock
- The intestine responds early to ischemia
- Translocation of LPS leads to the production of "bad stuff"
- Is the gut the source of all the "stuff," whatever the inciting event?
- Mediators in septic shock
- The systemic inflammatory response syndrome (SIRS) in severe infection
- What are superantigens?
- What are cytokines?
- TNF-α may be the major mediator
- TNF initiates a sequence of events
- Does TNF play a role in other forms of shock as a generic part of the SIRS?
- Does cytokine blockade help?
- How does all of this "stuff" interplay in septic shock? The inflammatory cascade.
- The bottom line

There are many similarities among the various types of shock, when one looks at damage to organs. The basic defect, regardless of the inciting event, is failure of oxygen delivery at the cell level. Let's look at what is known about human hypovolemic and septic shock, then "put it together" into a generic model of shock.

Human Hypovolemic Shock

The compensated stage — The body's initial response to hypovolemia is a reflex that results in the release of norepinephrine (NE) and epinephrine (E), and activation of the renin-angiotensin-aldosterone system (RAAS). NE and E cause tachycardia and increase the contractility of the heart. Additionally, there is venous and arteriolar constriction. The result is a decrease in the blood flow to skin, muscle, GI tract, and often, to the kidney, with a relative redistribution of blood to the brain and heart.

> **PRINCIPLE:** Many diseases occur when *normal* response systems are activated under *abnormal* circumstances.

Capillary hydrostatic pressure decreases in early shock, allowing fluid from the interstitium to flow into the vessels. This "autotransfusion" effect, along with the other mentioned mechanisms, allows the body to compensate adequately for up to a 25% volume loss. **[FIGURE 6-5]**

Decompensation — As the patient decompensates, perfusion of the brain and coronary arteries decreases. Cells switch to anaerobic metabolism, producing lactic acidosis. This shifts the oxygen-hemoglobin dissociation curve to the right and increases tissue oxygen delivery. The acidosis, though, also decreases cardiac function and makes the myocardium more susceptible to catecholamine effects (e.g., dysrhythmias).

Energy failure occurs — There is decreased synthesis of adenosine triphosphate (ATP), the major intracellular energy provider. This state of "energy failure" leads to increased intracellular sodium and water

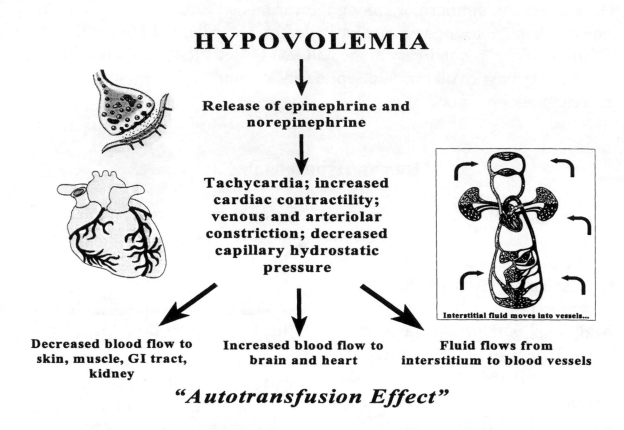

HYPOVOLEMIA

↓

Release of epinephrine and norepinephrine

↓

Tachycardia; increased cardiac contractility; venous and arteriolar constriction; decreased capillary hydrostatic pressure

Interstitial fluid moves into vessels...

Decreased blood flow to skin, muscle, GI tract, kidney

Increased blood flow to brain and heart

Fluid flows from interstitium to blood vessels

"Autotransfusion Effect"

Figure 6-5 — The compensated stage of human hypovolemic shock

accumulation (probably due to failure of ion channel regulatory mechanisms), and intracellular swelling. Calcium levels increase in the cytosol and mitochondria, further impairing ATP synthesis. The lysosomes then rupture, releasing enzymes that further increase cellular permeability. Other enzymes ("stuff"), including histamine, serotonin, kinins, and prostaglandins, are produced, leading to increased vascular permeability with subsequent fluid loss back to the interstitium.

Progressive cardiac failure follows. The effects of this microscopic energy failure are also evident on a gross level. There is progressive cardiac failure. Lung water increases, as does disruption of the epithelial integrity. Atelectasis (hypoaeration) and hemorrhages occur, leading to ventilation-perfusion mismatching, progressive shunting, and eventually, adult respiratory distress syndrome (ARDS).

Other organ systems are also affected. Hepatobiliary and pancreatic functions are hampered, including insulin release. The patient develops a diabetic-like state. Gastrointestinal motility is decreased and stress ulcers may form. Urine production tends to decrease and renal failure may follow, to which free radical formation in the kidneys may contribute.[9]

Coagulation abnormalities and disseminated intravascular coagulation (DIC) — Finally, function of the white blood cells and blood clotting system is impaired. There is decreased resistance to infection and disseminated intravascular coagulation (DIC) may occur spontaneously. Ninety-seven percent of patients who die of hemorrhagic shock have evidence of coagulation defects *prior* to fluid or blood administration. This occurs most often in patients with head trauma and suggests pre-existing DIC.[10] The most frequent laboratory abnormality is elevated protime (97%), followed by depressed platelet counts (72%), and elevated partial thromboplastin time (70%).

The important role of protein C — Protein C is a naturally-occurring anticoagulant that is activated by platelet-thrombin-thrombomodulin complexes. Activated protein C, in conjunction with the cofactor protein S, acts as an anticoagulant by inactivating clotting factors Va and VIIIa.[11] The result is reduced thrombin generation and decreased clot formation. Decreases in protein C concentrations and inhibition of the protein C anticoagulant system seem to play an important role in the development of the hypercoagulable state during DIC.

Tumor necrosis factor-alpha and interleukin 1 down-regulate the expression of thrombomodulin on endothelial cell surfaces. The result is decreased activation of protein C and a procoagulant state.[12] Animal studies show that administration of exogenous activated protein C prevents mortality and coagulopathy during sepsis.[13] Numerous human studies in sepsis reveal that low levels of protein C correlate with severity of illness.[14] Ongoing work using recombinant human activated protein C (rhAPC, Zovant®) found significant decreases in 28-day mortality in patients with sepsis.[15] Protein C plays a major role in the pathogenesis in both hypovolemic and septic shock.

Inflammation leads to coagulation, which leads to more inflammation. Eventually, this positive feedback loop leads to vascular collapse, organ failure, and death. **[FIGURE 6-5A]**

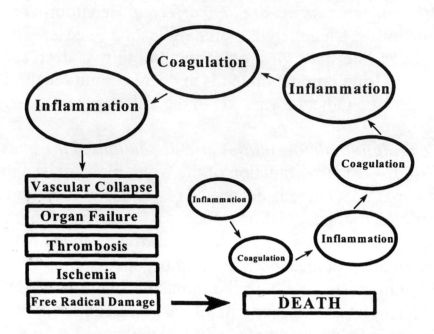

Figure 6-5A — The positive feedback loop of inflammation and coagulation, eventually leading to death.

The crucial point — The full-blown hypovolemic shock syndrome is a state of multiple system organ dysfunction, followed by multiple system organ failure with a metabolic acidosis, leaky capillaries, and widespread cellular dysfunction. As with septic shock, illustrated below, hypovolemic shock involves production and release of many mediators.[16] [17] **[FIGURE 6-6]**

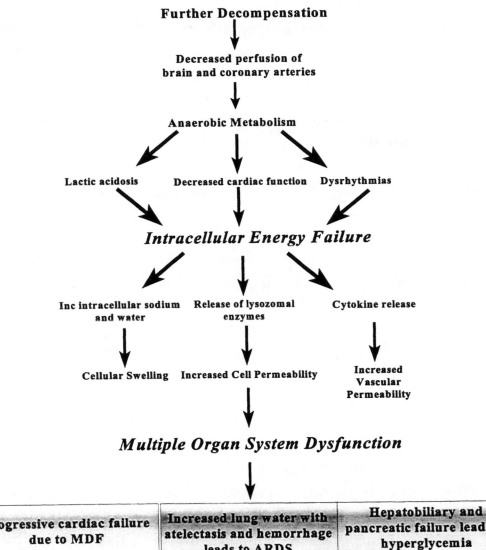

Further Decompensation

↓

Decreased perfusion of brain and coronary arteries

↓

Anaerobic Metabolism

Lactic acidosis   **Decreased cardiac function**   **Dysrhythmias**

Intracellular Energy Failure

Inc intracellular sodium and water   **Release of lysozomal enzymes**   **Cytokine release**

Cellular Swelling   **Increased Cell Permeability**   **Increased Vascular Permeability**

Multiple Organ System Dysfunction

Progressive cardiac failure due to MDF	Increased lung water with atelectasis and hemorrhage leads to ARDS	Hepatobiliary and pancreatic failure leads to hyperglycemia
Decreased GI motility leads to stress ulcers	Decreased urine output and renal failure	Impaired WBC and clotting function leads to infection and DIC

DEATH

Figure 6-6 — Decompensation in Hypovolemic Shock

6-17

Human Septic Shock

Human septic shock compared to hypovolemic shock — The pathogenesis of human septic shock is similar, following the initial infection, to that of hypovolemic shock:

- Infection occurs, resulting in the release of mediators. The likely source of mediators is the intestine.

- *Mediator release* leads to vasodilation and decreased myocardial function.

- Depressed myocardial function leads to cardiovascular insufficiency, followed by massive myocardial depression.

- Decreased tissue oxygenation because of massive myocardial depression leads to multiple system organ dysfunction (MSOD), then multiple system organ failure (MSOF).

- The result is unresponsive hypotension and death.

The intestine responds early to ischemia — The intestine is thought to be one of the first organs to respond to shock. Though this concept was originally advanced in septic shock, it probably applies to *all* types of shock. It should come as no surprise that sympathetic vasoconstriction of the mesenteric vessels is a normal regulatory mechanism to shunt flow to the more vital tissues, especially the brain and the heart. This stimulation may block splanchnic blood flow almost entirely for up to an hour.[18]

Ischemia increases permeability of the intestinal mucosal barriers, allowing bacteria and bacterial lipopolysaccharide coats (LPS) to translocate (spread through the bowel wall) into the blood. Even in cases where sepsis is not the inciting event, intestinal ischemia leads to translocation of normal gram-negative intestinal flora, whose polysaccharide coat has the same effect.

Translocation of bacteria or LPS from the intestinal tract likely represents the trigger event that eventually leads from early organ failure to late (septic) organ failure. **[FIGURE 6-7]**

Translocation of LPS leads to the production of "bad stuff" — LPS leads to production of mediators, such as tumor necrosis factor alpha (TNF-α).[19] LPS also induces the release of nitric oxide and glutamate.[20] These further decrease mesenteric flow. It appears that catecholamines are *not* primary mediators of LPS-induced decreases in mesenteric blood flow.[21]

Is the gut the source of all the initial "stuff," whatever the inciting event? Many experts would answer, "Probably so." In support of this theory is the fact that TNF-α causes *increased* endothelial permeability.[22] Experimental studies that have deliberately blocked endotoxin and bacterial translocation from bowel lumen to the systemic circulation show far lower levels of TNF-α and other mediators, even in patients who developed shock. Unfortunately, no human study to date has *proven* a definitive role of the gut in the pathogenesis of sepsis and multiple organ failure.[23]

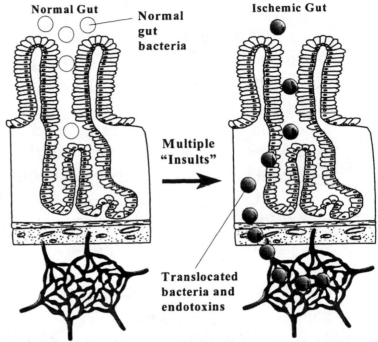

Figure 6-7 — Intestinal ischemia allows bacteria, either normal flora or exogenous infection, and endotoxin (LPS) to cross the bowel membrane and enter the systemic circulation. Once there, LPS initiates the "cascade" of the systemic inflammatory response syndrome.

However, three lines of evidence support a causative role for mesenteric ischemia in the "common denominator pathway" of shock:

1. Gastric pH monitoring (gastric tonometry) — Gastric tonometry has been shown to be useful in predicting outcomes of critically ill patients, monitoring the effectiveness of resuscitation, and predicting multiple organ dysfunction.[24] Limited data have raised the question whether the technique accurately indicates splanchnic perfusion.[25] Experts continue to disagree — in the absence of specific "splanchnic therapy," trauma patients whose gastric pH was greater than 7.32 at 24 hours following their initial injury had a significantly lower incidence of MSOF.[26] Another group of investigators show that use of specific "splanchnic therapy" to raise gastric pH resulted in a decreased incidence of MSOF.[27]

2. Morphological studies — Trauma patients with short periods (five to twenty minutes) of hypotension develop focal apoptosis of intestinal epithelial and lymphoid tissues extremely rapidly after injury (two to three hours). Apoptotic loss of intestinal epithelial cells may compromise bowel wall integrity and serve as a mechanism for translocation of bacterial LPS into the systemic circulation.[28]

3. Early post-surgical refeeding studies — Studies have shown early enteral feeding of post-surgical patients results in a lower incidence of adult respiratory distress syndrome (ARDS) and improved outcomes in persons with already established ARDS.[29] Similar results have been noted in post-surgical sepsis.[30]

Mediators in septic shock. The systemic inflammatory response syndrome (SIRS) is an acute illness characterized by generalized activation of the endothelium. SIRS is a great term because it describes *generically* a syndrome resulting in the release of mediators ("stuff") due to a *variety* of causes. First, let's look at the systemic inflammatory response syndrome in severe infection.

> **REMEMBER: Though the SIRS was first described in sepsis, it is a *generic* response to a *variety* of circumstances.**

The systemic inflammatory response syndrome in severe infection — The most severe form of the syndrome is found in patients with shock due to gram-negative sepsis. Sepsis may also occur from gram-positive organisms. The primary pathway is identical in most ways to that of hypovolemic shock.[31] Both animal and clinical data suggest that, unlike endotoxin-mediated shock, gram-positive infection produces only a modest tumor necrosis factor (TNF-α) response and does not respond well to anti-TNF-α therapies.[32] Nonetheless, gram-positive infections may still be deadly due to "superantigens."

Now I really feel like a comic-book character; what are "superantigens?" The pyogenic exotoxins of Group A Streptococci and enterotoxins of Staphylococcus aureus are a family of related toxins that act as "superantigens" because of their ability to stimulate many T-cell subsets. These toxins have been implicated in gastrointestinal food poisoning, toxic shock syndromes, gram-positive sepsis, and, possibly, septic shock. There is increasing evidence that gram-positive infections frequently coexist in septic shock and that bacterial superantigens play a major role. This explains why the systemic inflammatory response system is still activated in gram-positive infection, despite the lower levels of TNF-α.[33]

What are cytokines? Cytokines are endogenously produced small molecular weight proteins with multiple biological effects. Cytokines such as interleukin-1 (IL-1) and tumor necrosis factor (TNF-α), as well as interferon-gamma and interleukin-6 (IL-6), may play a critical role in the SIRS. The biochemical changes induced by TNF-α and IL-1 include increased synthesis of nitric oxide, prostaglandins, platelet-activating factor, and endothelial cell adhesion molecules. Remember, all cytokines that are present in disease states also have a *normal* function in the body. They are deleterious only when released at an inappropriate time. Changes in blood levels of these mediators during treatment are valuable for monitoring septic patients.[34]

> **REMEMBER**: All cytokines that are present in disease states have a *normal* function in the body. They are deleterious only when released at an inappropriate time.

TNF-α may be the major mediator. TNF-α is most likely the major mediator involved in the pathogenesis of the SIRS and septic shock.

- ***TNF-α causes*** in vivo ***depression of heart muscle*** — TNF-α injected *in vivo* to guinea pigs causes myocardial depression and alters cardiac responsiveness to norepinephrine (NE).[35] Though TNF-α stimulates an early beneficial effect on myocardial function, it impairs myocardial performance some 18 to 22 hours later. This effect is serum transferable. Since the serum half life of TNF-α is six to seven minutes, it appears that the cardiac effects of TNF-α are long-lasting since cardiac dysfunction is evident long after the injected TNF-α is absent.

TNF-α initiates a sequence of events. TNF-α has been shown to stimulate the production of mediators implicated in the pathogenesis of septic shock, including interleukin-1, interleukin-6, leukotrienes, and platelet activating factor. These findings suggest that TNF-α initiates a sequence of immunologic events, culminating in impaired cardiac performance 18 to 22 hours later.[36] As noted previously, TNF-α also appears to lower levels of protein C.

Does TNF-α play a role in other forms of shock? TNF-α is released from both the heart and the kidney in response to ischemia and reperfusion. TNF-α released during cardiopulmonary bypass induces glomerular fibrin deposition, cellular infiltration, and vasoconstriction, leading to a reduction in glomerular filtration rate (GFR). Thus, its role as a mediator is a generic one in the SIRS, rather than sepsis-specific.[37]

Does cytokine blockade help? It seems reasonable that antibodies to TNF-α may abate its initiation of a downward spiral. Specific blockade of TNF-α using neutralizing antibodies or soluble receptors to TNF-α in animal models of SIRS reduces mortality and severity of disease. Similar results have been observed by blocking IL-1 with soluble IL-1 receptors or IL-1 receptor antagonists. Experimental work has

> **REMEMBER: Cytokines and other mediators are produced *any time* the SIRS is present, not just in sepsis.**

also shown that LPS antagonists block lipopolysaccharide-induced release of tumor necrosis factor-alpha and other cellular mediators and may be an effective therapeutic agent for human septic shock.[38]

- Preliminary clinical studies suggest that blockade may be useful in treating human SIRS.[39] A murine (rodent) anti-TNF-α monoclonal antibody, CB0006, is safe in a human clinical trial and may be useful in septic patients with increased circulating TNF-α concentrations. Further studies are needed to determine efficacy and the ultimate clinical utility of this immunotherapeutic agent in sepsis.[40] Published data from on-going studies should appear soon, and look promising in preliminary reports.

How does all of this "stuff" interplay in septic shock? Enter the "inflammatory cascade" of septic shock; if unabated, the cascade occurs in three stages: **[FIGURE 6-8]**

- **Induction phase** — Bacterial lipopolysaccharides (LPSs) are released into the blood. Endotoxin itself does not cause the hemodynamic manifestations of sepsis; further interactions between lipopolysaccharide and the host immune system are required for cytokine secretion and subsequent shock.

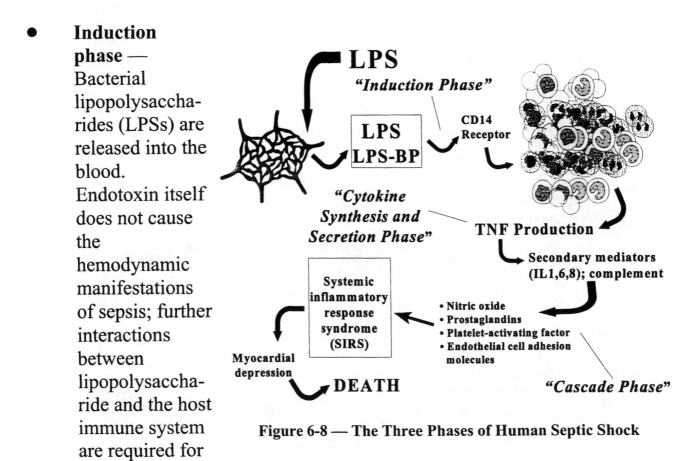

Figure 6-8 — The Three Phases of Human Septic Shock

- LPS-binding protein (LPS-BP) binds to LPS and enhances neutrophil and RE cell function. The LPS-LPS-BP complex induces TNF-α production by macrophages. The receptor for this complex is the CD14 molecule on the macrophage/monocyte membrane.

Recognition of gram-negative bacterial lipopolysaccharide by CD14, a glycoprotein expressed at the surface of monocytes, plays a major role in shock. There is increasing evidence that CD14 also serves as a receptor for other microbial products, including peptidoglycan of gram-positive bacteria. Host cells recognize microbial products, activate, and produce a large array of mediators needed for the development of controlled inflammatory processes. When the activation process is out of control, such as in septic shock, these mediators can be detrimental to the host.[41]

PRINCIPLE: All mediators in disease also have normal roles.

- **Cytokine synthesis and secretion phase** — Once the LPS-LPS-BP complex binds to the CD14 molecule, the synthesis of TNF-α begins. After translation of mRNA into TNF-α, post translational modifications generate the mature secreted form. Transcription of TNF-α is inhibited by agents that increase the intracellular cAMP concentration. Translation of TNF-α mRNA is inhibited by corticosteroids. After secretion of TNF-α, toxicity may be inhibited by monoclonal antibodies directed against TNF-α or by artificial protein inhibitors of TNF-α. **[FIGURE 6-9]**

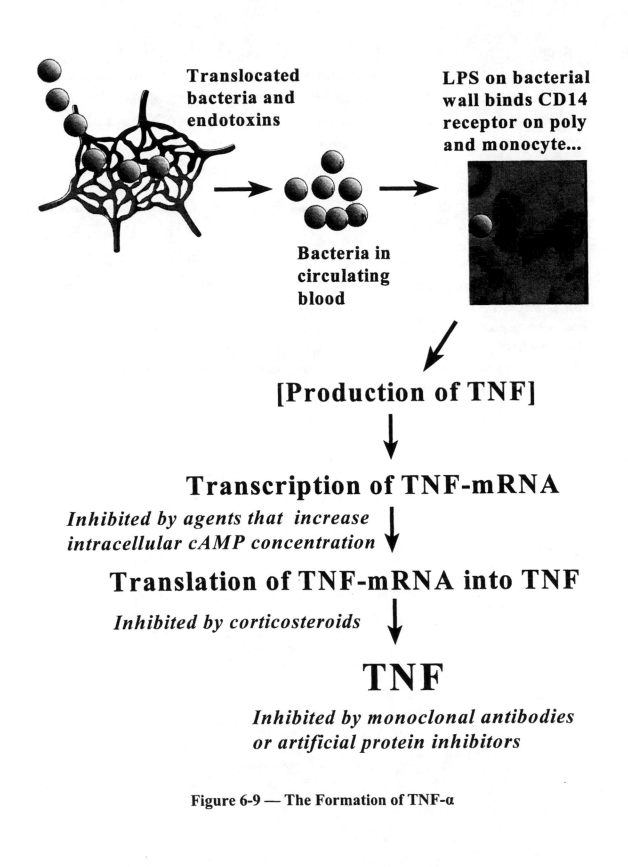

Translocated bacteria and endotoxins

Bacteria in circulating blood

LPS on bacterial wall binds CD14 receptor on poly and monocyte...

[Production of TNF]

Transcription of TNF-mRNA

Inhibited by agents that increase intracellular cAMP concentration

Translation of TNF-mRNA into TNF

Inhibited by corticosteroids

TNF

Inhibited by monoclonal antibodies or artificial protein inhibitors

Figure 6-9 — The Formation of TNF-α

- **Cascade phase** — Once TNF-α is secreted, the cascade of inflammation erupts with secondary secretion of other mediators (including IL 1, IL 6, IL 8, platelet activating factor, prostaglandins, and leukotrienes), activation of neutrophils and endothelial cells, synthesis of acute phase reactants, and onset of coagulopathy.

Free-radical formation likely plays a role in mediating direct membrane damage.[42] Melatonin is a scavenger of oxyradicals and peroxynitrite (a free radical byproduct), and an inhibitor of nitric oxide (NO) production. It has been used to prevent development of chemical peritonitis (non-septic shock) induced in rats by administration of the drug, zymosan.[43]

> **REMEMBER:** Septic shock is only *one* manifestation of the generic systemic inflammatory response syndrome. Once triggered, the SIRS cascade is similar, regardless of the inciting cause.

The bottom line — In both human hypovolemic *and* septic shock there is a common pathway of patient death once a certain point is reached. Many animal models suggest the same in just about every type of shock imaginable.

PATHOGENESIS OF HUMAN SEPTIC SHOCK

Nidus of infection
(Abscess, peritonitis, pneumonitis, cellulitis, etc.)
|
Bloodstream Invasion or Local Production and Release of Mediator
|
MEDIATORS RELEASED:
Complement derived anaphylatoxins (C5a, C3a)
Kinins
Eicosanoids (prostaglandins, leukotrienes, thromboxane)
Platelet activating factor (PAF)
Histamine
Myocardial depressant factor (MDF)
Tumor necrosis factor (TNF-α)
Endotoxin
Interleukin-1, Interleukin-2, Interleukin-6
Beta-endorphin
Other lymphokines or monokines
| |
PERIPHERAL AND PULMONARY   **DIRECT MYOCARDIAL**
VASCULAR EFFECTS   **EFFECTS**
| |
Vasodilation of arteriolar/venular beds   **Decreased LV ejection fraction**
Vasoconstriction   **LV dilatation**
Leukocyte aggregation   **Dec ventricular compliance**
Vascular endothelial cell dysfunction |
| |
CARDIOVASCULAR INSUFFICIENCY
Maldistribution of blood flow
Reduced resistance to blood flow
Lactic acidemia
Increased mixed venous O2
|
Severe decrease in SVR (40%) **Severe myocardial**   **Severe multiple**
                                 depression (10%)   **system organ**
                                                            dysfunction (50%)
                                        |
                                        |
Multiple System Organ Failure
|
Unresponsive hypotension, then DEATH

The systemic inflammatory response syndrome

"Classic Examples"
WBC Dysfunction in the SIRS
- What are the normal vascular changes in early inflammation?
- WBC dysfunction is universal in the SIRS
- What are adhesion molecules?

An Alternative Hypothesis in the Development of MSOD
The Bottom Line — A Generic Model of Shock

OBJECTIVE: Define and describe the systemic inflammatory response syndrome (SIRS).

This systemic inflammatory response syndrome (SIRS) is a *generic* total body response to many insults. It likely represents the "tie that binds" all types of shock together, once a certain point is reached. The historical development of these concepts is fascinating. Besides the infectious causes that may produce systemic inflammatory response syndrome, noninfectious pathologic causes include pancreatitis, ischemia, multitrauma and tissue injury, hemorrhagic shock, immune-mediated organ injury, and the exogenous administration of putative inflammatory mediators such as tumor necrosis factor or other cytokines.

PRINCIPLE: Bad "stuff" begets more bad "stuff."

REMEMBER: A common end point is reached where a "systemic inflammatory response syndrome" develops. From here on, the pathways are nearly identical, regardless of the original instigating event.

"Classic examples" — Acute pancreatitis is the classic example of a noninfectious process that leads to hemodynamic features identical to sepsis: cardiovascular instability, reduced ejection fraction, and decreased systemic vascular resistance. In addition, there are many striking similarities in the cytokine and inflammatory mediator profiles, suggesting that the hemodynamic abnormalities may result from the same pathogenic mechanisms, but because of different inflammatory stimuli.[44] Hemorrhagic shock is another classic example. The crucial link — a common point is reached where a "systemic inflammatory response syndrome" develops. From here on, the pathways are nearly identical, whatever the original instigating event.

WBC Dysfunction in the SIRS

What are the normal vascular changes in early inflammation? Acute inflammation has three major components:

1. *Vascular alterations* increase blood flow to the inflamed area. Vasodilation leads to the initial red color (*rubor*) noted in an inflamed area.

2. *Structural changes in the vessel walls* allow plasma proteins and leukocytes to leave the circulation and form an inflammatory exudate. Increasing vascular permeability leads to stasis of circulation in the involved area. Leukocytes first line the endothelium of vessels (**margination**), and then pass through vessel walls in a process known as **diapedesis**. Once in the interstitium, they follow a chemotactic stimulus to the inflamed area.

3. *Emigration of leukocytes* from the microcirculation to the injury occurs when various chemotactic agents aid in the movement of leukocytes from the blood vessel to the injured area. These agents include bacterial products, complement (e.g., C5a), leukotrienes, and interleukins. These also result in activation of leukocytes, which release enzymes that phagocytose and kill foreign cells.

WBC dysfunction is universal in the SIRS. Endotoxin exposure renders polymorphonuclear cells (PMNs) hyperadhesive to the blood vessel endothelium. This produces activated inflammatory cells that are incapable of leaving the vessels. As such, the PMN is more likely to promote tissue injury from *within* microvascular beds than to clear pathogens from extravascular sites. Moreover, the functional characteristics of activated PMNs are similar during trauma, burn injury, sepsis, surgery, and other inflammatory conditions. This suggests that several clinical conditions might have a common effector in the activated, yet dysfunctional (unable to migrate) PMN.[45] But wait, there's more . . . Why do the PMNs "adhere" to blood vessel walls anyway?

What are adhesion molecules? One of the most important events in the reaction to all forms of injury is adhesion of leukocytes to endothelium, a prelude to their emigration into tissues (see immediately above). The leukocyte adhesion process is central to inflammation, atherosclerosis, and immune reactions. WBC adhesion is governed largely by the interaction of complementary adhesion molecules on endothelia and on leukocytes.

The most important adhesion molecule pairs are the selectins, the cellular adhesion molecules (ICAM-1 and VCAM-1), and the β_1 and β_2 integrins. Studies in experimental animals and humans have confirmed a role for these

---

CELLULAR ADHESION MOLECULES:

- **Selectins**
- **ICAM-1 and VCAM-1 (immunoglobulins)**
- **β_1 and β_2 integrins**

---

molecules in a number of pathological processes, including transplant rejection, septic shock, atherosclerosis, late phase hypersensitivity reactions, immunologically-mediated lung and kidney disease, and reperfusion injury. Overactivity of adhesion molecules prevents normal WBC emigration into the tissues. **[FIGURE 6-10]**

1. **Selectins** (E, P, L) bind to cell surface glycoproteins. They facilitate movement of white blood cells ("rolling") toward the vessel wall.

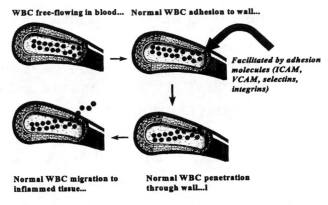

WBC free-flowing in blood... Normal WBC adhesion to wall...

Facilitated by adhesion molecules (ICAM, VCAM, selectins, integrins)

2. **Cellular adhesion molecules** (ICAM-1 [intercellular adhesion molecule 1], and VCAM-1 [vascular cell adhesion molecule 1]) facilitate the binding of leukocytes to the endothelial lining of blood vessels.

Normal WBC migration to inflammed tissue...

Normal WBC penetration through wall...l

Figure 6-10 — Adhesion molecules (lectins) facilitate adhesion of WBCs to the vessel's endothelial surface as a prelude to migration through the wall.

3. **Integrins** function as receptors for the cellular adhesion molecules. The principal integrin receptors for ICAM-1 are the β_2-integrins LFA-1 and MAC-1. Those for VCAM-1 are the integrins $\alpha_4\beta_1$ and $\alpha_4\beta_7$.

Selectins, cellular adhesion molecules, and integrins belong to a category of molecules known as **lectins**. These are proteins that bind carbohydrates with high affinity and specificity. They are located in the vascular endothelium and serve in a wide variety of cell to cell recognition and adhesion processes.

An Alternative Hypothesis

An alternative hypothesis in the development of MSOD — Some experts have proposed an alternative stage by stage development cycle for multiple organ dysfunction syndrome:[46] **[FIGURE 6-11]**

*   **Stage 1** — The patient develops a nidus of infection, an injury, or organ disease (e.g., pancreatitis). The body's initial response is a proinflammatory state with release of multiple mediators on a local level. Shortly, a compensatory anti-inflammatory response occurs to

prevent the proinflammatory mediators from becoming overly destructive (i.e., a "yin-yang" effect).

- **Stage 2** — If the original insult is severe enough and not "dealt with" on a local level during Stage 1, proinflammatory and later anti-inflammatory mediators appear in the systemic circulation. Proinflammatory mediators are part of the body's normal response and help recruit neutrophils, T cells, platelets, and coagulation factors to the site of injury or infection. The anti-inflammatory response is designed to down-regulate the initial proinflammatory response. At this stage, significant organ dysfunction is rare.

- **Stage 3** — At this point, the body loses control of the proinflammatory response, resulting in the clinical findings of the systemic inflammatory response syndrome (SIRS). Pathologic changes occur that lead to microcirculatory abnormalities, ischemia, profound vasodilation, redistribution of blood flow, and often, shock. Unless homeostasis is restored rapidly, organ dysfunction and failure occur.

- **Stage 4** — Without treatment, the patient then develops what has been called the "**compensatory anti-inflammatory response syndrome**" (CARS). Anti-inflammatory mediators flood the systemic circulation. The result is immunosuppression — some have referred to this as a period of "immune paralysis." Treatment with interferon has been shown to up-regulate the "paralyzed" immune system in some patients.[47]

- **Stage 5** — This stage is referred to as "**immunologic dissonance**." Basically, the patient has inappropriate and unbalanced normal regulatory systems. This is the final stage of multiple organ dysfunction syndrome (MODS). Death often occurs, unless the body regains homeostatic control.

Not all experts "buy into" the above cascade. It is the only model, though, that proposes a "yin-yang" approach to the problem. At each stage, there is a proinflammatory, followed by an anti-inflammatory, response. Initially (Stages 1 and 2), these are appropriate. As things get out of balance, normal homeostasis fails, and normal regulatory systems produce "stuff" that ends up becoming harmful (Stages 3-5).

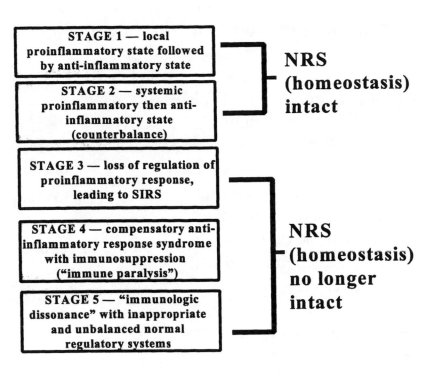

Figure 6-11 — Proposed stages in development of multiple organ dysfunction syndrome

---

OBJECTIVE: Draw a summary diagram for the proposed "final common mechanism" for all forms of shock.

The Bottom Line — A Generic Model of Shock

Investigators have proposed different models for shock. Don't feel bad if you are as confused as I am. I learned from one of my mentors many years ago two concepts that ring true, regardless of which model you like:

1.   "All roads in shock, regardless of the type, ultimately lead to heaven."

2.   "All forms of shock end in cardiogenic shock and death."

Though many details need to be filled in, the following represents a reasonable combination of current thinking regarding shock: (See **Figure 6-11A**)

1.   Regardless of the initial inciting event, sufficient tissue hypoxia leads to a *single common pathway* of deterioration.

2.   The most likely initial event common to all types of shock is mesenteric ischemia.

3.   Mesenteric ischemia leads to translocation of lipopolysaccharide coats (LPS) from our own *normal endogenous* E. coli to the blood.

Tissue hypoxia

↓

Mesenteric ischemia

↓

Translocation of LPS to bloodstream

↓

Mediator release (TNF-α, IL-1, IL-6)

↓

Loss of protein C anticoagulant activity

↓

MSOD — organs dysfunction

↓

MSOF — organs fail

↓

Cardiogenic shock

↓

DEATH

Figure 6-11A — Generic model for all forms of shock, regardless of initial instigating cause. "All roads lead to shock heaven . . ."

4.   LPS stimulates production of mediators. At a minimum, these include TNF-α, IL-1, and IL-6. Current evidence suggests that TNF-α is the "ringleader."

5.   TNF-α (and maybe the interleukins) inhibits the anticoagulant activity of the protein C system, leading to a hypercoagulable state.

6.   Tissue ischemia due to microvascular coagulation leads to multiple system organ dysfunction (MSOD).

7.   When MSOD becomes severe enough, multiple system organ failure (MSOF) results.

8.   When enough organs fail, so does the heart. The result is terminal cardiogenic shock — complete energy failure of the myocardium — and death.

Standard treatments

Is anything really "standard" in the treatment of shock? You bet — as for *any* condition, always pay careful attention to Airway, Breathing, and Circulation. Most agree that the following are *still* in order for patients with shock:

- Oxygen with any required ventilatory assistance; airway maintenance.

- Attention to the possibility of cervical spine injury in trauma.

- Stop exsanguinating hemorrhage if present.

- Apply MAST suit (pneumatic antishock trousers) — inflate as necessary; may need to avoid in cardiogenic shock. In some circles, the use of MAST is controversial.

- Trendelenburg positioning unless shortness of breath predominates or the patient becomes worse.

"STANDARD" TREATMENT FOR SHOCK"

- **ABC's**
- **Attention to possible C-spine injury**
- **Stop hemorrhage**
- **MAST suit**
- **Trendelenburg position**
- **IV fluids**
- **Pressors**

- Two intravenous lines — the fluid of choice is debatable; either Ringer's lactate or normal saline is fairly safe under most circumstances. Warmed fluids are better, if possible. A fluid challenge (250-1000 cc over 10-15 minutes) is reasonable unless the patient is in fulminant cardiac failure.

- Pressors — these agents elevate blood pressure. If possible, the patient should be euvolemic prior to initiating pressor therapy. A combination of pressors (e.g., dopamine and norepinephrine) as a "catecholamine cocktail" may be more effective than a single agent.

Pressor Agents

What's new on the "standard" pressor drugs? Below is a summary of current data on the three most common pressor agents.[48] Please note that dobutamine is actually a positive inotropic agent, and that its pressor effect is indirect (increasing the cardiac output).

- **Dopamine** (DA) is a naturally occurring catecholamine that is the immediate precursor of norepinephrine (NE). It is indicated in hypotension unresponsive to fluids, and in oliguric states. DA inhibits insulin secretion and may contribute to the hyperglycemia frequently found in critically ill patients. DA stimulates dopaminergic, α, and β-1 receptors.

  There are two known dopaminergic (DA) receptors. The **DA-1 receptor** is linked to adenyl cyclase. Its activation leads to increased levels of intracellular cAMP, causing smooth muscle relaxation. The greatest number of DA1 receptors are in the renal and mesenteric vascular beds but are also found in cerebral, coronary, and skeletal muscle, and also cutaneous vessels. Activation of **DA-2 receptors**, on the other hand, inhibits adenyl cyclase, reducing NE release from cardiac and vascular nerves. DA-2 receptors also inhibit sympathetic activity by reducing ganglionic transmission.

*[**NOTE**: Several other DA receptors have been described in the neurology literature. They are not relevant to the use of DA as a pressor agent and have been excluded here.]*

DOPAMINE RECEPTORS

Receptor	Location	Actions
DA-1	Renal, mesenteric vascular beds; also in cerebral, coronary, skeletal muscle; skin vessels	Increases cAMP by activation of adenyl cyclase, causing smooth muscle relaxation
DA-2	Heart, blood vessels	Inhibits adenyl cyclase, reduces NE release from nerves; inhibits sympathetic activity by reducing ganglionic transmission

The DA-1 receptor agonist fenoldopam (Corlopam®) has been shown to be of benefit experimentally in managing hypertension and heart failure, and in preserving renal function.[49] However, most studies in humans have not demonstrated prevention of acute renal failure in high-risk patients or improved outcome in those with established acute renal failure.[50]

- **Dobutamine** (DBT) is a synthetic catecholamine that acts as a relatively powerful inotrope. It is indicated in low cardiac output states where adequate preload is present. DBT is contraindicated in patients with asymmetrical septal hypertrophy (ASH), since increased contractility may worsen obstruction. DBT primarily stimulates β-1 receptors with a small β-2 and α effect.

- **Norepinephrine** (NE) is a naturally occurring catecholamine that directly stimulates β-1 and α-adrenergic receptors. NE is primarily indicated in tricyclic antidepressant overdose patients who do not respond to dopamine. In addition, data show that low dose NE increases BP and urine flow, often with reversal of shock in patients with septic shock.[51]

• **Epinephrine** (E) is a naturally occurring catecholamine with α, β-1, and β-2 effects. It is used in cardiac arrest, anaphylactic shock, and asthma and may be helpful in dopamine-resistant septic shock.[52]

SUMMARY OF "PRESSORS"

DRUG:	RECEPTORS STIMULATED:
Dopamine	Dopaminergic, α, β-1
Dobutamine	Primarily β-1; some β-2, α
Norepinephrine	β-1, α
Epinephrine	α, β-1, β-2

Controversial treatments — the fluid debate

OBJECTIVE: **Defend the following statements:**
- **"Shock does not necessarily equal hypotension."**
- **"Raising the blood pressure in shock may worsen bleeding."**
- **"We really don't know how best to monitor a patient in shock."**
- **"There are no compelling data to change fluid therapy at this time."**

Colloid versus Crystalloid

Which fluid, colloid or crystalloid? The debate whether to use colloid (e.g., albumin, dextran, hypertonic saline), crystalloid (e.g., normal saline, Ringer's Lactate), or a combination continues. In general, colloid therapy restores intravascular volume more effectively and requires only about one half the fluid volume of a crystalloid. Frequently, patients treated with crystalloid are inadequately fluid resuscitated. If significant anemia is present, red blood cells should be transfused to optimize oxygen carrying capacity, whatever the fluid chosen.

Crystalloids do not contribute to colloid oncotic pressure. They rapidly equilibrate with interstitial water so that only about 20 to 30% of the administered fluid remains within the vascular system after three to four hours. Advocates of crystalloids, on the other hand, point out that colloids may leak from capillaries in shock and that a significant amount ends up in the interstitium anyway. Other data suggest that colloid administration, while it increases colloid osmotic pressure, neither increases nor decreases the leakage of water or albumin from the pulmonary capillaries into the lung interstitium.[53]

The following conclusions may be reached safely regarding colloids versus crystalloids: **[FIGURE 6-13]**

- Hemodynamic stability and cardiac function can be restored to the same physiologic end points using crystalloid or colloid, but two to four times the volume of crystalloid must be infused compared with colloid.

- Blood and colloid solutions are more efficient in rapidly expanding intravascular volume.

- Infusion of large amounts of saline during resuscitation results in marked reduction of colloid oncotic pressure and hematocrit.[54] Patients resuscitated with crystalloid tend to develop peripheral edema that may be mistaken as fluid overload. The result may be inadequate restoration of volume.

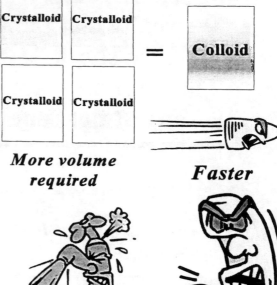

Figure 6-13 — Summary of Colloids vs Crystalloids

- There is no consistent evidence that either fluid regimen reliably affects morbidity or mortality more favorably than the other, particularly if patients are closely monitored for signs of improvement or complications of therapy.

- Therapy with colloids is significantly more costly than therapy with crystalloids. If one chooses colloid, two reasonable alternatives in sepsis are albumin-containing solutions

REMEMBER: There is no consistent evidence that *either* fluid regimen affects morbidity or mortality more favorably than the other.

or hydroxyethyl starch (HES). Due to significant cost savings and approximately equal efficacy to 5% albumin infusion, HES seems an excellent alternative. HES continues to expand plasma volume for 24 to 36 hours.[55]

Are Fluids Harmful in Shock?

What about raising the BP; won't this increase hemorrhage? In animal models of uncontrolled hemorrhage, immediate IV administration of hypertonic saline/dextran significantly increased hemorrhage volume and mortality. However, the accentuation of hemorrhage and reduction in survival were not as great as that produced by the standard practice of replacing the lost blood with three times that volume of Ringer's lactate.[56] Another study demonstrated that small-volume hypertonic saline administration led to increased bleeding and hemodynamic instability but no increased mortality. The animals with no treatment, which best simulates the "scoop-and-run policy" of EMS in the field, were hemodynamically most stable, with minimal blood loss.[57]

Can fluids be delayed safely until the time of operation? Apparently the answer is "yes," *if* you live in Houston, Texas. In a controversial study, victims of penetrating truncal injury received IV fluid resuscitation either in the ambulance and in the ED before surgery, or received IV fluid resuscitation only at the time of surgical intervention. There were no significant differences in the rate of survival until hospital discharge.

The data did not include patients with blunt trauma. The "nonfluid" patients actually ended up receiving nearly as much as the "fluid patients" by the time surgery took place. In addition, investigators claimed a five minute transport time to a single major trauma center in Houston from anywhere in the city — all I can say is, "Have you ever driven in Houston?" Further study is necessary to determine if it is advantageous to delay fluid resuscitation until surgical intervention.[58]

Isn't the question really, "Should we give fluids at all?" Based on animal experiments performed three decades ago, the traditional management of hypovolemic hemorrhagic shock includes adequate circulatory volume with aggressive initial infusion of crystalloid solution. However, in several recent animal studies, investigators have found that aggressive treatment with fluids before control of bleeding results in a higher mortality rate, especially if blood pressure is elevated.[59] This notion has been supported, to some extent, by the Houston data on patients with penetrating injuries to the torso.[60] Often, even significant injuries clot and stop bleeding. It is probably disadvantageous to vigorously resuscitate with either fluids, a MAST suit, or pressors to artificially elevate the blood pressure, as this may dislodge a soft clot and increase bleeding.[61]

REMEMBER: Unless the patient has penetrating truncal trauma, "standard" fluid therapy is still considered appropriate by most experts.

What's the "bottom line?" The situation is far less clear for blunt trauma. As a general rule, unless the patient has penetrating truncal trauma, "standard" fluid therapy is still considered appropriate by most experts. This may change in the near future, as further research becomes available. We really don't know the best parameter to monitor in shock anyway (blood pressure, cardiac output, and tissue perfusion do not necessarily correlate).[62] It is perfectly logical that some level of perfusion maintains tissue viability pending more definitive treatment, if necessary, without furthering bleeding. We just need to figure out what that level is and how to monitor it. It's probably *not* "normal BP."

REMEMBER: We really don't know the best parameter to monitor in shock.

Newer treatments

Naloxone
- Naloxone
- Why does naloxone work, even if just in animal models?
- Endorphins block sympathetic discharge, leading to hypotension
- What are the clinical data?
- Why not try naloxone in acute CHF or cardiogenic shock?
- The bottom line on naloxone in shock

Corticosteroids
- Why corticosteroids?
- Might lower physiologic doses be helpful?
- What do the data show regarding adrenal insufficiency and shock?
- The bottom line on corticosteroids in shock

Pentoxifylline
- Pentoxifylline (PTX)
- Animal studies of pentoxifylline
- Human studies of pentoxifylline
- What's the bottom line regarding PTX?

Fibronectin

Thyroid Releasing Hormone (TRH)
- TRH
- Is there actual thyroid hormone deficiency in shock?
- What data support a role for TRH in treatment of shock?
- What if I'm not a rat; will TRH help?

ACTH
- ACTH
- What do the data show?
- What about ACTH in septic shock?
- What's the bottom line?

Numerous trials are underway evaluating a variety of potentially promising anti-shock therapies.[63] Besides immune therapy, discussed earlier, the most interesting include naloxone, corticosteroids, pentoxifylline, fibronectin, TRH, and ACTH.

Naloxone

Naloxone — The narcotic antagonist naloxone (Narcan®) produced excellent results in a variety of animal studies.[64] Unfortunately, human studies have shown severe adverse reactions including pulmonary edema, seizures, severe hypotension, and asystole.[65] Naloxone is considered investigational at this time.

Newer Treatments for Shock:

- Naloxone
- Corticosteroids
- Pentoxifylline
- Fibronectin
- TRH
- ACTH

Why does naloxone work, even if just in animal models? Theoretically, naloxone may be helpful in shock because the stress leads to production of adrenocorticotropic hormone (ACTH). ACTH is a cleavage product of a larger molecule. The remaining products of ACTH production are endorphins, endogenous morphine-like compounds. So, ACTH production in shock is accompanied by endorphin production, which may lead to hypotension. **[FIGURE 6-14]**

- Experimental findings show that morphine pellet implantation in mice results in the escape of gram-negative organisms from the gastrointestinal tract (remember the role of the intestine in shock?). This leads to the hypothesis that morphine used postoperatively or chronically for analgesia may serve as a cofactor in the precipitation of sepsis and shock.[66] So, reversing deleterious effects of either morphine or endorphin by naloxone makes good pharmacological sense.

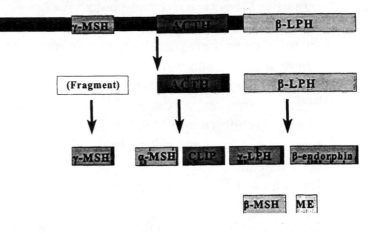

Figure 6-14 — A large promolecule is cleaved into ACTH, endorphins, and met-enkephalin (ME), and MSH fragments.

Endorphins block sympathetic discharge, leading to hypotension. In hemorrhage, when blood loss exceeds approximately 20% of total blood volume, hypotension develops abruptly due to a decrease in vascular resistance. This vasodilation is accompanied by decreased plasma NE levels and decreased sympathetic nerve activity. Therefore, the transition from normotension to hypotension during hemorrhage involves a decrease in vascular resistance, associated with a decrease in sympathetic nerve activity. Opioid receptor blockade with naloxone reverses acute hemorrhagic hypotension by increasing vascular resistance. The increase in resistance is accompanied by increased plasma NE and increased sympathetic nerve activity.[67] Naloxone's reversal of the hypotension suggests that central involvement of endogenous opioid peptides is the cause of hypotension during blood loss.[68]

REMEMBER: Release of endorphins is a normal regulatory system to alleviate pain and modulate discharge of the sympathetic nervous system during stress (e.g., hemorrhage).

What are the clinical data?
Naloxone infusion is clinically effective in improving the hemodynamic profile of a subgroup of patients with severe early hyperdynamic septic shock, but does not appear to improve the overall survival rate.[69]

- In one study, patients with documented septic shock resistant to a one-liter fluid challenge were given naloxone, initial bolus 0.03 mg/kg, followed by infusion at a rate of 0.2 mg/kg/h over one hour. A significant increase in mean arterial pressure (MAP) over baseline was noted at five minutes, as well as a significant increase in systolic arterial pressure over pre-naloxone levels at five minutes and at one hour. There was a nonsignificant increase in cardiac index, pulmonary capillary wedge pressure, and systemic vascular resistance (SVR). No side effects were noted. No effect on survival was demonstrated, but there was no negative effect on mortality, either. By increasing MAP, naloxone may serve as a temporizing agent during the treatment of patients critically ill with septic shock.[70] In a Chinese study, naloxone was also shown to decrease production of lactic acid in patients with shock, though no differences in patient mortality were noted.[71]

- In another study, thirteen consecutive patients with documented septic shock and resistance to a one-liter fluid challenge underwent invasive hemodynamic monitoring and the administration of naloxone by initial bolus of 0.03 mg/kg followed by infusion at a rate of 0.2 mg/kg. over one hour. Naloxone resulted in a significant rise in mean arterial pressure (MAP) over baseline at both 5 minutes and at 30 minutes. There was also a significant increase in systolic arterial pressure over the same time frame. There was a moderate, nonsignificant increase in cardiac index, pulmonary capillary wedge pressure, and systemic vascular resistance. Though no side effects were noted, there was no effect on survival or mortality. The authors suggested that naloxone may serve as a temporizing agent during the treatment of patients critically ill with septic shock.[72] Similar findings were also noted in a related study.[73]

Naloxone has been tried experimentally in:

- **Hemorrhagic shock (good results)**
- **Septic shock (no survival benefit)**
- **Chronic CHF (no effect)**

Why not try naloxone in acute CHF or cardiogenic shock? It's tempting to try giving naloxone in patients with acute CHF, but I think we face a potential dilemma. Remember that endorphins suppress sympathetic nervous system action. In a sense, the release of beta endorphin is nature's way of modulating excessive sympathetic stimulation that occurs in CHF (see **Chapter 3**). The effects of opioid antagonism are mediated, in part, by enhancing endogenous beta-adrenergic actions *in vivo*.[74] Blocking endorphins with naloxone might have the equivalent physiological effect of giving an epinephrine bolus to patients — and I doubt that any of us would seriously consider this as "routine care."

The bottom line on naloxone in shock — Only a few studies have investigated the use of naloxone in human septic shock. In experimental studies, and in some patients in early septic shock, naloxone has caused a transient pressor effect. Of these studies, most have not been able to show a beneficial effect regarding survival. A recent meta-analysis of five naloxone trials showed that the drug was associated with significant hemodynamic improvement, but that the case fatality rate was not changed. The investigators concluded that the clinical usefulness of naloxone to treat shock remains to be determined and that additional randomized clinical trials are needed to assess its usefulness.[75]

REPORTED SIDE EFFECTS OF NALOXONE IN SHOCK:

- **Hypotension**
- **Hypertension**
- **Ventricular arrhythmias**
- **Acute pulmonary edema**

Treatment is not completely free of side effects, some of which are life threatening. Episodes of hypotension, hypertension, ventricular arrhythmias, and acute pulmonary edema have been reported. These adverse effects are thought to be caused by centrally mediated catecholamine responses to exogenous opiate reversal. In the opinion of most clinicians, the use of naloxone should currently be considered investigational, until further studies clarify the role of opiate antagonism in septic shock.[76]

REMEMBER: Naloxone should currently be considered investigational, until further studies clarify the role of opiate antagonism in septic shock.

Corticosteroids

Why corticosteroids? The basis for use of corticosteroids in shock originated in the studies of Schumer and colleagues, who showed that large doses of steroids (e.g., methylprednisolone, 30 mg/kg IV, one or more times daily) led to significant improvement in survival of patients with septic shock.[77] Others were unable to replicate their excellent results.

Results of three large clinical studies failed to demonstrate a direct benefit of corticosteroids in shock, especially when used in "superpharmacological doses." None demonstrated a direct increase in mortality but morbidity from secondary infection *was* increased. There is also an increased risk of liver and kidney dysfunction following high dose steroid therapy in shock.[78] Though theoretically sound and experimentally attractive, the emerging consensus among clinicians is that currently, high-dose corticosteroids should not be used for treatment of septic shock.[79]

Might lower physiologic replacement doses be helpful? On the other hand, physiologic replacement doses of steroids *may* be beneficial. A significant number of patients with septic shock have an inadequate corticotropin stimulation test result. These patients tend to do poorly when compared with septic patients who have an adequate response. These findings suggest that some patients with septic shock may have

> ***REMEMBER:* Critically ill patients often have acquired adrenal insufficiency; physiologic corticosteroid replacement may be helpful.**

relative adrenocortical insufficiency that should respond to a trial of *replacement* steroids instead of *high* dose steroids.[80] If direct tests of corticotropin reserve are impractical, treatment with glucocorticoids is warranted.[81]

What do the data show regarding adrenal insufficiency and shock? Over time, more and more data have supported the contention of acquired adrenal insufficiency in shock. The adrenocortical response to corticotropin (synthetic ACTH) is attenuated in patients with septic shock and circulatory failure. This attenuated adrenocortical responsiveness is likely due to effects of circulating mediators from the systemic inflammatory response.[82] Besides adults, recent studies document that adrenal insufficiency is common in children with septic shock. It is associated with an increased vasopressor requirement and duration of shock.[83]

Suspect adrenal insufficiency in patients with septic shock who do not respond to conventional treatment. Performing the ACTH infusion test and initiating a trial of stress doses of glucocorticoids pending the results is a reasonable strategy in this situation.[84] The standard-dose (250 micrograms) rapid ACTH infusion test appears to be adequate for detection of adrenal insufficiency.

> *REMEMBER:* **Performing an ACTH infusion test and initiating a trial of stress doses of glucocorticoids pending the results is a reasonable strategy in patients with shock.**

- A recent prospective study in adults demonstrated that infusion of "stress doses" of hydrocortisone reduced the time to cessation of vasopressor therapy in human septic shock (loading dose of 100 mg given within 30 min and followed by a continuous infusion of 0.18 mg/ kg/h; when septic shock had been reversed, the dose of hydrocortisone was reduced to 0.08 mg/kg/h; this dose was kept constant for six days). This was associated with a trend to earlier resolution of sepsis-induced organ dysfunctions. Overall shock reversal and mortality were not significantly different between the steroid and nonsteroid groups.[85]

- Other data suggest that hydrocortisone improves the pressor response to NE. This effect appears to be more marked in patients with impaired adrenal function reserve. Since impaired adrenal function reserve may partly be accounted for by the depressed pressor sensitivity to NE, addition of physiological doses of hydrocortisone (50 mg IV bolus) appears to be beneficial.[86]

- Other investigators found that moderate doses of hydrocortisone (100 mg IV, three times daily for five days) may be beneficial, even in the absence of adrenal insufficiency. Shock reversal within seven days after the onset of corticosteroid therapy was a very strong predictor of survival. Administration of modest doses of hydrocortisone in the setting of pressor-dependent septic shock for a mean of 96 hours resulted in a significant improvement in hemodynamics and a beneficial effect on survival. There were no significant differences in outcome in responders and nonresponders to a short corticotropin test. Thus, the beneficial effects do not appear related to adrenocortical insufficiency.[87]

The bottom line on corticosteroids in shock. A recent meta-analysis of studies on *high-dose* steroids demonstrated:

- Corticosteroids appear to increase mortality in patients with overwhelming infection.

- There are no beneficial effects in persons with septic shock.

- Patients who received steroids had a trend toward increased mortality overall. A similar trend was observed for patients with septic shock.

> *REMEMBER:* High-dose steroids in shock are unwarranted at this time.

- No difference in secondary infection rates was demonstrated in corticosteroid-treated patients with sepsis or septic shock. However, there was a trend toward increased mortality from secondary infections in patients receiving corticosteroids.

- The occurrence rate of gastrointestinal bleeding was increased slightly in the steroid treatment group.

The study concluded: "Current evidence provides no support for the use of [high dose] corticosteroids in patients with sepsis or septic shock, and suggests that their use may be harmful."[88] These results were similar to those found in other studies.[89]

However, recent work, cited above and involving mostly hydrocortisone, now suggests two intriguing possibilities:

- Acquired adrenal insufficiency may occur in shock and respond to physiologic or moderate doses of steroids (unlike the "megadoses" used in the earlier work).

- Even some patients without significant adrenal insufficiency appeared to respond to moderate doses of hydrocortisone, *without* any of the severe side effects noted in the high-dose methylprednisolone studies.

Putting it all together, I think we will see a resurgence of moderate doses of hydrocortisone used routinely in shock. No, it's not yet a "standard of care," but may well be, depending on how the data pan out. Certainly, if a patient has acquired adrenal insufficiency, and we fail to treat it appropriately (read my lips — hydrocortisone), we've committed negligence. The potential legal implications are (and this is *not legal advice*):

REMEMBER:

- **Physiologic or moderate doses of steroids may treat acquired adrenal insufficiency in shock.**

- **Some patients without adrenal insufficiency respond to moderate doses of hydrocortisone, *without* any of the severe side effects noted in the high-dose methylprednisolone studies.**

- Either we test all patients in shock for acquired adrenal insufficiency **OR**

Welcome Back Steroids (whether we like it or not!)

- We empirically give physiologic to moderate doses of hydrocortisone to all patients with shock.

Pentoxifylline

Pentoxifylline — Used in intermittent claudication for years, the methylxanthine drug pentoxifylline (PTX; Trental®) is thought to improve microcirculatory flow by influencing red blood cell deformity in hypoxic areas. PTX potentiates the anti-inflammatory actions of adenosine, prostacyclin, and prostaglandins of the E series by its synergistic action on intracellular cyclic AMP. It may have additional effects as well, including modification of platelet aggregation.[90]

PRINCIPLE: If you're going to block "stuff," you need to block *all* the stuff.

Several studies indicate that PTX is also a potent inhibitor of tumor necrosis factor (TNF-α) release. It is uncertain whether this occurs via the drug's methylxanthine action (inhibition of phosphodiesterase, leading to increased levels of cAMP). Suggestive is the fact that another methylxanthine derivative, amrinone, also decreases production of TNF-α during sepsis.[91]

PTX inhibits oxygen free-radical production by polymorphonuclear leukocytes, the aggregation of platelets, disseminated intravascular coagulation, and the production of cytokines. Consequently, PTX improves perfusion in the microcirculation as well as tissue oxygenation.[92]

Potential Beneficial Actions of Pentoxifylline in Shock:

- **Improves microcirculatory flow**
- **Potentiates anti-inflammatory action of adenosine, prostacyclin, and E-prostaglandins**
- **Inhibits TNF-α**
- **Decreasea neutrophil action**
- **Inhibits free radicals**
- **Antifibrogenic action**
- **Decreases cytokine production**

Animal studies of pentoxifylline — Pentoxifylline (PTX) appears to have a "therapeutic window." It only works when given within a specific, and as yet undefined, period of time. Animal work suggests that once full-blown septic shock is established, PTX by itself is not curative.[93]

- In a rat study of hemorrhagic shock, PTX treatment led to significantly increased survival, possibly by blocking adhesion of leukocytes to the endothelium of blood vessels.[94]

- PTX restored the impaired Ca^{2+} influx movement and prevented increased hepatocyte lipid peroxidation in a rat model. Since altered cellular Ca^{2+} regulation is a key event of cellular dysfunction, resuscitation with PTX after hemorrhagic shock may provide an adjuvant therapeutic tool to prevent postischemic hepatic failure.[95]

- PTX inhibits endotoxemia and lipopolysaccharide (LPS)-induced release of TNF-α. In addition, in a rat model, it inhibited production of bacterial superantigens like staphylococcal enterotoxin B (SEB) and toxic shock syndrome toxin 1 (TSST-1).[96]

- When compared with controls, treatment with PTX plus thalidomide reduced mortality in a model of septic shock. The tissue damage was less severe in animals from the groups that received PTX or PTX plus thalidomide. PTX seems to potentiate the beneficial effects of thalidomide, reducing mortality and attenuating the pathological changes produced by septic shock.[97] (Yes, it's the same thalidomide that caused birth defects, but now it's being re-evaluated as an anti-inflammatory and anti-tumor agent!)

- PTX, used as a long-term continuous infusion, can be harmful during gram-negative septic shock. The relative risk of death was significantly increased with PTX therapy in a dose-dependent fashion. Investigators suggest that high PTX levels slowed endotoxin clearance, resulting in high levels of endotoxin and increased proinflammatory mediator release and death.[98]

- PTX ameliorated some of the deleterious hemodynamic manifestations of streptococcal sepsis and resulted in improved survival in a piglet model, without significantly modifying plasma TNF-α levels.[99]

- PTX improves survival and reduces blood concentrations of TNF-α, IL-6, lactate, and endothelin-1 in fulminant intra-abdominal sepsis in rats. The primary effect of PTX in this sequence is probably reduction of TNF-α.[100]

Human studies of pentoxifylline — Though human studies are exciting, some of the "hype" needs to be tempered by the ongoing debate as to whether PTX inhibits production of only TNF-α, or if other cytokines are also affected.

- Continuous intravenous administration of PTX (1 mg/kg/h; maximum, 1800 mg/d) beneficially influenced cardiopulmonary dysfunction in patients with sepsis. The 28-day mortality rate was 30% in PTX-treated patients and 33% in the placebo group. Hospital mortality was 41% in the PTX group and 54% in the placebo group.[101]

- PTX at 1 mg/kg/h over 24 hours led to significant decreases in TNF-α levels. At the same time, IL-6 levels were significantly increased. In the therapy group, the systemic vascular resistance was significantly higher after 24 hours, whereas the cardiac index declined. These data suggest that inhibiting a single mediator in severe septic shock cannot stop the inflammatory overreaction process.[102]

- Patients were randomly assigned to receive either PTX (1 mg/kg) followed by an infusion of 1.5 mg/kg/h for 24 hours or placebo. In PTX-treated patients, at 24 hours, serum concentrations of TNF-α were significantly lower compared with controls. Serum concentrations of IL-6 and IL-8 did not differ between the two treatment groups. Five patients in the PTX group and four patients in the placebo group died.[103]

Not all data suggest that the sole effect of PTX involves suppression of TNF-α. In one study, PTX was shown to diminish strongly production of IL-2, interferon-gamma, IL-1, IL-10, and TNF-α. The most profound effects *were*, however, on TNF-α.[104] Additionally, PTX inhibits expression of the inflammatory adhesion molecule ICAM-1 in human mononuclear cells.[105] Taken together, these data demonstrate that PTX possesses a much broader spectrum of activity on cytokine production than was initially described.

What's the bottom line regarding PTX? My "crystal ball" tells me that we will be using PTX in many patients with shock, especially due to sepsis, *in combination* with other agents.

Fibronectin

Fibronectin — Fibronectin is an α-2 globulin, also known as cold-insoluble globulin or surface-binding glycoprotein. It is thought to modulate the phagocytic response of hepatic macrophage cells. Fibronectin deficiency has been demonstrated repeatedly in trauma and postoperative patients with sepsis, and correlates temporally with diminished phagocytic activity, increased vascular permeability, impaired wound healing, and pulmonary failure. Both plasma fibronectin and tissue fibronectin have been postulated as contributing to systemic defense against invasive infection.

Cryoprecipitate was found to correct fibronectin deficiency, thus leading to experimental and clinical trials of cryoprecipitate and fibronectin infusion. Overall, plasma fibronectin has been consistently shown to decrease in critically ill patients with sepsis, multiple organ failure, and coagulopathy, though a single measurement of plasma level cannot be used as a marker or prognostic factor. Plasma fibronectin levels are decreased in children with meningococcemia, especially those with shock who die. This decrease is associated with high IL-6 levels.[106]

FIBRONECTIN:

- **Modulates phagocytic response of hepatic macrophages**

- **Low levels in trauma, postoperative sepsis**

- **Low levels correlate with diminished phagocytic activity, increased vascular permeability, impaired wound healing, and pulmonary failure**

In some instances, fibronectin might improve target organ function in septic states. However, the clinical use of cryoprecipitate or fibronectin for the prophylaxis or treatment of sepsis or septic shock is not supported by present data.[107]

Thyroid Releasing Hormone (TRH)

Thyroid releasing hormone (TRH) — Although the mechanism of action of TRH in shock is not completely understood, it clearly acts by an antagonism of the endorphin system, but perhaps *not* at the opiate receptor.[108] This hypothesis is based on the fact that TRH reverses the pharmacologic and physiologic effects of endorphins without modifying analgesia. Not all experts agree, however, suggesting that instead of working via an alternative pathway, TRH somehow modifies opiate receptors.[109]

Limited work in head injured animals also suggests that TRH's ability to antagonize many pathophysiological effects of endogenous opioids or exogenous opiates *except* their analgesic effects is highly beneficial.[110] The complete mechanism is probably a combination of opiate receptor antagonism and autonomic nervous system stimulation.[111]

Potential Mechanisms of TRH in Shock:

- **Endorphin antagonism**
- **Sympathetic stimulation**
- **Vagal stimulation**
- **Free radical antagonism**

Recent studies have shown that afferent vagal fibers, brain cholinergic neurons, and central muscarinic receptors play a role in the mechanism of the anti-shock effect of TRH.[112] In addition, it is also thought to antagonize directly the deleterious actions of free radicals.[113]

Is there actual thyroid hormone deficiency in shock? Data indicate that patients with septic shock present an altered hypothalamic-pituitary-thyroid axis. There are significant differences in thyroid function between survivors and nonsurvivors. Survivors are characterized by a greater thyroid-stimulating hormone (TSH) response to TRH, indicating a less deranged hypothalamic-pituitary-thyroid axis. Thyroid function improves in survivors, but not in non-survivors.[114]

What data support a potential role for TRH in treatment of shock? The value of TRH in improving hemodynamic function has been documented in animal models of both hemorrhagic and endotoxic shock including primates. Survival improvement has been documented for hemorrhagic shock, but not consistently for endotoxic shock. Here are some of the data:

• TRH significantly improved 3-day survival in a canine model of hemorrhagic shock. During uncompensated shock, TRH-treated dogs had significantly higher mean arterial pressure, cardiac index, stroke index, right and left ventricular stroke work indexes, and arterial pH than control animals. At the conclusion of the experiment, however, there were few differences between control and TRH-treated animals. These results suggest that improved 3-day survival in canine hemorrhagic shock might be related to hemodynamic improvement by TRH at a critical stage of circulatory collapse.[115]

REMEMBER: TRH appears to be a physiologic opiate antagonist without effects on pain responsiveness.

• TRH was beneficial in a canine model of hemorrhagic shock. Animals receiving TRH manifested improved hemodynamics, despite increased levels of beta-endorphin, suggesting an endorphin-blocking effect of TRH.[116]

• Although no difference in survival existed, TRH had a slower onset, but more sustained effect, on MAP than did epinephrine and normal saline in a rabbit model of anaphylactic shock.[117]

• TRH significantly improved cardiovascular function when it was injected intravenously into conscious rats subjected to experimental endotoxic or hemorrhagic shock. It appears to be a physiologic opiate antagonist without effects on pain responsiveness.[118]

• TRH has been reported to reduce endotoxin-induced hypotension and mortality rate in conscious rats. These effects may be transient, especially when TRH is used as monotherapy.[119]

• In a rat model of volume-controlled hemorrhagic shock with 100% mortality in saline-treated animals, TRH injection led to significant improvement. Four mg/kg induced the prompt and sustained disappearance of the EKG and EEG signs of heart and brain ischemia, along with the reversal of hypotension and respiratory depression and with 100% survival rate at the end of the two hour observation period.[120]

- The thyrotropin releasing hormone analogue, RGH 2202, reverses experimental hemorrhagic shock in rats.[121]

What if I'm not a rat; will TRH help? Unfortunately, there are no studies in humans that, at this point, support the therapeutic use of TRH in shock.

<u>ACTH</u>

ACTH — Adrenocorticotrophic hormone (ACTH) is secreted by the anterior pituitary gland and stimulates production of corticosteroids by the adrenal cortex. Interesting and impressive effects have been noted in experimental studies. While having negligible effects on cardiovascular function in the normal animal, ACTH induces a potent and sustained reversal of otherwise rapidly fatal hemorrhage-induced hypovolemic shock in rats and dogs. The main sites of action are thought to be at the peripheral level.

ACTH-induced reversal of hemorrhagic shock is an extra-hormonal, adrenal-independent effect, because it is not affected by adrenalectomy. ACTH is antagonized by morphine, and requires the functional integrity of the sympathetic nervous system and afferent vagal fibers to work. The response is associated with a massive increase in the circulating blood volume, likely due to a mobilization from peripheral pooling sites. In addition, venous blood flow in peripheral vascular beds is restored and the venous pO_2 normalized.[122]

> **REMEMBER: ACTH appears to mobilize blood from peripherally pooled sites leading to rapid restoration of circulating blood volume. Inhibition of nitric oxide production, an intrinsic vasodilator, may be the key mechanism by which ACTH works.**

What do the data show? Relatively few studies on ACTH exist, compared to some of the other compounds we've discussed. Here are some of the most interesting:

- Sustained increase in plasma corticosterone levels following hemorrhage and resuscitation have been shown in animal models. Depression of hepatic function during hemorrhage leads to decreased hepatic production of 11β-hydroxysteroid dehydrogenase (11β-HSD), a microsomal enzyme responsible for the degradation of bioactive corticosterone. The high level of corticosterone negatively regulates corticotropin release, further reducing adrenal responsiveness to corticotropin stimulation. Thus, the liver appears to play an important role in regulating adrenal function following trauma and severe hemorrhage.[123] This mechanism may explain observed abnormalities in corticotropin stimulation tests noted in patients with shock.

- Anesthetized rats subjected to hemorrhagic shock developed a massive increase in nitric oxide (NO)-hemoglobin, associated with a fall in mean arterial pressure, pulse pressure, respiratory rate and heart rate. Levels of NO-hemoglobin continued to increase despite IV saline and 100% of the animals died within thirty minutes. IV ACTH led to prompt disappearance of NO-hemoglobin and a parallel improvement of cardiovascular and respiratory functions.[124]

- In a model of volume-controlled hemorrhagic shock in rats, invariably leading to death within 30 minutes of bleeding termination, the intravenous injection of ACTH restored cardiovascular and respiratory functions and greatly prolonged survival. Pretreatment with nitric oxidase synthetase (NOS) inhibitors potentiated the effects of ACTH. On the other hand, pretreatment with L-arginine, the substrate of NOS, blocked beneficial actions of ACTH. These findings suggest that inhibition of NO overproduction is involved in the mechanism of action of ACTH in shock reversal.[125]

- In another rat model of hemorrhagic shock, ACTH bolus led to an improvement in cardiovascular and respiratory parameters similar to improvement using "standard dose" norepinephrine.[126]

- The cardiovascular and metabolic responses to treatment with ACTH(1-24) were investigated in a porcine model of septicemia. Infusion of ACTH appeared to have no beneficial effects in this study.[127]

- In a single case report, a 45 year-old woman sustained a spontaneous rupture of the right atrium in the intensive care unit after mitral valve replacement. During the surgery, in addition to fluids, 10 mg ACTH (1-24) was injected into a peripheral vein. Although the blood loss was significant, the authors note that the patient's condition improved rapidly after the occlusion of the atrial tear with an initial small volume of transfusion.[128]

What about ACTH in septic shock? As noted below, the data are sparse for ACTH, but better for so-called ACTH "fragments," such as MSH. Native ACTH and "fragments" work equally well in hemorrhagic shock, however.[129] The reason so much research has been devoted to ACTH in hemorrhagic shock might be a big hint — it works best here. Current thinking is that the mechanism of ACTH in hemorrhage is to rapidly

REMEMBER: Current data suggests that ACTH leads to rapid mobilization of pooled blood into the peripheral circulation.

mobilize blood pooled in peripheral reserve organs, such as the liver. In fact, hepatectomized animals fail to respond to ACTH in experimental hemorrhagic shock. Similar results have been noted following experimental splenectomy.[130]

Alpha (α)-melanostimulating hormone (MSH) and ACTH have identical amino acid sequences at positions 1 through 13 because MSH is formed from ACTH cleavage. **[FIGURE 6-15]** It should come as no surprise

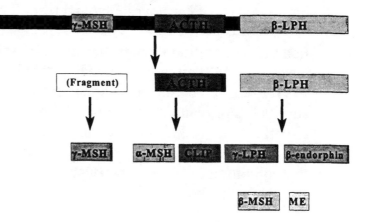

Figure 6-15 — A large promolecule is cleaved into ACTH, endorphins, met-enkephalin (ME), and MSH fragments.

that the two molecules have similar physiological activity.[131] Collectively, ACTH and all of its cleavage byproducts are known as "melanocortins." ACTH is the most potent.[132]

Studies using ACTH (amino acids 1 through 24) in sepsis have been few and far between. The one noted immediately above showed no beneficial effect. This appears not to be the case with α-MSH. Current data suggests:

- α-MSH reduces signs of systemic inflammation in mice with endotoxemia, including increased levels of serum tumor necrosis factor-alpha and nitric oxide.[133]

- α-MSH prevents LPS-induced hepatic inflammation by inhibiting production of chemoattractant molecules (chemokines), which then modulate infiltration of inflammatory cells.[134]

What's the bottom line? Again, a "wait and see" attitude is necessary as studies in humans are seriously lacking in this area. The **TABLE** below summarizes the proposed mechanisms of these newer therapeutic modalities.

TABLE — SUMMARY OF NEWER THERAPEUTIC MODALITIES

TREATMENT:	PROPOSED MECHANISM(S):
Naloxone	• Opiod receptor blockade
Corticosteroids	• High dose = empirical use (*not recommended*) • Physiologic doses = replacement of acquired adrenal insufficiency
Pentoxifylline	• Blocks release of TNF-α • Inhibits free radical generation • Decreases cytokine production
Fibronectin	• Modulates phagocytic response of macrophages
TRH	• Antagonism of endorphin system • Likely *not* at opiod receptor • Free radical antagonism
ACTH	• Mobilization of pooled peripheral blood • Inhibition of nitric oxide production • Melanocortin production (α-MSH) inhibits cytokines

Summary

Shock is a clinical syndrome involving widespread cellular dysfunction as a result of inadequate delivery and use of oxygen at the cellular level. The resultant production of mediators leads to a potentially fatal cycle, regardless of the initial inciting event.

The "classic" clinical picture of shock is a diaphoretic patient who is pale, tachycardic, tachypneic, and hypotensive. As expected, most patients in shock don't "read the book first," prior to becoming ill.

> **PRINCIPLE:** If a finding is present, it helps you; if not, IDM — it don't matter! A negative test does *not* mean a *normal* patient.

Hypotension is a late sign of shock — by the time it becomes evident, the process may have become irreversible. Even tachycardia, a reliable sign when present, is absent in nearly one-half of patients with hemorrhagic shock. Reasons for this are unclear, though a vagal mechanism probably plays some role, especially in persons with intra-abdominal pathology.

Mechanistically, shock is classified into four types: hypovolemic, cardiogenic, obstructive, and distributive. Central shock occurs when the central circulation (heart

> **PRINCIPLE:** One way or another, everyone dies in cardiogenic shock.

and great vessels) is unable to pump sufficient blood to maintain tissue oxygen needs. This results from an impairment in cardiac emptying, either due to direct myocardial dysfunction (cardiogenic shock) or obstruction to normal blood flow in one of the great vessels (obstructive shock). Peripheral shock occurs at the level of the vascular bed and may be due

> **PRINCIPLE:** Bad "stuff" begets more bad "stuff."

to either hypovolemia (hypovolemic shock) or loss of vascular tone (distributive shock).

The systemic inflammatory response syndrome (SIRS) is a generic set of typical reactions of the body to a variety of stimuli. The most common stimulus is severe infection. Regardless of the nidus, though, the SIRS always results in the production of vasoactive mediators, such as tumor necrosis factor (TNF-α) and interleukin-6 (IL-6).

Human models of both hypovolemic and hemorrhagic shock suggest that mediator production follows a common pathway in all types of shock, eventually leading to death. This generic trigger point is known as the "systemic inflammatory response syndrome (SIRS)." Mediators are responsible for ongoing interactions of different cell types, finally leading to a sustained inflammation and multiple organ damage in the body. In the setting of trauma or shock, many activators including bacterial as well as non-bacterial factors may be present that induce local and systemic inflammatory responses. Some experts argue that a true state of immunologic dissonance exists with complete imbalance between proinflammatory and anti-inflammatory mediators.

> **REMEMBER: Cytokines and other mediators are produced *any time* the SIRS is present, not just in sepsis.**

> **REMEMBER: Though the SIRS was first described in sepsis, it is a *generic* response to a variety of circumstances.**

Many lines of evidence support the concept that the gut may be the reservoir for systemic sepsis and subsequent MSOD/MSOF in a number of pathophysiologic states. TNF-α release somehow initiates a sequence of events leading to the full-blown syndrome — a state of multiple system organ dysfunction, followed by multiple system organ failure with metabolic acidosis, leaky capillaries, and widespread cellular dysfunction. So far, immunologic attempts to block mediators have met with little success in humans.

> **PRINCIPLE: If "stuff" causes the problem, then give "anti-stuff" to improve things.**

"Standard" treatment for shock involves careful attention to Airway, Breathing, and Circulation. Though controversial in some experts' minds, most routinely give 250 to 1000 cc of either normal saline or Ringer's lactate as a fluid challenge over 10 to 15 minutes. The MAST garment may be helpful, particularly if the patient's blood pressure is below 50 mm Hg. Pressors are of most potential benefit once the patient is euvolemic.

The colloid versus crystalloid debate is unlikely to end any time soon. A summary of the major conclusions suggests:

- Two to four times the volume of crystalloid must be infused to get the equivalent hemodynamic effect of colloid.

- Blood and colloid solutions are more efficient in rapidly expanding intravascular volume.

- Infusion of large amounts of saline during resuscitation results in marked reduction of colloid oncotic pressure and hematocrit. Edema may develop, which may be mistaken as fluid overload, resulting in inadequate volume restoration.

- There is no consistent evidence that either fluid regimen (colloid versus crystalloid) reliably affects morbidity/mortality more favorably than the other.

- Therapy with colloids is significantly more costly than therapy with crystalloids.

Some experts argue that the real question is not which fluid, but rather, "How much, *if any*, fluid to give?" Several animal models have shown that:

1. Animals with the highest post-resuscitation BP have the highest mortality.

2. Those with either the lowest or moderately-low BP have a better outcome.

These data suggest that normotension, at least when there is ongoing bleeding, worsens the situation. Allowing severe hypotension may not be as good as allowing the patient to remain only *moderately* hypotensive. This approach avoids worsening the "bleeding head" and permits at least enough tissue oxygenation to prevent significant ischemia.

In addition to immunotherapy directed toward various mediators, the following have been the subject of much research attention in recent years: naloxone, corticosteroids, pentoxifylline, fibronectin, TRH, and ACTH. Though insufficient data currently exist to suggest routine use, several (e.g., pentoxifylline, ACTH) hold clinical promise.

> **PRINCIPLE**: A multi-flanked attack works better than just a one-pronged one.

Crossword Puzzle Review

Path Chap 6 -- Shock

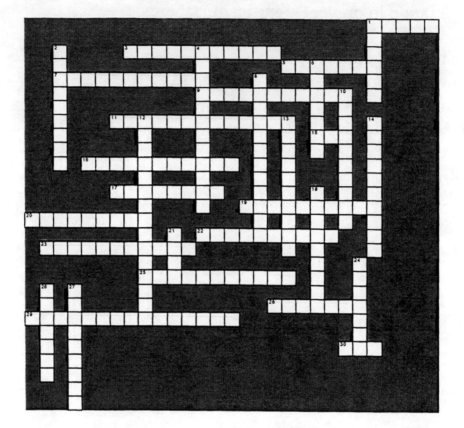

Across

1. Syndrome of inadequate delivery and use of oxygen at the cellular level.
3. The body's initial response to hypovolemia results in the release of norepinephrine and _____.
5. General term for proteins that bind carbohydrates with high affinity and specificity.
7. WBC _____ is common in the SIRS.
9. Type of shock when the cardiac pump cannot adequately circulate the available volume.
11. Phase of shock where cells switch to anaerobic metabolism.
15. Decreased production of _____ (abbrev) leads to intracellular energy failure.
16. _____ is not necessary to diagnose shock.
17. Many times, a catecholamine _____ is preferable to a single agent.
19. Immunologic _____ occurs because the patient has inappropriate and unbalanced normal regulatory systems.
20. Endogenously produced proteins of small molecular weight with multiple biological effects.
22. Molecular _____ prevent misfolding and aggregations of proteins.
23. Type of shock where the intravascular compartment is inadequately filled for proper tissue perfusion.
25. Type of shock where physical obstruction to blood flow in the heart or great vessels is present.
28. A significant number of patients with shock have acquired _____ insufficiency.
29. Capillary hydrostatic pressure decreases in early shock, allowing fluid from the interstitium to flow into the vessels.
30. General term (abbrev) for compounds produced in shock that ultimately result in cardiogenic shock and death.

Down

1. The systemic response to infection.
2. In shock, TRH acts by an antagonism of the _____ system.
4. Acute _____ is the "classic" example of a noninfectious process that leads to identical hemodynamic features of septic shock.
6. Form of shock when the heart and great vessels are unable to pump sufficient blood to maintain tissue oxygen needs.
8. Type of shock due to a major defect in arterial resistance, venous capacitance, or both with loss of vascular tone.
10. Activation leads to formation of the membrane attack complex.
12. High-dose _____ should not be used for treatment of septic shock.
13. Profound myocardial _____ has been described in the end stages of most forms of shock.
14. Type of shock that occurs at the level of the peripheral vascular bed.
18. The _____ is thought to be one of the first organs to respond to shock.
21. Acute illness characterized by generalized activation of the endothelium (abbrev).
24. Two to four times the volume of crystalloid must be infused compared with _____.
26. Unless the patient has penetrating truncal trauma, "standard" fluid therapy is still considered appropriate.
27. Neutrophil _____ is altered in the SIRS.

References

1.	Johnson, B.A. and Weil, M.H. *Redefining ischemia due to circulatory failure as dual defects of oxygen deficits and of carbon dioxide excesses.* Crit Care Med 1991; 19:1432-8.

2.	Wo, C.C.J., et. al. *Unreliability of blood pressure and heart rate to evaluate cardiac output in emergency resuscitation and critical illness.* Crit Care Med 1993; 21:218-23.

3.	Snyder, H.S. and Dresnick, S.J. *Lack of a tachycardic response to hypotension in penetrating abdominal injuries.* J Emerg Med 1989; 7:335-9.

4.	Emerson, C.P. and Ebert, R.V. *A study of shock in battle casualties: measurements of the blood volume changes occurring in response to therapy.* Ann Surg 1945; 122:745-72.

5.	Snyder, H.S. *Lack of a tachycardic response to hypotension with ruptured ectopic pregnancy.* Am J Emerg Med 1990; 8:23-6.

6.	Weil, M.H. and Henning, R.J. *New concepts in the diagnosis and fluid treatment of circulatory shock.* Thirteenth annual Becton, Dickinson and Company Oscar Schwidetsky Memorial Lecture. Anesth Analg 1979 Mar-Apr; 58(2):124-32; Weil, M.H. and Gazmuri, R.J. *Shock: new developments in the management of shock.* Appl Cardiopulm Pathophysiol 1991; 4(2):103-7.

7.	Hollenberg, S.M., et al. *Cardiogenic shock.* Ann Intern Med 1999 Jul 6; 131(1):47-59.

8.	Hands, M.E., et. al. *The in-hospital development of cardiogenic shock after myocardial infarction: incidence, predictors of occurrence, outcome and prognostic factors.* J Am Coll Cardiol 1989; 14:40-6.

9.	Burke, T.J., et al. *Renal response to shock.* Ann Emerg Med 1986; 15:1397.

10. Ordog, G.J., et al. *Coagulation abnormalities in traumatic shock.* Ann Emerg Med 1985; 14: 650-5.

11. Marlar, R.A., et al. *Mechanism of action of human activated protein C, a thrombin-dependent anti-coagulant enzyme.* Blood 1982; 257:859-64.

12. Moore, K.L., et al. *Endotoxin enhances tissue factor and suppresses thrombomodulin expression of human vascular endothelium* in vitro. J Clin Invest 1987; 79:124-30; Nawroth, P.O. and Stern, D.M. *Modulation of endothelial cell hemostatic properties by tumor necrosis factor.* J Exp Med 1986; 163:740-5.

13. Taylor, F.B., et al. *Protein C prevents the coagulopathic and lethal effects of* Escherichia coli *infusion in the baboons.* J Clin Invest 1987; 79:918-25.

14. Mesters, R.M., et al. *Prognostic value of protein C concentrations in neutropenic patients at high risk of severe septic complications.* Crit Care Med 2000; 28:2209-16.

15. Elchisa, M.A. *Zovant (rhAPC) clinical trial for sepsis stopped by Eli Lilly.* June 29/2000; http://pharmacology.about.com/health/pharmacology/library/0daily/00news/blnews000629.

16. Seekamp, A.J., et al. *Cytokines and adhesion molecules in elective and accidental trauma-related ischemia/reperfusion.* J Trauma 1998 May; 44(5):874-82.

17. Hierholzer, C., et al. *Rapid and simultaneous activation of Stat3 and production of interleukin 6 in resuscitated hemorrhagic shock.* Arch Orthop Trauma Surg 1999; 119(5-6):332-6.

18. Guyton, A.C. and Hall, J.E. Pocket Companion to Textbook of Medical Physiology, Sixth Edition. WB Saunders: Philadelphia, 1999; p. 551.

19. Schlag, G., et. al., *The cell in shock: the origin of multiple organ failure.* Resuscitation 1991; 21:137-80.

20. Lin, H.C., et al. *Systemic administration of lipopolysaccharide induces release of nitric oxide and glutamate and c-fos expression in the nucleus tractus solitarii of rats.* Hypertension 1999 May; 33(5):1218-24.

21. Baykal, A., et al. *Effects of adrenaline or endotoxin tolerance states on mesenteric blood flow in endotoxaemia.* Aust NZ J Surg 1999 Feb; 69(2):134-7.

22. Worrall, N.K., et al. *TNF-alpha causes reversible* in vivo *systemic vascular barrier dysfunction via NO-dependent and -independent mechanisms.* Am J Physiol 1997 Dec; 273(6 Pt 2):H2565-74.

23. Hachenbert, T. and Grundling, M. *Acute failure of the intestinal barrier: pathophysiology, diagnosis, prophylaxis and therapy.* Anaesthesiol Reanim 1999; 24(1):4-12.

24. Miller, P.R., et al. *Threshold values of intramucosal pH and mucosal-arterial CO_2 gap during shock resuscitation.* J Trauma 1998; 45:868-72.

25. Creteur, J.J. *Does gastric tonometry monitor splanchnic perfusion?* Crit Care Med 1999 Nov; 27(11):2480-4.

26. Kirton, O.C., et al. *Failure of splanchnic resuscitation in the acutely injured trauma patient correlates with multiple organ system failure and length of stay in the ICU.* Chest 1998; 113:1069-74.

27. Barquist, E., et al. *The impact of antioxidant and splanchnic-directed therapy on persistent uncorrected gastric mucosal pH in the critically injured trauma patient.* J Trauma 1998; 44:355-60.

28. Hotchkiss, R.S., et al. *Rapid onset of intestinal epithelial and lymphocyte apoptotic cell death in patients with trauma and shock.* Crit Care Med 2000; 28:3207-17.

29. Gadek, J.E., et al. *Effect of enteral feeding with eicosapentaenoic acid, gamma-linolenic acid, and antioxidants in patients with acute*

respiratory distress syndrome. Enteral Nutrition in ARDS Study Group. Crit Care Med 1999 Aug; 27(8):1409-20.

30. Galban, C.C. *An immune-enhancing enteral diet reduces mortality rate and episodes of bacteremia in septic intensive care unit patients.* Crit Care Med 2000 Mar; 28(3):643-8.

31. Opam, S.M., et al. *Clinical gram-positive sepsis: does it fundamentally differ from gram-negative bacterial sepsis?* Crit Care Med 1999 Aug; 27(8):1608-16.

32. Sriskandan, S. and Cohen J. *Gram-positive sepsis: mechanisms and differences from gram-negative sepsis.* Infect Dis Clin North Am 1999 Jun; 13(2):397-412.

33. Bannan, J., et al. *Structure and function of streptococcal and staphylococcal superantigens in septic shock.* Infect Dis Clin North Am 1999 Jun; 13(2):387-96.

34. Dofferhoff, A.S.M., et al. *Patterns of cytokines, plasma endotoxin, plasminogen activator inhibitor, and acute-phase proteins during the treatment of severe sepsis in humans.* Crit Care Med 1992; 20:185-192.

35. Heart, S.O., et al. *Tumor necrosis factor-alpha causes myocardial depression in guinea pigs.* Crit Care Med 1992; 20:523-7.

36. DeMeules, J.E., et al. *Tumor necrosis factor and cardiac function.* J Trauma 1992; 32:686-92.

37. Meldrum, D.R. and Donnahoo, K.K. *Role of TNF-α in mediating renal insufficiency following cardiac surgery: evidence of a postbypass cardiorenal syndrome.* J Surg Res 1999 Aug; 85(2):185-99.

38. Kawata, T., et al. *E5531, a synthetic non-toxic lipid A derivative blocks the immunobiological activities of lipopolysaccharide.* Br J Pharmacol 1999 Jun; 127(4):853-62.

39. Dinarello, C.A., et. al. *Anticytokine strategies in the treatment of the systemic inflammatory response syndrome.* JAMA 1993; 269:1829-35.

40. Fisher, C.J., et al. *Influence of an anti-tumor necrosis factor monoclonal antibody on cytokine levels in patients with sepsis.* Crit Care Med 1993; 21:318-27.

41. Heumann, D., et al. *Molecular basis of host-pathogen interaction in septic shock.* Curr Opin Microbiol 1998 Feb; 1(1):49-55.

42. Novelli, G.P. *Role of free radicals in septic shock.* J Physiol Pharmacol 1997 Dec; 48(4):517-27.

43. Cuzzocrea, S., et al. *Protective effect of melatonin in a non-septic shock model induced by zymosan in the rat.* J Pineal Res 1998 Aug; 25(1):24-33.

44. Wilson, P.G., et al. *Acute pancreatitis as a model of sepsis.* J Antimicrob Chemother 1998 Jan; 41 Suppl A:51-63.

45. Wagner, J.G. and Roth, R.A. *Neutrophil migration during endotoxemia.* J Leukoc Biol 1999 Jul; 66(1):10-24.

46. Bone, R.C., et al. *Sepsis: a new hypothesis for pathogenesis of the disease process.* Chest 1997; 112:235-43.

47. Fisher, C.J. Jr., et al. *Influence of an anti-tumor necrosis factor monoclonal antibody on cytokine levels in patients with sepsis.* Crit Care Med 1993; 21:318-27; Kox, W.J., et al. *Interferon-gamma in the treatment of the compensatory anti-inflammatory response syndrome (CARS) — a new approach: proof of principle.* Arch Intern Med 1997; 157:389-93.

48. Peters, J.I. and Utset, O.M. *Vasopressors in shock management: choosing and using wisely.* J Crit Illness 1989; 4:62-8.

49. Murphy, M.B. and Elliot, W.J. *Dopamine and dopamine receptor agonists in cardiovascular therapy.* Crit Care Med 1990; 18:S14.

50. Power, D.A., et al. *Renal-dose (low-dose) dopamine for the treatment of sepsis-related and other forms of acute renal failure: ineffective and probably dangerous.* Clin Exp Pharmacol Physiol Suppl 1999 Apr;

26:S23-8.

51.   Hesselvik, J.F. and Brodin, B. *Low dose norepinephrine in patients with septic shock and oliguria: effects on afterload, urine flow, and oxygen transport.* Crit Care Med 17; 1989:179-81.

52.   Bollaert, P.E., et al. *Effects of epinephrine on hemodynamics and oxygen metabolism in dopamine-resistant septic shock.* Chest 1990; 98:949-53.

53.   Sibbald, W.J., et al. *The short-term effects of increasing plasma colloid osmotic pressure in patients with noncardiac pulmonary edema.* Surgery 1983; 93:620.

54.   Stamler, K.D. *Effect of crystalloid infusion on hematocrit in nonbleeding patients, with applications to clinical traumatology.* Ann Emerg Med July 1989; 18:747-9; Greenfield, R.H., et al. *Effect of crystalloid infusion on hematocrit and intravascular volume in healthy, nonbleeding subjects.* Ann Emerg Med January 1989; 18:51-5.

55.   Hankeln, K., et al. *Comparison of hydroxyethyl startch and lactated Ringer's solution on hemodynamics and oxygen transport of critically ill patients in prospective crossover studies.* Crit Care Med 1991; 17:133.

56.   Bickwell, W.H., et al. *Use of hypertonic saline/dextran versus lactated Ringer's solution as a resuscitation fluid after uncontrolled aortic hemorrhage in anesthetized swine.* Ann Emerg Med September 1992; 21:1077-85.

57.   Krausz, M.M., et al. *"Scoop and run" or stabilize hemorrhagic shock with normal saline or small-volume hypertonic saline.* J Trauma 1992; 33:6-10.

58.   Martin, R.R., et al. *Prospective evaluation of preoperative fluid resuscitation in hypotensive patients with penetrating truncal injury: a preliminary report.* J Trauma 1992; 33:354-62.

59.   Bickell, W.H., et al. *The detrimental effects of intravenous crystalloid after aortotomy in swine.* Surgery 1991; 110:529-36; Stern S.A., et al. *Effect of blood pressure on hemorrhage volume and survival in a near-fatal hemorrhage model incorporating a vascular injury.* Ann Emerg Med 1993; 22:155-63; Stern S.A., et al. *Multiple resuscitation regimens in a near fatal porcine aortic injury hemorrhage model.* Acad Emerg Med 1995; 2:89-97.

60.   De Guzman, E., et al. *Limited volume resuscitation in penetrating thoracoabdominal trauma.* AACN Clin Issues 1999 Feb; 10(1):61-8.

61.   Bickell, W.H., et al. *Immediate versus delayed fluid resuscitation for hypotensive patients with penetrating torso injuries.* N Engl J Med 1994; 331:1105.

62.   Shoemaker, W.C., et al. *Hemodynamic patterns of survivors and nonsurvivors during high risk elective surgical operations.* World J Surg 1999 Dec; 23(12):1264-71.

63.   Faist, E. and Kim, C. *Therapeutic immunomodulatory approaches for the control of systemic inflammatory response syndrome and the prevention of sepsis.* New Horiz 1998; 6(suppl 2):97-102; Opal, S.M. and Yu, R. *Anti-endotoxin strategies for the prevention and treatment of septic shock.* Drugs 1998; 55:497-508; Opal, S.M. *New strategies in the management of sepsis.* Biomed Prog 1998; 11:52-6.

64.   Tseng, C.S., et al. *Effects of opioid agonists and opioid antagonists in endotoxic shock in rats.* Ma Tsui Hsueh Tsa Chi 1993 Mar; 31(1):1-8; Haglind, E. *Effects of continuous naloxone infusion in intestinal ischemia shock in the rat.* Circ Shock 1992 Nov; 38(3):195-201; Reynolds, D.G., et al. *The therapeutic efficacy of opiate antagonists in hemorrhagic shock.* Resuscitation 1989 Dec; 18(2-3):243-51; Schadt, J.C. *Sympathetic and hemodynamic adjustments to hemorrhage: a possible role for endogenous opioid peptides.* Resuscitation 1989 Dec; 18(2-3):219-28; Tuggle, D.R. and Horton, J.W. *Effects of naloxone on splanchnic perfusion in hemorrhagic shock.* J Trauma 1989 Oct; 29(10):1341-5.

65.   Rock P., et al. *Efficacy and safety of naloxone in septic shock.* Crit Care Med 1985; 13:28-33.

66.   Hilburger, M.E., et al. *Morphine induces sepsis in mice.* J Infect Dis 1997 Jul; 176(1):183-8.

67.   Baker, C.H., et al. *Reduced microvascular adrenergic receptor activity due to opioids in endotoxin shock.* Circ Shock 1990 Oct; 32(2):101-12.

68.   Schadt, J.C. *Sympathetic and hemodynamic adjustments to hemorrhage: a possible role for endogenous opioid peptides.* Resuscitation 1989; 18:219-28.

69.   Safani, M., et al. *Prospective, controlled, randomized trial of naloxone infusion in early hyperdynamic septic shock.* Crit Care Med 1989 Oct; 17(10):1004-9.

70.   Hackshaw, K.V., et al. *Naloxone in septic shock.* Crit Care Med 1990 Jan; 18(1):47-51.

71.   Lu, H., et al. *Clinical effects of naloxone on hemorrhagic shock.* Chung Hua Wai Ko Tsa Chih 1995 Jun; 33(6):355-8.

72.   Hackshaw, K.V., et al. *Naloxone in septic shock.* Crit Care Med 1990 Jan; 18(1):47-51.

73.   Safani, M., et al. *Prospective, controlled, randomized trial of naloxone infusion in early hyperdynamic septic shock.* Crit Care Med 1989 Oct; 17(10):1004-9.

74.   Dziki, A.J., et al. *Beta-adrenergic-dependent and -independent actions of naloxone on perfusion during endotoxin shock.* Circ Shock 1993 Jan; 39(1):29-38.

75.   Boeuf, B., et al. *Therapy of shock with naloxone: a meta-analysis.* Crit Care Med 1998 Nov; 26(11):1910-6.

76.   Putterman, C. *Modern approaches to the therapy of septic shock.* Am J Emerg Med 1990; 8:152-61, 1990.

77. Schumer, W. *Steroids in the treatment of clinical septic shock.* Ann Surg 1976 Sep; 184(3):333-41.

78. Slotman, G.J., et al. *Detrimental effects of high-dose methylprednisolone sodium succinate on serum concentrations of hepatic and renal function indicators in severe sepsis and septic shock.* Crit Care Med 1993; 21:191-5.

79. Bone, R.C., et al. *A controlled clinical trial of high-dose methylprednisolone in the treatment of severe sepsis and septic shock.* N Engl J Med 1987 Sep 10; 317(11):653-8.

80. Rothwell, P.M., et al. *Cortisol response to corticotropin and survival in septic shock.* Lancet 1991; 337:582-3.

81. Kidess, A.I., et al. *Transient corticotropin deficiency in critical illness.* Mayo Clin Proc 1993; 68:435-41.

82. Briegel, J., et al. *A comparison of the adrenocortical response during septic shock and after complete recovery.* Intensive Care Med 1996 Sep; 22(9):894-9.

83. Hatherill, M., et al. *Adrenal insufficiency in septic shock.* Arch Dis Child 1999 Jan; 80(1):51-5.

84. Soni, A., et al. *Adrenal insufficiency occurring during septic shock: incidence, outcome, and relationship to peripheral cytokine levels.* Am J Med 1995 Mar; 98(3):266-71.

85. Briegel, J., et al. *Stress doses of hydrocortisone reverse hyperdynamic septic shock: a prospective, randomized, double-blind, single-center study.* Crit Care Med 1999 Apr; 27(4):723-32.

86. Annane, D., et al. *Impaired pressor sensitivity to noradrenaline in septic shock patients with and without impaired adrenal function reserve.* Br J Clin Pharmacol 1998 Dec; 46(6):589-97.

87. Bollaert, P.E., et al. *Reversal of late septic shock with supraphysiologic doses of hydrocortisone.* Crit Care Med 1998 Apr; 26(4):645-50.

88. Cronin, L., et al. *Corticosteroid treatment for sepsis: a critical appraisal and meta-analysis of the literature.* Crit Care Med 1995 Aug; 23(8):1430-9.

89. Lefering, R. and Neugebauer, F.A. *Steroid controversy in sepsis and septic shock: a meta-analysis.* Crit Care Med 1995 Jul; 23(7):1294-303.

90. Ambrus, J.L., et al. *Platelet aggregation in septic shock: effect of pentoxifylline.* J Med 1990; 21(1-2):121-8.

91. Biroir, B.P. and Beutler, B. *Effect of amrinone on tumor necrosis factor production in endotoxic shock.* Circ Shock 1992 Mar; 36(3):200-7.

92. Thiel, M. and Bardenheuer, H.J. *Drug therapy of sepsis: an indication for pentoxifylline?* Anaesthesist 1994 Apr; 43(4):249-56.

93. Ridings, P.C., et al. *Beneficial cardiopulmonary effects of pentoxifylline in experimental sepsis are lost once septic shock is established.* Arch Surg 1994 Nov; 129(11):1144-52.

94. Tighe, D., et al. *Pretreatment with pentoxifylline improves the hemodynamic and histologic changes in decreased neutrophil adhesiveness in a pig fecal peritonitis model.* Crit Care Med 1990; 18:184; Waxman, K., et al. *Pentoxifylline in resuscitation of experimental hemorrhagic shock.* Crit Care Med 1991; 19:728; Bone, R.C. *Inhibitors of complement and neutrophils: a critical evaluation of their role in the treatment of sepsis.* Crit Care Med 1992; 20:891-8.

95. Silomon, M., et al. *Pentoxifylline prevention of altered hepatocyte calcium regulation during hemorrhagic shock/resuscitation.* Crit Care Med 1998 Mar; 26(3):494-500.

96. Krahauer, T., et al. *Pentoxifylline inhibits superantigen-induced toxic shock and cytokine release.* Clin Diagn Lab Immunol 1999 Jul; 6(4):594-8.

97. Arrieta, O., et al. *Protective effect of pentoxifylline plus thalidomide against septic shock in mice.* Int J Exp Pathol 1999 Feb; 80(1):11-16.

98. Quezado, Z.M., et al. *Increasing doses of pentoxifylline as a continuous infusion in canine septic shock.* J Pharmacol Exp Ther 1999 Jan; 288(1):107-13.

99. Del Moral, T., et al. *Effects of treatment with pentoxifylline on the cardiovascular manifestations of group B streptococcal sepsis in the piglet.* Pediatr Res 1996 Sep; 40(3):469-74.

100. Lundblad, R., et al. *Pentoxifylline improves survival and reduces tumor necrosis factor, interleukin-6, and endothelin-1 in fulminant intra-abdominal sepsis in rats.* Shock 1995 Mar; 3(3):210-5.

101. Staubach, K.H., et al. *Effect of pentoxifylline in severe sepsis: results of a randomized, double-blind, placebo-controlled study.* Arch Surg 1998 Jan; 133(1):94-100.

102. Staudinger, T., et al. *Influence of pentoxifylline on cytokine levels and inflammatory parameters in septic shock.* Intensive Care Med 1996 Sep; 22(9):888-93.

103. Zeni, F., et al. *Effects of pentoxifylline on circulating cytokine concentrations and hemodynamics in patients with septic shock: results from a double-blind, randomized, placebo-controlled study.* Crit Care Med 1996 Feb; 24(2):207-14.

104. Bienvenu, J., et al. *Production of proinflammatory cytokines and cytokines involved in the TH1/TH2 balance is modulated by pentoxifylline.* J Cardiovasc Pharmacol 1995; 25 Suppl 2:S80-4.

105. Mandi, Y., et al. *Inhibition of tumor necrosis factor production and ICAM-1 expression by pentoxifylline: beneficial effects in sepsis syndrome.* Res Exp Med (Berl) 1995; 195(5):297-307.

106. Riodan, F.A., et al. *Plasma fibronectin levels in meningococcal disease.* Eur J Pediatr 1997 Jun; 156(6):451-3.

107. Putterman, C. *Modern Approaches to the therapy of septic shock*. Am J Emerg Med 1990; 8:152-161.

108. McCabe, J.B. *New prospects for shock treatment: symposium closing remarks*. Resuscitation 1989; 18:321-6.

109. Liu, L.M., et al. *The importance of delta and kappa opioid receptors in the property of thyrotropin-releasing hormone against hemorrhagic shock*. Shock 1997 Jan; 7(1):60-4.

110. Wang, G.L. and Zhu, C. *Effects of thyrotropin-releasing hormone on acute experimental traumatic head injury in cats*. Chin Med J (Engl) 1991 Nov; 104(11):939-44.

111. Guarini, S., et al. *A pharmacological study of the cardiovascular effects of TRH-T in haemorrhagic shock in rats*. Arch Int Pharmacodyn Ther 1989 May-Jun; 299:65-76.

112. Vergoni, A.V., et al. *Afferent vagal fibres and central cholinergic mechanisms are involved in the TRH-induced reversal of haemorrhagic shock*. Pharmacol Res 1991 Apr; 23(3):271-8.

113. Chen, H. *Protective effect of thyrotropin-releasing hormone against lipid peroxidation injury during traumatic shock in rats*. Chung Hua I Hsueh Tsa Chih (Taipei) 1991 Aug; 71(8):438-40.

114. Leon-Sanz, D., et al. *Pituitary-thyroid function in patients with septic shock and its relation with outcome*. Eur J Med Res 1997 Nov 28; 2(11):477-82.

115. Sugiura, A., et al. *Thyrotropin-releasing hormone increases survival in canine hemorrhagic shock*. J Surg Res 1986 Jan; 40(1):63-8.

116. Teba, L., et al. *Beneficial effect of thyrotropin-releasing hormone in canine hemorrhagic shock*. Circ Shock 1987; 21(1):51-7.

117. Muelleman, R.L., et al. *Blood pressure effects of thyrotropin-releasing hormone and epinephrine in anaphylactic shock*. Ann Emerg Med 1988 Apr; 17(4):309-13.

118. Holaday, J.W., et al. *Thyrotropin-releasing hormone improves cardiovascular function in experimental endotoxic and hemorrhagic shock.* Science 1981 Jul 10; 213(4504):216-8.

119. Brackett, D.J., et al. *Evaluation of thyrotropin releasing hormone as a therapeutic intervention for endotoxemia.* Regul Pept 1990 Jul 30; 29(2-3):153-62.

120. Tagliavini, S., et al. *TRH reverses the ECG and EEG ischemic changes induced by massive hemorrhage in rats.* Life Sci 1991; 49(24):1815-21.

121. Coppi, G., et al. *The thyrotropin releasing hormone analogue, RGH 2202, reverses experimental haemorrhagic shock in rats.* Eur J Pharmacol 1990 Jun 21; 182(1):185-8.

122. Bertolini, A., et al. *The adrenocorticortropic hormone [acth]-induced reversal of hemorrhagic shock.* Resuscitation 1989; 18:253-67.

123. Wang, P., et al. *Mechanism of adrenal insufficiency following trauma and severe hemorrhage: role of hepatic 11beta-hydroxysteroid dehydrogenase.* Arch Surg 1999 Apr; 134(4):394-401.

124. Guarini, S., et al. *Adrenocorticotropin normalizes the blood levels of nitric oxide in hemorrhage-shocked rats.* Eur J Pharmacol 1997 Oct 1; 336(1):15-21.

125. Bazzini, C., et al. *Inhibition of nitric oxide synthases enhances the effect of ACTH in hemorrhagic shock.* Life Sci 1997; 61(19):1889-97.

126. Bazzini, C., et al. *Comparison of the effects of ACTH-(1-24), methylprednisolone, aprotinin, and norepinephrine in a model of hemorrhagic shock in rats.* Resuscitation 1993 Jun; 25(3):219-26.

127. Donaldson, M.D., et al. *Lack of effect of ACTH in porcine Escherichia coli septic shock.* Circ Shock 1991 Nov; 35(3):152-8.

128. Noera, G., et al. *Haemorrhagic shock in cardiac surgery: pharmacological treatment with ACTH (1-24).* Resuscitation 1991 Oct; 22(2):123-7.

129. Coppi, G. and Falcone, A. *ACTH fragments reverse experimental haemorrhagic shock in rats.* Drugs Exp Clin Res 1992; 18(5):173-7.

130. Guarini, S., et al. *Anti-shock effect of ACTH-(1-24): influence of subtotal hepatectomy.* Pharmacol Res Commun 1988 May; 20(5):395-403; Guarini, S. *Anti-shock effect of ACTH: haematological changes and influence of splenectomy.* Arch Int Pharmacodyn Ther 1987 Oct; 289(2): 311-8.

131. Bertolini, A., et al. *Alpha-MSH and other ACTH fragments improve cardiovascular function and survival in experimental hemorrhagic shock.* Eur J Pharmacol 1986 Oct 14; 130(1-2):19-26.

132. Versteeg, D.H. *Melanocortins and cardiovascular regulation.* Eur J Pharmacol 1998 Oct 30; 360(1): 1-14.

133. Delgado Hernandez, R., et al. *Inhibition of systemic inflammation by central action of the neuropeptide alpha-melanocyte-stimulating hormone.* Neuroimmunomodulation 1999 May-Jun; 6(3):187-92.

134. Chiao, H., et al. *Alpha-melanocyte-stimulating hormone reduces endotoxin-induced liver inflammation.* J Clin Invest 1996 May 1; 97(9):2038-44.

CHAPTER 7
RENAL PROBLEMS

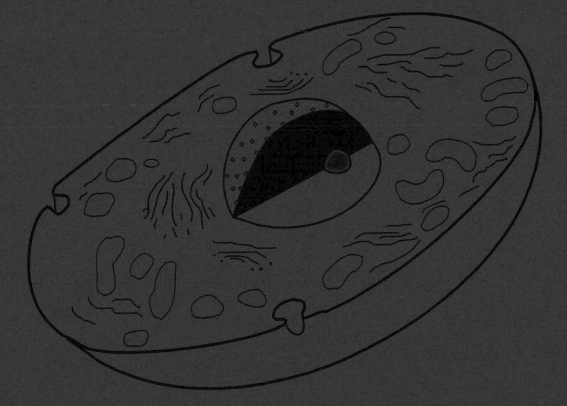

CHAPTER 7 — RENAL PROBLEMS

Contents

Objectives

After reading this chapter, you'll be able to:

- List and describe the major functions of the kidney.
- Summarize the three processes involved in urine formation.
- Describe the basic structure and function of a "generic" nephron.
- Summarize protein metabolism in the body and how it relates to the formation of urea.
- List and explain at least three causes of elevated blood urea nitrogen (BUN) levels.
- Describe and differentiate between pre-renal and renal azotemia.

Introduction

The kidneys play an essential role in regulation of many body functions. They are also involved in many cardiovascular conditions, such as hypertension and congestive heart failure. A fundamental understanding of normal renal physiology makes it far easier to understand what happens during disease states, such as renal failure.

PRINCIPLE: You must appreciate the *normal* to understand the *abnormal*.

There are numerous renal diseases that are not covered in this section. This deletion was deliberate. From a primary care point of view, the most important key to understanding kidney pathology is the ongoing interplay between it and the heart in congestive heart failure (**Chapter 3**).

Overview of Renal Function

OBJECTIVE: List and describe the major functions of the kidney.

Normal functions of the kidneys — The kidneys have multiple normal functions in the body. All serve to maintain homeostasis: **[FIGURE 7-1]**

- Regulation of fluid and electrolyte balance, as well as osmolarity.

- Excretion of metabolic waste products.

- Regulation of arterial pressure via excretion of sodium and water, as well as the production of renin.

- Regulation of acid-base balance.

- Regulation of erythrocyte production via the production of **erythropoietin** (stimulates RBC production in the bone marrow).

- Regulation of **vitamin D** metabolism.

- Synthesis of glucose from amino acids during prolonged fasting.

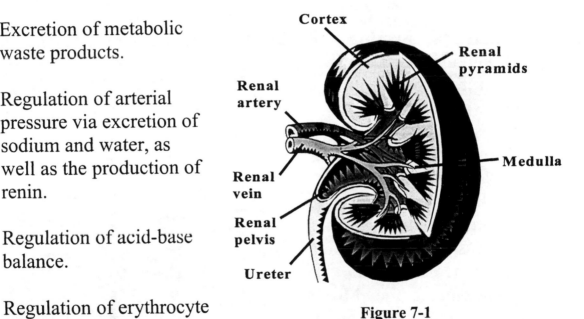

Figure 7-1

The basics of urine formation — The formation of urine results from the interplay of three separate, and related, renal processes that take place in the nephron: **[FIGURE 7-2]**

1.   **Glomerular filtration** — Filtering of fluid from the glomerular capillaries into the renal tubules (**1** in **Figure 7-2**).

2.   **Tubular reabsorption** — Return of water and solutes from the tubules back into the blood. Tubular reabsorption reduces urine volume and alters its composition. To be reabsorbed, a substance must first past through the renal epithelial cell membrane into the interstitial fluid. Then, it must pass back into the blood through the peritubular capillary membrane. Most plasma ions (e.g., sodium, chloride, bicarbonate), glucose, and amino acids are highly reabsorbed from the tubules. Metabolic waste products, such as urea and creatinine, are poorly reabsorbed and excreted in large amounts (**2** in **Figure 7-2**).

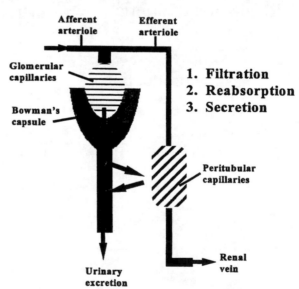

Basic Mechanisms of Renal Excretion

1. **Filtration**
2. **Reabsorption**
3. **Secretion**

Excretion = Filtration - Reabsorption + Secretion

Figure 7-2

3. **Tubular secretion** — Net movement of water and solutes into the tubules. Potassium and hydrogen ions, as well as certain organic acids and bases, are actively secreted into the urine (**3** in **Figure 7-2**).

Each of these processes is highly variable, depending upon the body's needs. All eventually lead to the excretion of urine. For any given substance, its urinary excretion rate can be mathematically expressed as follows:

Urinary excretion rate = Glomerular Filtration - Tubular Reabsorption + Tubular Secretion

---

OBJECTIVE: Describe the basic structure and function of a "generic" nephron.

The nephron is the structural and functional unit of the kidney. More than one million nephrons in each kidney form urine. The basic components of the nephron include: **[FIGURE 7-3]**

*   **Glomerulus** — Complex of capillaries (glomerular capillaries) in which fluid is filtered from the blood.

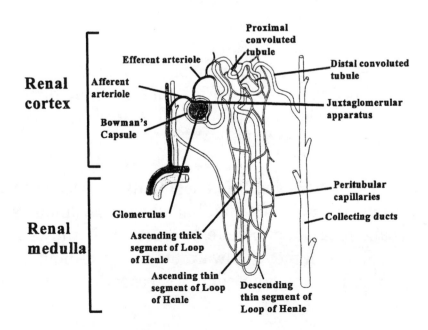

Figure 7-3 — The Nephron

- **Bowman's capsule** — Membrane surrounding the glomerulus.

- **Renal tubule** — Long tube in which fluid is converted into urine; the tubule empties into the renal pelvis, which receives urine from all the nephrons. The renal tubule is divided into four major structural and functional components: (numbers refer to locations marked on **FIGURE 7-4**).

1. **Proximal tubule** — Lies in the outer portion (cortex) of the kidney. Approximately 65% of water, sodium, chloride, and potassium are absorbed back into the body here. The proximal tubule is normally impermeable to waste products (**1**).

2. **Loop of Henle** — Has three functionally distinct segments (loops): the descending thin segment, ascending thin segment, and ascending thick segment. The **descending thin loop** is highly permeable to water, which is rapidly reabsorbed into the hyperosmotic interstitium. Tubular fluid becomes hyperosmotic as it moves toward the medulla. Roughly 15 to 20% of the glomerular filtrate volume is reabsorbed here (**2**).

   The great water permeability of the thin descending loop is due to the presence of water channels known as **aquaporins (AQP)**. There are four described types of aquaporins. AQP1 operate in the thin descending loop and the proximal tubule. AQP2-AQP4 function in the collecting ducts and principal cells. Mutations in aquaporins, especially in the collecting ducts, result in nephrogenic diabetes insipidus (loss of fluid from the kidneys).

   The **thin (3)** and **thick segments (4)** of the **ascending loop** are impermeable to water, but allow large amounts of sodium, chloride, and potassium to be reabsorbed. This allows the urine to become more dilute as it moves toward the cortex. About 25% of the filtered sodium, chloride, and potassium are reabsorbed in the thick ascending limb (**4**).

3. **Distal tubule** — Lies in the renal cortex and dilutes the tubular fluid. The first portion forms part of the **juxtaglomerular apparatus** that controls the glomerular filtration rate (GFR) and blood flow to each nephron (**5**). The initial portion of the distal tubule is impermeable to water, but highly permeable to sodium, chloride, and potassium (**6**). The result is further dilution of the urine. The second half of the distal duct and the cortical collecting tubule have similar functions (**7**).

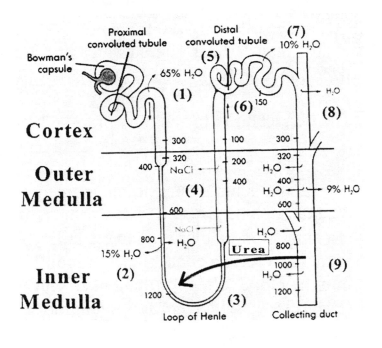

Figure 7-4 — Nephron Function

4. **Collecting tubules** — Include the cortical collecting tubule and associated cortical collecting ducts. Begin in the cortex and run toward the medulla, becoming the medullary collecting ducts. These empty into the renal pelvis.

Both the second half of the distal tubule and the cortical collecting tubule are nearly completely impermeable to urea. Their permeability to water is controlled by **anti-diuretic hormone** (ADH). High levels of ADH increase tubular permeability, increasing reabsorption of water (**8**). Collecting tubules contain two types of cells, with separate functions. **Principal cells** absorb sodium and water from the tubular fluid, and secrete potassium into the fluid. These functions are controlled by aldosterone, which stimulates the sodium-potassium pump to increase sodium reabsorption from the tubule and potassium secretion into the tubule. **Intercalated cells** absorb potassium ions from tubular fluid, and secrete hydrogen ions back into the tubule. Intercalated cells play an important role in regulation of acid-base balance.

The **medullary collecting ducts** are the final sites for processing of urine and reabsorb less than 10% of filtered water and sodium. They have several specialized functions (**9**):

- The permeability to water is controlled by anti-diuretic hormone (ADH).

- The tubule is highly permeable to urea. This allows some of the urea in the tubule to be absorbed into the interstitium. The result is an osmotic gradient from tubular fluid to medullary interstitium that allows the kidneys to form a concentrated urine. The reabsorbed urea then passes into the blood, often resulting in an elevation of the blood urea nitrogen (BUN) level, with a *normal* creatinine level (see "Pre-renal azotemia," below).

- The tubule secretes hydrogen ions into the urine to maintain acid-base balance in the body.

The final urine passes through the renal pyramids into the ureters and bladder, where it is excreted.

How and where do diuretics work? Diuretics block various membrane transporters and enzymes, leading to increased loss of electrolyte and water:

- Proximal tubule — Acetazolamide (Diamox®) inhibits carbonic anhydrase, decreasing HCO_3^- and Na^+ reabsorption; mannitol acts as an osmotic diuretic.

- Thick ascending limb — Furosemide and bumetanide inhibit the Na^+-K^+-2CL^- cotransporter by competing for the Cl^- receptor.

- Distal convoluted tubule — Thiazide diuretics compete for the Cl⁻ receptor on the NaCl transporter protein.

- Collecting duct — Amiloride and triamterene block the Na⁺ channel.

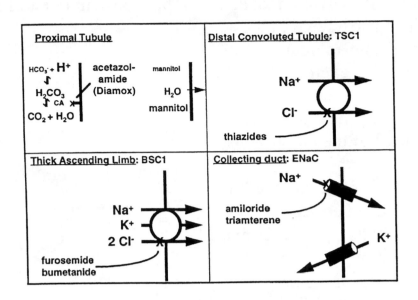

Sites of Actions of Various Diuretics

Acute Renal Failure — BUN and Creatinine

We commonly utilize the BUN (blood urea nitrogen) and Cr (creatinine) levels in patient evaluation. It's important (and fairly easy) to understand these two lab tests. Generally, we think of BUN and Cr as "kidney function" tests. True — and both, especially BUN, offer far *more* information than just "renal function," if you understand the normal production of blood urea nitrogen. BUN levels reflect protein metabolism; this is slightly reflected in the Cr as well, but Cr primarily reflects normal muscle metabolism. Let's look at creatinine, followed by BUN, to see their many uses in clinical decision making. Then, we'll talk more specifically about renal failure.

Where does creatinine come from and what does it mean? The protein **creatine** is synthesized from amino acids in the liver, kidney, and pancreas. After transport to muscle by **creatine transport protein**, creatine is reversibly phosphorylated to creatine phosphate (**phosphocreatine**) by the enzyme **creatine kinase (CK**, formerly known as creatine phosphokinase or **CPK** — yes, the same one used in diagnosis of MI). Phosphocreatine functions as a store of high-energy phosphate in muscle; the amount is proportional to a person's muscle mass. Creatine and phosphocreatine spontaneously interact at a slow but constant rate to form **creatinine**, most of which is excreted in the urine. The amount of creatinine excreted from the body is proportional to the total creatine phosphate content of the body. Thus:

Amino Acids

Creatine

Creatine kinase

Creatinine

Creatine phosphate (phosphocreatine)

- Urine creatinine levels can be used to estimate muscle mass.
- Any rise in blood creatinine levels is a sensitive indicator of kidney malfunction; normally, it is removed rapidly from the blood except for a small amount.

OBJECTIVE: Summarize protein metabolism in the body and how it relates to the formation of urea.

The BUN factory tour — The blood urea nitrogen (BUN) level reflects normal metabolism of protein and ammonia in the body. In the GI tract, protein foodstuffs are converted to amino acids, which are absorbed into the bloodstream. The primary role of dietary protein (amino acids) is to serve as building blocks in biosynthetic reactions, particularly protein synthesis. It is only used secondarily as "fuel." The majority of ingested amino acids are metabolized (deaminated) in the liver and kidneys to ammonia (NH_4^+ — actually, this formula represents the ammonium ion, which is the usual form in solution).

Though ammonia is essential for formation of urea by the liver, it is highly toxic to the central nervous system. Levels must be regulated closely. Sources of ammonia in the body include:

1. Amino acids — Many tissues, particularly the liver, form ammonia from amino acids.

2. Glutamine — The kidneys metabolize glutamine to glutamate, forming ammonia in the process. Most ammonia is excreted in the urine as NH_4^+. This is an important way that the body regulates acid-base balance. Glutamine is also hydrolyzed (broken down by the addition of a water molecule) in the intestine, forming ammonia as a byproduct.

3. Normal intestinal bacteria — Intestinal flora degrade urea to ammonia, which is absorbed via the portal vein, returned to the liver, and re-excreted as urea.

4. Amines — Dietary amines (digested into amino acids in the intestine) and amine hormones or neurotransmitters are metabolized to ammonia.

5. Purines and pyrimidines — The nitrogenous bases (e.g., those that make up DNA and RNA) contain amino groups. The bases are metabolized to ammonia.

The diet is not our only source of protein. Most body proteins have a high rate of normal turnover. They are constantly being synthesized and then degraded. Approximately 300 to 400 grams of body protein are hydrolyzed and resynthesized each day.

SOURCES OF AMMONIA:

- **Amino acids**
- **Glutamine**
- **Intestinal flora**
- **Amines**
- **Purines and pyrimidines**

Though some ammonia is excreted in the stool and urine, most is converted to urea in the liver. The process is known as the **urea cycle**. [FIGURE 7-5]. Most of the urea is excreted in the urine. Normally, a small amount remains in the blood as blood urea nitrogen (BUN). Variation within the normal range depends upon protein intake. A simplified version of the "BUN Factory" is illustrated in **FIGURE 7-6**.

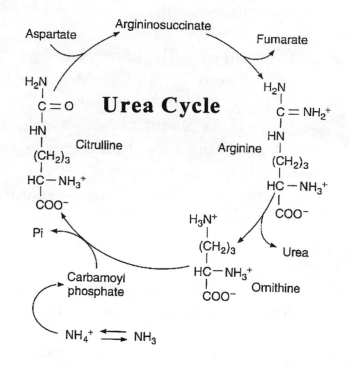

Figure 7-5 — The Urea Cycle

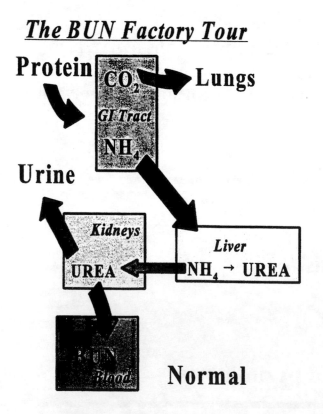

Figure 7-6

Causes of increased BUN — When the kidneys are unable to excrete urea as rapidly as it is produced, the BUN level rises. We'll discuss renal failure in combination with creatinine (Cr) levels later on. For now, let's concentrate on several *other* helpful uses for BUN levels. These include:

- GI bleeding.
- Starvation.
- Liver failure.

The "Porterhouse steak" metaphor — Remember that the BUN level reflects the small amount of urea that remains in the blood after the kidneys have excreted most of it. Let's imagine what would happen if we suddenly increased our oral protein intake — such as by eating two Porterhouse steaks. That's a lot of protein. Assuming the "BUN factory" is fully functional, additional "workers" will be recruited and the sudden protein overload metabolized via the normal "assembly line." The only difference is that there will be *more* of it to metabolize. Silly, I know, but please remember that there is a direct relationship between the *silliness level* and the *retention level*! [FIGURE 7-7]

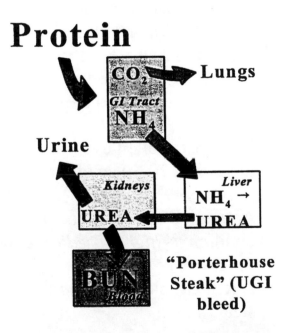

Figure 7-7 — In the case of protein overload (upper gastrointestinal [UGI] bleed), excess urea is manufactured by the liver; thus, more backs up in the blood, leading to an increase in the BUN level.

Follow the "Factory Tour," assuming that the workload has increased. The result? More NH_4 is made, so the liver must convert more to urea. Of course, the amount of urea to be excreted increases, as does the rate of urinary urea excretion. Based on the law of mass action (the more in, the more out — my paraphrase), there will therefore be *more* urea to "back up" into the blood, increasing the BUN with no change in the Cr level.

Good so far? I know you are wondering what all this has to do with pathology — answer, a lot. Metabolically, an upper GI bleed is very similar to eating two Porterhouse steaks. Globin (from hemoglobin) is released into the stomach and "overloads" the BUN factory, just as does any other ingested protein (e.g., Porterhouse steak). You guessed it — upper gastrointestinal bleeding (UGIB) results in an elevation of the BUN due to urea "backup," *without* a concomitant elevation of the Cr (unless renal failure or significant hypovolemia complicates the picture). In UGIB:

1.   BUN rises (often over 40 mg/dl) within four to six hours after loss of more than 20-30 cc of blood into the stomach.

2.   A serum BUN/creatinine ratio greater than 36 in adults, and 30 in children, is *highly predictive* for significant upper GI bleeding.[1]

3.   It remains elevated as long as the bleeding continues ("still eating steak").

4.   Once bleeding stops, the BUN level returns to normal within 24 hours.

5.   In the absence of other contributing factors, re-elevation of BUN after initially returning to normal levels suggests recurrent bleeding.

Absent other contributing factors, re-elevation of BUN is a reliable indication of rebleeding in over 90% of patients. On the other hand, positive return from a nasogastric (NG) tube is not terribly helpful in identifying candidates for endoscopic therapy. There is a 21% false-negative and 45% false-positive rate.[2]

So, BUN levels are an easy and scientifically valid way to help follow patients with UGIB. Of course, other labs (Hgb, Hct) and the clinical picture are very important as well!

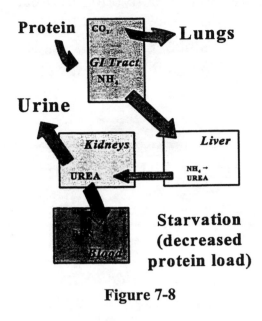

Figure 7-8

The "Steakhouse" is closed — starvation. The opposite of overloading the stomach with protein is, of course, *underloading* it. The most common way is poor dietary intake or starvation. And, the results are exactly the *opposite* of what we just outlined for protein overload (dietary or UGIB). The amounts of CO_2 and NH_4 produced in the colon are *decreased*. So, less urea is excreted by the kidneys, with less to "back up" into the blood. The BUN is *lower* than normal. **[FIGURE 7-8]** Now, think about it — other than "normal variation" or a lab error, is there another explanation for low BUN?

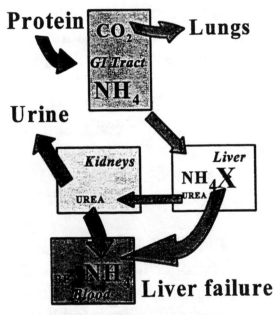

Figure 7-9 — Liver failure; note that the BUN is low, as in starvation, but for *different* reasons. In liver failure, the liver is *unable* to make urea ("X" in Figure). In starvation, liver function (urea production) is fine; there simply isn't enough substrate (ammonia) to make much urea.

Inquiring minds want to know (about liver failure). In hepatic failure, the amounts of NH_4 produced is unchanged (assuming no dietary modifications have been made). As a result of liver failure, however, NH_4 is not adequately converted to urea. The result — NH_4 "backs up," leading to elevated serum ammonia levels, and other signs of hepatic failure. In addition, since less urea is made by the liver, there is less to back up into the blood. The BUN *decreases* as a result. **[FIGURE 7-9]** The effect in liver failure (decreased BUN) is opposite to that in UGIB (increased BUN).

OBJECTIVE: Describe and differentiate between pre-renal and renal azotemia.

Now, please pass the beans (kidney, of course) — As we discussed earlier, BUN increases in renal failure, along with Cr. Though the term "azotemia" often refers simply to an elevation of the BUN, a more liberal use includes *both* BUN and Cr. While nephrologists use a three-part classification for renal failure, our modified two-part scheme is accurate in most patients: **[FIGURE 7-10]**

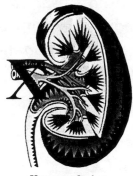 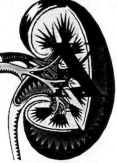

PRE-RENAL = "good beans, bad water supply"

RENAL = "good water supply, bad beans"

Hypoperfusion with intact glomerular function (hypovolemia, CHF)

Normal perfusion with altered glomerular function (renal failure, acute or chronic)

Figure 7-10 — Pre-renal versus renal azotemia

1.   **Prerenal azotemia** —
     Hypoperfusion of the kidneys (e.g., shock, hypovolemia, congestive heart failure) with *intact tubular function* ("bad water supply, good beans"). Note that patients with obstruction to urine flow distal to the bladder (e.g., kidney stones, prostate enlargement) also exhibit a similar initial biochemical picture. Nephrologists refer to this as **postrenal azotemia**. It will not be discussed further here.

2.   **Renal azotemia** — True renal failure of the renal parenchyma ("good water supply, bad beans"). This can occur acutely (e.g., following shock or nephrotoxins) or be chronic (e.g., diabetic nephropathy). We'll concentrate right now on acute renal failure.

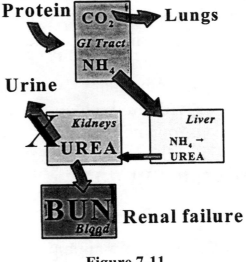

Figure 7-11

The rates of rise of BUN and Cr differ in prerenal and renal azotemia. These differences are reflected by different BUN-creatinine ratios (BUN/Cr): **[FIGURE 7-11]**

- In *prerenal azotemia*, BUN rises much *faster* than Cr. As a result, though both BUN/Cr are elevated, the BUN is usually greater than ten times the Cr level (e.g., BUN 25, Cr 2.0).

- In *renal azotemia*, the rates of rise of BUN and Cr are similar. Thus, both are elevated and the ratio is usually less than 10 (e.g., BUN 25, Cr 7.0).

Why is this ratio helpful? Serum BUN and Cr are increased in *both* renal and prerenal azotemia. In renal azotemia, the reason is because of actual tubular damage. In prerenal azotemia, tubular function is intact, but there is *hypoperfusion* to the nephron.

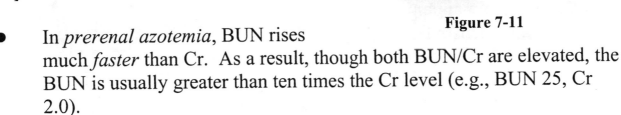

Renal hypoperfusion

Activation of renin-aldosterone system

Fluid and sodium retention

Increased BUN
(Direct physiologic consequence of decreased GFR)

Figure 7-12 — Increased BUN in pre-renal azotemia is a direct reflection of a normal attempt by the kidney to retain fluid in the face of decreased glomerular filtration rate (GFR).

The differential rate of rise in BUN and Cr in prerenal azotemia reflects a "normal response system." In prerenal azotemia, decreased renal perfusion is sensed as *hypovolemia* (regardless of the reason) by the kidneys, with subsequent activation of the renin-angiotensin-aldosterone system. The result is decreased glomerular filtration with fluid retention that leads to increased levels of BUN and creatinine in the blood. **[FIGURE 7-12]**

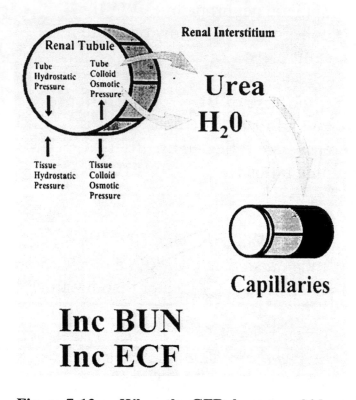

In addition, as part of the body's attempt to maintain euvolemia, angiotensin II exerts a direct renal effect that causes urea to pass from the medullary collecting duct into the renal interstitium. This forms an osmotic gradient that favors reabsorption of water. Since interstitial urea is then reabsorbed into the blood, the BUN level rises. This increase is *in addition* to any "backup" that has already occurred due to decreased renal perfusion. This retention of urea and water by the kidney is a normal physiological response to hypoperfusion. **[FIGURE 7-13]**

Figure 7-13 — When the GFR decreases, kidney tubules allow urea to flow into the interstitial tissue. The osmotic effect draws fluid from the tubules as well. Together, the urea and fluid are reabsorbed into the blood vessels. The result — increased circulatory volume and blood urea levels. The latter is manifested as an elevation of the BUN. This rise is a direct reflection of a *normal regulatory mechanism* and occurs whenever the juxtaglomerular apparatus is hypoperfused (regardless of the reason).

On the other hand, the renal tubules are *impermeable* to creatinine. In prerenal azotemia, the Cr level rises *only* as a function of decreased glomerular filtration, which is determined by renal blood flow. So, both BUN and Cr levels increase. In prerenal azotemia versus true renal failure, *more* urea is reabsorbed by the kidney's "normal" attempt to form concentrated urine. As a result, the BUN is elevated *out of proportion* to the Cr. The BUN/Cr ratio is not always diagnostic, but neither is any other test (remember, you are smarter than the "test").

Summary

The kidneys serve numerous functions, including regulation of fluid and electrolytes, as well as acid-base balance. The nephron is the structural and functional unit of the kidney and carries out three basic processes: glomerular filtration, tubular secretion, and tubular reabsorption. Though the details of renal failure and nephrology are beyond the scope of this text, the BUN Factory Tour allows us to understand that the BUN represents normal metabolism of protein by the GI tract and liver. With this knowledge, BUN becomes helpful not only in diagnosing renal failure, but in upper GI bleeding, starvation, and liver failure as well. The BUN/Cr ratio is often, but not always, helpful in differentiating prerenal from renal azotemia, due to different rates of rise of BUN and creatinine (Cr) in each state.

Crossword Puzzle Review

Path Chap 7 -- Renal

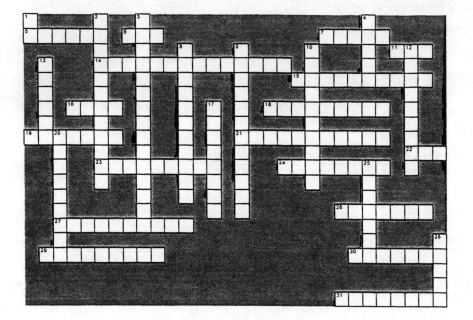

Across

5. Any rise in blood creatinine levels is a sensitive indicator of _____ malfunction.
6. A small amount of urea remains in the blood and is measured as the _____ (abbrev) level.
7. A BUN to Cr _____ of greater than 10:1 suggests prerenal azotemia.
11. The permeability to water of collecting tubules is controlled by _____ (abbrev).
14. Stimulates RBC production in the bone marrow.
15. Complex of capillaries in which fluid is filtered from the blood.
16. Urine creatinine levels can be used to estimate muscle _____.

18. Starvation leads to _____ BUN levels in the serum.
19. Structural and functional unit of the kidney.
21. Long tube in which fluid is converted into urine.
22. Ammonia is highly toxic to the _____ (abbrev).
23. Increased GI protein loads leads to _____ BUN levels in the serum.
24. The _____ tubule is normally impermeable to waste products.
26. BUN levels reflect _____ metabolism.
27. The great water permeability of the thin descending loop is due to the presence of water channels known as _____.

29. Net movement of water and solutes into the tubules.
30. Bowman's _____ is a membrane around the glomerulus.
31. "Good beans, bad water supply."

Down

1. Creatine is reversibly phosphorylated to creatine phosphate (phosphocreatine) by the enzyme _____ (abbrev).
2. Tubular fluid becomes _____ as it moves toward the medulla.
3. The first part of the distal tubule forms the _____ apparatus.
4. The majority of ammonia is converted to urea in the _____.
8. All normal renal functions serve to maintain _____.

9. Return of water and solutes from the tubules back into the blood.
10. Filtering of fluid from the glomerular capillaries into the renal tubules.
12. _____ block various membrane transporters and enzymes, leading to increased loss of electrolyte and water.
13. Creatinine levels reflect _____ metabolism.
17. An elevated BUN in the face of a normal creatinine level suggests GI _____.
20. Phosphocreatine serves as a store of high-energy _____ in muscle.
25. Accumulates during liver failure.
28. "Bad beans, good water supply."

References

1.   Ernst, A.A., et al. *Usefulness of the blood urea nitrogen/creatinine ratio in gastrointestinal bleeding.* Am J Emerg Med 1999 Jan; 17:134; Urashima, M., et al. *BUN/Cr ratio as an index of gastrointestinal bleeding mass in children.* J Pediatr Gastroenterol Nutr 1992 Jul; 15(1):89-92; Richards, R.Jj, et al. *Can the blood urea nitrogen/creatinine ratio distinguish upper from lower gastrointestinal bleeding?* J Clin Gastroenterol 1990 Oct; 12(5):500-4.

2.   Cuellar, R.E., et al. *Gastrointestinal tract hemorrhage. The value of a nasogastric aspirate.* Arch Intern Med 1990 Jul; 150(7):1381-4.

CHAPTER 8
"GOLDEN RULES OF PATHOPHYSIOLOGY"
A SUMMARY

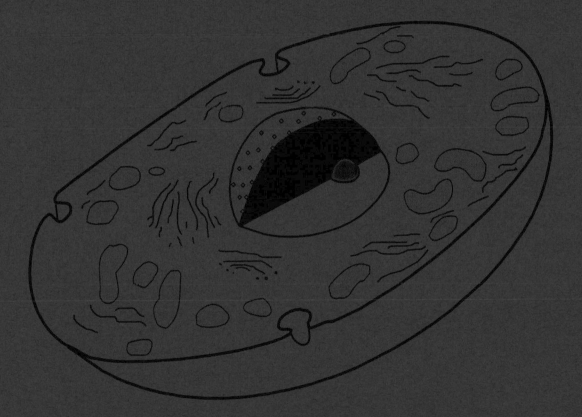

CHAPTER 8 — "GOLDEN RULES OF PATHOPHYSIOLOGY" — A SUMMARY

Contents

Introduction
Basic principles of medical science
Homeostasis and normal regulatory systems (NRS)
"Stuff"
The Basics — Airway, Breathing, Circulation
"Tests"
Crossword Puzzle Review

[*NOTE: There is no Summary or References in this chapter.*]

Introduction

This chapter contains a compilation of all generic principles discussed in the previous chapters. They are divided into categories, as noted above. I have listed the principles in order of importance, at least in my opinion. Each includes at least one example, discussed earlier in the text. I have included parenthetical initial page references wherever possible.

> ***Note to educators*** — These principles form an outline of the basic mechanisms and important considerations for all disease. Each principle could serve easily as the basis for a review or examination question. For example: *"Defend, using principles and examples, the concept that all human disease is 'autoimmune' in nature."* In fact, if I were limited to one essay question on the entire topic of pathophysiology, that would be it!

BASIC PRINCIPLES OF MEDICAL SCIENCE

PRINCIPLE: **Much of medicine follows simple, yet elegant principles. Once you learn the principle, it's easy to fill in the specifics for many different conditions.**

> *EXAMPLE*: Failure of normal regulatory systems (NRSs) to "fire" at the proper time, or a NRS's firing at the wrong time, but in response to an *appropriate* stimulus, is a common underlying theme in most human diseases [p. 1-6]. Congestive heart failure is a prime example — the kidney *thinks* we are hypovolemic, and responds in kind . . . The problem is that we are actually *hypervolemic* but the kidney doesn't know it, due to renal hypoperfusion [p. 3-42].

PRINCIPLE: **There are far more *similarities* than *differences* among the body's cells and organs.**

> *COROLLARY*: **By concentrating on *similarities* rather than *differences*, you need only to learn the underlying principles once. The rest involves *applying* the principle *with understanding* to various diseases.**

> *EXAMPLE*: The electrophysiology of ventricular fibrillation in the heart is nearly identical, down to a molecular level, to that of a generalized seizure in the brain. Causes and treatments also overlap significantly [p. 5-4].

PRINCIPLE: **You must appreciate the *normal* to understand the abnormal.**

> *EXAMPLE*: Diabetic ketoacidosis (DKA) occurs when the normal "yin-yang" balance of glucose is disrupted. Normally, insulin has anabolic effects, while the counterregulatory hormones (CRHs) (glucagon, epinephrine) have catabolic actions. DKA occurs when there are *decreased* levels of insulin (decreased anabolism) and *increased* levels of CRH (increased catabolism) [p. 2-32].

PRINCIPLE: **To understand what's new, you must be comfortable first with what's old.**

> *EXAMPLE*: The majority of intercellular communications occur via G-protein mediated reactions and cell surface receptors. Our current model, which includes second messengers and transfer of high-energy phosphate groups via G-proteins, is merely an updated version of the "lock and key" enzyme-substrate model described many years ago [p. 1-18].

PRINCIPLE: **Much of what we used to call "basic science" *directly impacts* our clinical practice and we must understand it to be our best.**

> *EXAMPLE*: Some antidysrhythmic agents (e.g., procainamide) exert their effects directly on ion channels. The aldosterone blocker, spironolactone (Aldactone®), affects ion channels in the kidneys, colon, and sweat glands [p. 3-53]. Ion channels are "gated" by G-proteins [p. 1-20]. Thus, what we do *clinically* directly affects events on a *molecular* level. In the past, these events were usually thought to be the bailiwick of basic science research only. Now, they impact directly on our clinical practice.

PRINCIPLE: **An apple fell from the tree, hitting Sir Isaac Newton, because of *gravity*. Like all laws of Nature, we're not about to change this fact any time soon.**

EXAMPLE: The beauty of medical science is that it follows simple, yet elegant, rules. If we use these appropriately, our patients benefit. Moving a patient with a free-flowing pleural effusion causes the fluid to move within the pleural space, due to gravity.

PRINCIPLE: **Water goes *down*, air goes *up*. This is a fixed law of nature.**

COROLLARY: **The main reason we don't understand concepts is that we try to rewrite the Laws of Nature.**

EXAMPLE: The "zones of the lungs" diagram merely reiterates, in a scientific fashion, the fact that "water goes down, air goes up" due to gravity. Though the diagram is often drawn in the shape of lungs, with the apices at the top, the principle holds, no matter what the patient's position. This explains why we don't become cyanotic when changing positions — unless congenital heart disease (e.g., pulmonic stenosis, tetralogy of Fallot) interferes with normal pulmonic blood flow and "rewrites" the laws of physics [p. 3-24].

PRINCIPLE: **Patients don't always "read the textbook" before they get sick.**

EXAMPLE: It's relatively easy to suspect an ailment when the patient has a "textbook" presentation. The presence of atypical signs and symptoms are the real challenge. It's relatively safe to assume that somewhere between 70% and 80% of all patients will have "typical" presentations of their problem. The rest require a "thinking cook." For example, hypoglycemia in an elderly patient may present as stroke-like symptoms or disorientation. It's easy to assume the patient has had a stroke or suffers from dementia (e.g., Alzheimer's disease). The "thinking cook" would also check the blood sugar — if it's low, the therapeutic response to glucose may be quite gratifying [p. 2-25].

PRINCIPLE: **The left brain seems to exist, at times, to overthink something that is *perfectly clear* into something *totally incomprehensible*.**

> *COROLLARY*: **Be open-minded; use your *right brain* first, to consider many possibilities. Then, refine them into an educationally-sound, medically-correct, and legally-defensible list of "probabilities," using the *left brain*.**

> *EXAMPLE*: If we look at a patient's chest x-ray and see a large infiltrate, our left brain immediately wants to jump to a diagnostic conclusion (e.g., "the patient has pneumonia"). In reality, the only thing we can safely conclude from the film itself is that the *finding* of an infiltrate is present. Pneumonia is a *diagnosis*. Humans, not tests, make diagnoses [p. 1-79]. The diagnostic triangle approach forces us to use our right brain first, then integrate other information using the left brain [p. xi].

PRINCIPLE: **There's nothing wrong with a "cookbook approach" as long as there's a "thinking cook."**

> *EXAMPLE*: The "four fixes" (oxygen, fluids, sugar, electricity) is a list of common causes of many different medical problems (e.g., altered mental status, seizures). Three of four of these "fixes" may be tried with relative safety in most patients. And the fourth, electricity, should always be considered (e.g., tachycardia, bradycardia requiring electrical treatment). No one should follow this, or any other protocol, empirically. The "thinking cook" approach assumes that we *consider* the alternatives first, and then judiciously choose the best for the patient [p. 1-71].

PRINCIPLE: **Sometimes the *best* treatment is *no* treatment at all.**

> *EXAMPLE*: One of the most difficult things for health care providers to do is nothing, in the face of abnormal lab values or vital signs. The "thinking cook," for example, asks why the blood pressure is high following a stroke. If it represents normal responsive hypertension due to a loss of cerebral autoregulation, acute lowering of the "abnormal number" may actually worsen the patient's condition. Watchful waiting is the most appropriate therapy in many situations [p. 3-61].

PRINCIPLE: **A multi-flanked attack works better than just a one-pronged one.**

> *EXAMPLE*: There are numerous conditions whose mechanisms are now clear enough that several avenues of attack are available. In many cases, this multi-flanked attack offers synergistic benefits. Congestive heart failure (ACE blockers, ARBS, β-blockers) [p. 3-4] and asthma [p. 4-4] (steroids, leukotriene blockers) are two conditions where this approach has been applied successfully.

HOMEOSTASIS AND NORMAL REGULATORY SYSTEMS (NRSs)

PRINCIPLE: **All human disease, in a strict sense, is "autoimmune" in nature.**

EXAMPLE: When we think of autoimmune disease, visions of HLA-B27 and ankylosing spondylitis come to mind. By "autoimmune" in this text, I refer to a broader interpretation — the body's own normal regulatory systems either fail to operate when they should, or "fire" when they shouldn't. The past several chapters have given many illustrations of normal mediators' having a double-edged sword effect. Under normal homeostatic conditions, mediators are of great benefit. If they fail to work, problems occur. Yet, if they are activated under inappropriate circumstances, these very same "normal" mediators may kill us.

EXAMPLE: An easy-to-remember example is free radicals. Remember, this is the major mechanism by which white blood cells kill bacteria. If free radicals were not produced (e.g., chronic granulomatous disease), we would have frequent and potentially life-threatening bacterial infections. If, however, they are produced inappropriately (post-ischemia, hypoglycemia), they indiscriminately destroy *our own* cells, much as they were normally intended to destroy bacteria [p. 1-44].

EXAMPLE: A similar situation occurs when the renin-angiotensin-aldosterone-ANP (atrial natriuretic protein) system is activated during congestive heart failure (CHF). Hypoperfusion of the kidney activates the system, whether we are really hypovolemic or not (obviously, not the case in CHF). Continued production of angiotensin II and ANP has deleterious effects (fibrosis, hypervolemia, ventricular remodeling, inhibition of excitation-contraction coupling) [p. 3-42].

EXAMPLE: The mediators produced in shock *all* have normal proinflammatory and anti-inflammatory functions. However, when produced in excess or at an inappropriate time, "immunologic dissonance" results, leading to the systemic inflammatory response syndrome, multiple organ dysfunction, failure, and eventually, death due to cardiogenic shock [p. 6-32].

PRINCIPLE: **Homeostasis is maintained by interactions of numerous "normal regulatory systems" (NRSs) of the body.**

EXAMPLE: NRSs are not autonomous — they interact and communicate with each other continuously. When the balance in one system is disrupted, others are necessarily affected. The heart-lung-brain triangle illustrates this principle. When a person suffers a stroke, he or she typically hypoventilates and may develop cardiac dysrhythmias. Treatment of the initiating event ("imbalance") may lead to resolution of the others. Of course, hypoventilation and cardiac dysrhythmias cannot be ignored, "pending" outcome of the stroke [p. 5-2]!

PRINCIPLE: **Many diseases arise from *loss* of a normal regulatory system (NRS) or *normal activation* of a NRS under *abnormal* circumstances, with untoward results.**

EXAMPLE: Severe hypoglycemia in diabetics occurs because they have lost a significant part of their counterregulatory "early warning" system (glucagon, epinephrine). Similarly, one of the reasons for an ever-increasing death rate from asthma is a loss of the early pulmonary "stretch response." Normally, the response would result in dyspnea early in the course of an attack. Without this normal regulatory system, patients present with far advanced disease, unaware of the severity of their condition [p. 2-15].

COROLLARY: **A** *normal response* **to an** *abnormal situation* **may lead to problems.**

EXAMPLE: As mentioned earlier, congestive heart failure is the classic example of activation of a NRS under abnormal circumstances [p. 3-51]. Another is anaphylaxis — the purpose of our immune system is to prevent attack from foreign materials and agents [p. 3-66]. Under many circumstances, this is beneficial. When the cascade is activated during anaphylaxis, the very same mediators are potentially lethal to us.

"STUFF"

PRINCIPLE: **Normal regulatory systems produce "stuff" that has a normal "job description." Under abnormal circumstances, this normal "stuff" may become "bad stuff" and hurt us.**

> *COROLLARY*: **The absence of "good stuff" and/or the production of "bad stuff" leads to disease.**

> *EXAMPLE*: Type I diabetes mellitus results from an absolute insulin deficiency due to autoimmune destruction of pancreatic beta cells. This same response is also thought to be responsible for the loss of glucagon counterregulation with the progression of disease (glucagon is made by alpha cells in the pancreas) [p. 2-17].

> *EXAMPLE*: Tumor necrosis factor (TNF) is an important normal inflammatory mediator. Its inappropriate release during congestive heart failure, though, is responsible for a series of anatomic changes (ventricular remodeling) that make a bad situation even worse. It becomes "bad stuff" [p. 3-22].

PRINCIPLE: **If the lack of "stuff" causes the problem, replace the missing "stuff" to fix it.**

> *EXAMPLE*: Recent data have shown that caffeine (2-3 cups of caffeinated coffee per day) effectively restores the "early warning system" in diabetics with previously severe hypoglycemic spells. The result is fewer severe attacks, without a loss of glucose control or hypertriglyceridemia [p. 2-17].

PRINCIPLE: **If "stuff" leads to problems, give "anti-stuff" to stop the formation of "stuff," block its action, or both.**

> *EXAMPLE*: Inflammatory mediators underlie the pathophysiology of both asthma and COPD. Treatment with inhaled steroids ("anti-stuff") is considered routine in most settings. Leukotriene blockers, parasympathetic nervous system blockers, and anti-IgE antibodies also offer benefit [p. 4-5].

> *EXAMPLE*: Catecholamines are produced when the heart is stretched, such as in hypervolemia or congestive heart failure. Though part of a normal regulatory mechanism under usual circumstances (the Bainbridge reflex), persistence of the stimulus leads to continued production of epinephrine, high levels of which are cardiotoxic. This finding has led to a radical change in our approach to chronic heart failure. The use of β-blockers has become routine. Suppression of high catecholamine levels improves patient well-being and survival [p. 3--22].

PRINCIPLE: **As long as the "stuff" that caused the problem in the first place is *still* present, so is the problem.**

> *COROLLARY*: **If you block only some of the "stuff," the patient *still* has a potentially severe problem.**

> *EXAMPLE*: Multiple mediators are produced during anaphylaxis, including histamine. The initial release of histamine causes the release of numerous additional mediators from mast cells and eosinophils (e.g., leukotrienes, prostaglandins, slow reacting substance of anaphylaxis, eosinophilic chemotactic factor). Most antihistamines block only histamine. It's easy to see how, if other mediators are also present, blocking histamine alone hasn't really solved the problem [p. 3-71].

PRINCIPLE: **If the "stuff" outlasts the treatment, there's still a problem.**

COROLLARY: **Some "stuff" outlasts "anti-stuff."**

EXAMPLE: The duration of "stuff" produced in many conditions is greater than that of our typical treatments. Intravenous DW50 only lasts one and one-half hours in the typical patient. If hypoglycemia should occur due to long-acting insulin, an oral agent , or an insulin overdose,, the patient initially will improve and then may worsen [p. 2-30].

EXAMPLE: Intravenous naloxone (Narcan®) lasts less than two hours in most people. However, most narcotics (legal and illicit) work for at least three to four hours. The implications are obvious — the patient is initially resuscitated, only to have a similar problem (e.g., respiratory arrest) recur once the naloxone has worn off. Intramuscular (IM) administration of naloxone, 2 mg, seems to alleviate this problem because it lasts up to six hours.

EXAMPLE: Late-phase reactions occur in 20% of patients with anaphylactic reactions. It is impossible to predict who will be affected. Though the mediators of the late phase reaction are somewhat different from those of the early reaction, their appearance still depends upon the IgE-antigen interaction that occurs initially, leading to degranulation of mast cells. Since aqueous epinephrine alone, regardless of the dose or route of administration, is short-lived (less than one hour), the patient is "unprotected" against the late reaction. Thus, pharmacologic prophylaxis is necessary in most patients (e.g., steroids, long-acting epinephrine [Susphrine®], cetirizine [Zyrtec®]) [p. 3-77].

PRINCIPLE: **If you're going to block "stuff," you need to block *all* the stuff.**

> **EXAMPLE**: Leukotriene blockers in asthma are effective in only 30% to 40% of patients. The most likely reason is that leukotrienes aren't the *only* mediators released. Corticosteroids block only one of two paths in leukotriene synthesis, so by themselves they may not be 100% effective, either. A combination of these drugs may prove the most beneficial [p. 4-7]. And, research continues on other "stuff" blockers in obstructive lung disease.

PRINCIPLE: **Bad "stuff" begets more bad "stuff."**

> **EXAMPLE**: When homeostatic systems are thrown out of balance, the result is gradually increasing chaos. Typically, mediator release leads not to an arithmetic progression of events (e.g., 1, 2, 3, 4 . . .) but a geometric one (1, 2, 4, 8, 16, 32 . . .). Following infection or injury, the inflammatory cascade leads to release of anti-inflammatory mediators on a local level. If the mediator combination fails to halt the process, the same cascade occurs systemically. Unstopped, the normal systems are overwhelmed as production of mediators continues, worsening an already bad situation [p. 6-32].

> **EXAMPLE**: In congestive heart failure, release of tumor necrosis factor initiates ventricular remodeling (in combination with angiotensin II). The result is a change in the geometry of the heart from a cylinder to a sphere. The greater radius of a spherical configuration means that the heart must work harder (due to LaPlace's Law) to maintain the same ventricular pressure [p. 3-24]. And, this must take place in the face of decreased oxygen and "food," due to TNF downregulation of nitric oxide and creatine transport protein receptors (loss of vasodilator effect and decreased availability of creatine). The failing heart then works even worse, leading to a vicious cycle of increasing dysfunction, renal hypoperfusion, and ventricular remodeling [p. 3-22].

THE BASICS: AIRWAY, BREATHING, CIRCULATION

PRINCIPLE: **All physiology and pathophysiology starts and ends with the ABCs.**

> *EXAMPLE*: Our current knowledge of biochemistry and cell biology has linked cell surface receptors, G-proteins, and second messengers to a variety of major chemical reactions in the body [p. 1-20]. Despite our understanding of these and the ability to modify their actions pharmacologically, all is lost if Airway, Breathing, and Circulation are not intact.

PRINCIPLE: **Patients live or die due to adequacy or failure of Airway, Breathing, and Circulation.**

> *EXAMPLE*: The major "clinical lesion" in diabetic ketoacidosis (DKA) is hypovolemia. The average fluid deficit in an adult is six to nine liters over a 24-hour period. The main treatment priority is fluid administration. Insulin, though important, becomes secondary. Studies have shown that insulin may be withheld initially, in favor of adequate fluid replacement, without injury. On the other hand, no human ethics committee in the world would approve a practice of withholding fluids and just giving insulin [p. 2-36].

PRINCIPLE: **When it "hits the fan," go back to basics.**

> *EXAMPLE*: Our understanding of the "yin-yang" balance between insulin and the counterregulatory hormones in DKA is highly refined. On the other hand, over-attention to this sophisticated biochemistry causes inattention to the major underlying problem — hypovolemia. When patients are not getting better as you'd expect, look for a problem in the basics, not in the "fancy" stuff [p. 2-36].

EXAMPLE: We'd all agree that insulin is supposed to lower the blood sugar. So, if we are manipulating a person's insulin dose according to the fasting blood sugar (FBS), we would *increase* the appropriate insulin if the FBS is up. If it continues to increase on subsequent days, we would also increase the insulin, figuring that more is needed. With me so far? Now, after three or four days of this, it becomes obvious that insulin is not doing what we originally intended — *lowering* the sugar. Now, it's time to go back to the basics — is it possible that by increasing the insulin dose, we are actually *worsening* nocturnal hypoglycemia, leading to counterregulatory hormone release and an *increased* FBS (Somogyi effect, or "dawn phenomenon") [p. 2-20]?

PRINCIPLE: **Always think "Oxygen, fluids, sugar, and electricity" (the "four fixes").**

EXAMPLE: When the going gets rough, always reassess the adequacy of Airway, Breathing, and Circulation. If these are intact, then consider empiric administration of oxygen, a fluid bolus, or glucose (of course, as a "thinking cook"). Hypoglycemia, for example, may present with a wide variety of signs and symptoms, ranging from cardiac dysrhythmias to respiratory arrest [p. 1-71].

PRINCIPLE: **The treatment of hypoxia is oxygen, not a "brown paper bag."**

EXAMPLE: "Anxiety-hyperventilation" is a diagnosis of exclusion. Else, we run the very real risk of harming the patient. The FIO_2 in a "brown paper bag" after 30 seconds of rebreathing is only 10% (versus 21% in room air). If the patient has any underlying problem that would normally require oxygen (e.g., pulmonary embolism, angina, myocardial infarction), we've impaired "Breathing" [p. 4-34].

PRINCIPLE: **Hyperventilation is a normal respiratory mechanism to compensate for metabolic acidosis. Having the patient rebreathe CO_2 by breathing through a "brown paper bag" does little to improve the pH.**

> *EXAMPLE*: Even if we were to give nasal oxygen prior to utilizing "brown paper bag" rebreathing, there are dangers. The first is the attitude of complacency that usually accompanies this approach. Second, and more important, is the fact that we are increasing the patient's pCO_2 level by rebreathing. If he or she is hyperventilating to compensate for a metabolic acidosis (by creating a respiratory alkalosis), we will have worsened the situation [p. 4-34].

PRINCIPLE: **Apparent "anxiety hyperventilators" have something *seriously wrong* until proven otherwise.**

> *COROLLARY*: **Give the patient the benefit of the doubt and administer oxygen first.**

> *EXAMPLE*: Many diseases, some potentially fatal (e.g., MI, pulmonary embolism, DKA), result in hyperventilation. Whether these are present is initially nearly impossible to tell, either in or out of the hospital setting. As noted above, "brown paper bag" treatment is potentially deadly. The "thinking cook" approach is to administer oxygen, withhold the brown paper bag, and consider *why* the problem is present [p. 4-34].

"TESTS"

PRINCIPLE: **You're only as good as the information you have to work with.**

EXAMPLE: The quality of decisions we are able to make depends upon the data on which we rely. In upper gastrointestinal bleeding, for example, aspiration of bright red blood (BRB) from a nasogastric (NG) tube suggests ongoing bleeding. However, the *absence* of BRB is only 70% sensitive — meaning that 30% of patients will have ongoing bleeding with a negative NG aspirate. This is why the BUN, hematocrit and hemoglobin levels, at least in a relatively stable patient, are more sensitive tests. Of course, the patient's clinical appearance and vital signs provide important information as well [p. 7-15].

PRINCIPLE: **If a finding is present, it helps you; if not, IDM — it doesn't matter. A negative test does *not* mean a *normal* patient.**

EXAMPLE: Test results that confirm what we *already suspect* are the most helpful. The "negative predictive value" or "rule-out" rate of many tests is less helpful. Take, for example, the patient with one hour of crushing, substernal chest pain. ST-segment elevation of 5 mm in contiguous EKG leads is compatible with acute myocardial ischemia — agreed? What if the clinical picture is the same, but the EKG, normal or nonspecific? Is the patient any less likely to have an acute cardiac event? Probably not — the only thing that the lack of ST-segment changes means is that the patient may not be a candidate for acute reperfusion therapy. Similarly, an elevated CK-MB level is compatible with acute MI, but a negative test in the first four to six hours does not *rule out* either myocardial infarction or acute myocardial ischemia.

PRINCIPLE: **If the patient looks *sick* and the test looks good, the patient is still *sick*.**

> *EXAMPLE*: When pulse oximeters became widely available, many intelligent health care providers let their brains take a leave of absence. Suddenly, we tended to assume (at least until reality resurfaced) that if the SpO_2 was more than 90%, the patient was doing all right. We forgot the rule that, in humans, blue is not a normal skin color! Always look at the patient first, not the test [p. 1-67].

> *EXAMPLE*: "STAT" portable chest x-ray films are routine in many Emergency Departments for patient with acute shortness of breath. Though I'm not knocking the potential value of a chest film, I am criticizing the practice of waiting for a test result to determine whether the patient is sick. I've seen radiographers enter an ED to take a portable film, only to stop and request rightly that the patient be given oxygen *prior* to their taking the film. Remember — there is very little therapeutic benefit of acute x-radiation on hypoxia!

PRINCIPLE: **"Borderline abnormal" lab results are the *most* dangerous for the patient because they encourage us to become complacent.**

> *EXAMPLE*: Lab results that are only a "little bit" on the high or low side don't generate a "**PANIC VALUE**" mark or an urgent phone call from the lab. As a result, we sometimes overlook them. And, some of these "borderline results" represent conditions that are potentially deadly.

Take the example of a patient with normal electrolytes except for a slightly low HCO_3^- value, say 15 (normal range = 22-25). Recall that metabolic acidosis results in intracellular movement of hydrogen. As a result, potassium shifts out of the cells, into the serum — this occurs *irrespective* of the total serum pH. So, whatever the patient's potassium level while the acidosis is present, it is *higher* than when the acidosis was not there. In other words, the potassium level is expected to *fall* when the acidosis corrects. If the patient's baseline potassium (before correction of the acidosis) was borderline low, it could easily fall into the hypokalemic range when the acidosis normalizes. The result, since *small* changes in serum K^+ levels lead to *large* changes in cardiac membrane potential, could be a fatal cardiac dysrhythmia. By understanding these electrolyte kinetics, you can see how dangerous it is to "blow off" a mildly decreased HCO_3^- value, especially if all else is normal [p. 2-42].

PRINCIPLE: **There is a *big* difference between *baseline* and *normal*.**

COROLLARY: **Trying to achieve *normal* levels in chronically compensated patients, rather than just returning them to their usual *baseline*, is often dangerous.**

EXAMPLE: COPD patients who are chronic CO_2 retainers have a chronic *respiratory acidosis* (high pCO_2) accompanied by a chronic compensatory *metabolic alkalosis* (high HCO_3). If these patients are placed on mechanical ventilation and we try to normalize their blood gases by hyperventilating the patient (lowering the high pCO_2), an acute and severe metabolic alkalosis remains (now *uncompensated* by CO_2 retention). Due to its effect on the oxyhemoglobin dissociation curve (Bohr effect), tissue oxygen delivery is hampered and metabolic shock may result [p. 4-35]. Even if the patient survives this event, weaning from the ventilator is usually incredibly difficult because the patient's normal regulatory systems are used to a "baseline" of high pCO_2 and high HCO_3. A better approach is to utilize "permissive hypercapnia," allowing the pCO_2 to remain somewhat high. The goal, then, becomes ventilating the patient back to his or her *baseline level*, not to normal [p. 4-15].

CROSSWORD PUZZLE REVIEW

Path Chap 8 -- Summary

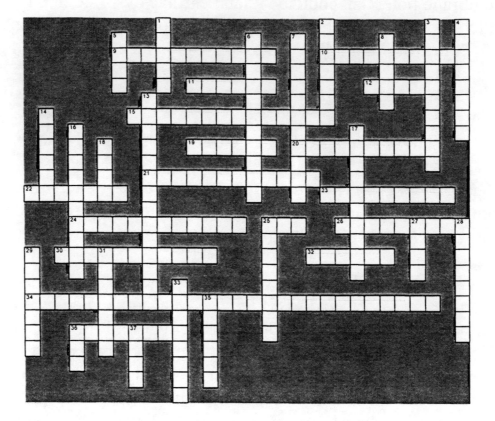

Across

9. You're only as good as the _____ you have to work with.
10. The absence of "good stuff" and /or the _____ of "bad stuff" leads to disease.
11. The treatment of hypoxia is _____ not a "brown paper bag."
12. Much of what we used to call _____ science directly impacts our clinical practice.
15. A _____ _____ (2 words) to an abnormal situation may lead to problems.
19. A negative test does not mean a _____ patient.
20. All human disease, in a strict sense, is _____ in nature.
21. There are far more _____ than differences among the body's cells and organs.
22. An apple fell from the tree, hitting Sir Isaac Newton, because of _____.
23. Hyperventilation is a normal respiratory compensatory mechanism for _____ acidosis.
24. There's nothing wrong with a "cookbook approach" as long as there's a _____.
25. If you're going to block "stuff," you need to block _____ the stuff.
26. If the "stuff" outlasts the _____, there's still a problem.
30. Sometimes the best treatment is _____ _____ (2 words).
32. When it "hits the fan," go back to _____.
34.
36. Some "stuff" _____ "anti-stuff."

Down

1. If "stuff" leads to problems, give "anti-stuff" to stop the formation of "stuff," _____ its action, or both.
2. If the lack of "stuff" causes the problem, _____ the missing "stuff" to fix it.
3. Much of medicine follows simple, yet elegant _____.
4. You must appreciate the normal to understand the _____.
5. If the patient looks sick and the test looks good, the patient is still _____.
6. _____ is maintained by interactions of numerous "normal regulatory systems" (NRS) of the body.
7. Trying to achieve normal levels in chronically _____ patients, rather than just return them to their usual baseline, is dangerous.
8. Always think oxygen, fluids, _____, and electricity (the "four fixes").
13. Normal regulatory systems produce "stuff" that has a normal _____ _____ (2 words).
14. A multi-flanked attack works _____ than just a one-pronged one.
16. Many diseases arise from loss of a NRS or normal _____ of a NRS under abnormal circumstances
17. Be open-minded; use your _____ _____ (2 words) first to consider many possibilities.
18. The _____ brain seems to exist, at times, to over think something that is perfectly clear into being totally incomprehensible.
25. Patients live or die due to _____ or failure of Airway, Breathing, and Circulation.
27. Bad "stuff" begets _____ bad "stuff."
28. Patients don't always read the _____ before they get sick.
29. As long as the "stuff" that caused the problem in the first place is still present, so is the _____.
31. The main reason we don't understand concepts is that we try to _____ the Laws of Nature.
33. Under abnormal circumstances, normal "stuff" may become _____ _____ (2 words) and hurt us.
35. Water goes down, air goes up. This is a fixed law of _____.
36. To understand what's new, you must be comfortable first with what's _____.
37. All physiology and pathophysiology starts and ends with the _____.

CROSSWORD PUZZLE REVIEW

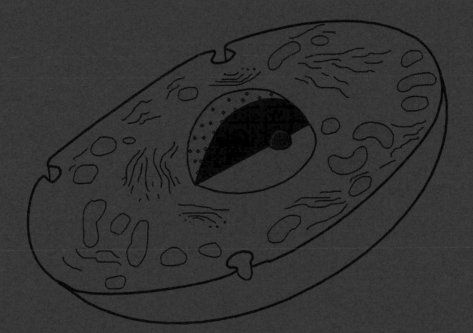

THE ANSWERS

Path Chap 1 -- The Basics

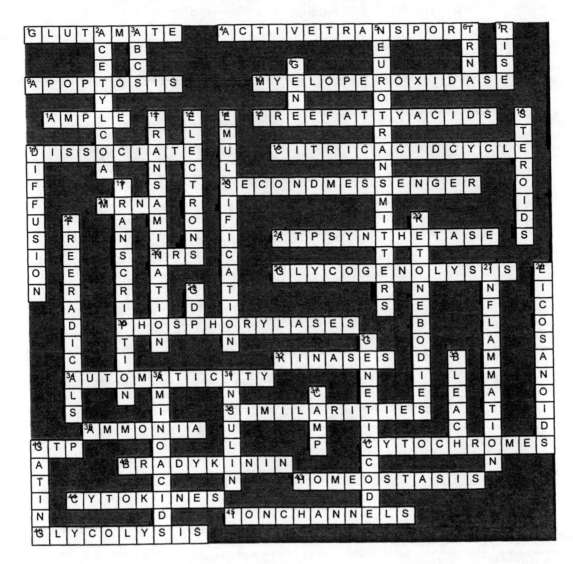

Across

The amino groups of most amino acids are ultimately funneled to _____.

_____. Movement of substances across a membrane in combination with a carrier protein against an energy gradient.

Genetically-programmed cell death.

0. Chronic granulomatosis results from congenital deficiency of sufficient _____.

1. Always take an _____ history.

5. _____ are eventually broken down to acetyl CoA from fat digestion, which enters into the citric acid cycle.

7. Ketones _____ in the blood, resulting in free hydrogen ions.

8. During the _____ _____ _____ (3 words), acetyl CoA is converted to water and carbon dioxide, and ATP is produced.

0. Compound that becomes activated by the triplex of ligand-receptor and G-protein (two words).

1. Carries the genetic code to the cytoplasm to control the formation of proteins (abbrev).

4. Catalyzes conversion of ADP to ATP during oxidative phosphorylation.

5. The myriad of "checks and balances" in the body (abbrev).

26. Process where glycogen is broken down into glucose.

30. Remove phosphate groups from molecules.

32. Add phosphate groups to molecules.

34. Each cell contributes to and benefits from normal on-going processes.

38. There are more _____ among the body's systems than differences.

39. Main toxic product of the urea cycle.

40. Attached to activated G-proteins.

41. Electrons are shuttled between compounds known as _____ as they pass through the electron transport chain.

42. Potent stimulator of increased vascular permeability, vasodilation, and bronchoconstriction.

43. _____ is a steady state in the internal environment.

44. Proteins produced by activated lymphocytes and macrophages that modulate the function of other cells.

45. Carry sodium, potassium, chloride, and calcium ions between cells.

46. _____ splits glucose into two molecules of pyruvic acid (pyruvate).

46. Glycerol released from the metabolism of triglycerides is eventually metabolized via _____.

Down

2. Pyruvate is converted to _____.

3. All physiology and pathophysiology begins and ends with the _____.

5. Use cell membrane receptors, G-proteins, and second messengers.

6. Transports amino acids to the ribosomes to be used in the assembly of proteins (abbrev).

7. During starvation, ingestion of a ketogenic diet, or DKA, levels of ketone bodies _____ in the blood.

8. Each _____ is a double-stranded helical molecule of deoxyribonucleic acid (DNA) that controls formation of ribonucleic acid (RNA).

12. _____ is the first step in the catabolism of most amino acids.

13. During oxidative phosphorylation, _____ from hydrogen enter a series of reactions, known as the electron transport chain.

14. The first step in digestion of fat.

16. Typically use intracellular receptors, leading to de novo synthesis of new proteins.

17. Random movement of molecules through spaces in the membrane.

19. Process of making RNA from DNA.

22. _____ are highly-reactive chemical intermediates that are short one electron in their outer orbital shell.

23. Excess acetyl CoA from fat breakdown is converted to _____ _____ (2 words).

27. Characteristically lacking in cells that have undergone apoptosis.

28. General term for products made from arachadonic acid.

29. Attached to inactivated G-proteins.

31. The _____ consists of triplets of three successive bases on a DNA strand, each coding for a specific protein.

33. The "respiratory burst" results in the formation of hypochlorous acid, more commonly known as _____.

35. The main digestive product of proteins.

36. Carbohydrates do not require _____ to be absorbed through the intestinal mucosa.

37. Intracellular calcium and _____ are the two most common second messengers.

40. Stimuli that open or close ion channels.

Path Chap 2 -- Endocrine/Metabolic

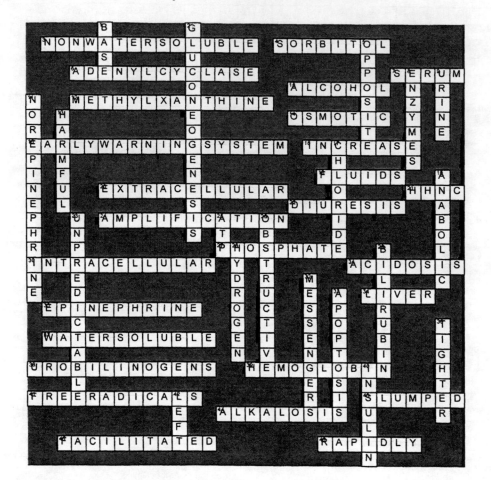

Across

3. Unconjugated (indirect) bilirubin is _____.
4. Chronic complications of diabetes probably occur from a combination of protein glycosylation and accumulations of intracellular _____.
6. Epinephrine leads to the G-protein mediated activatation of _____.
7. The _____ potassium exerts a major effect on membrane electrical potential.
10. Other drugs associated with hypoglycemia include _____, fluoxetine (Prozac), and glyburide (Micronase) when combined with ciprofloxacin (Cipro).
12. Caffeine is a _____ drug, much like aminophylline.
14. The main role of sodium is to maintain _____ balance between the extracellular and intracellular compartments of the body.
15. Diabetics who have lost part of their _____ _____ _____ (3 words) are more likely to have severe hypoglycemic spells.
16. Acidosis results in an _____ in the serum potassium level.
18. The major initial treatment in DKA.
20. Sodium is the major _____ fluid electrolyte.
21. Compared to DKA, _____ (abbrev) results in significant elevations of serum osmolality.
22. Exposure of the body to cold usually results in a cold _____.
24. Mechanism by which very low concentrations of epinephrine or glucagon are required for a significant hormonal effect to occur.
27. Many important biochemical reactions involve the addition or removal of _____ to or from a substance.
30. Potassium is the major _____ fluid electrolyte.
31. A low serum bicarbonate level indicates a metabolic _____.
34. The presence of bilirubin on the dip UA indicates a _____ or hepatobiliary problem.
34. Unconjugated (indirect) bilirubin is converted to conjugated (direct) bilirubin by the _____.
35. Second most important counterregulatory hormone of glucose metabolism.
37. Conjugated (direct) bilirubin is _____.
38. Bilirubin is converted to _____ in the colon and either excreted in the stool or filtered by the kidneys and excreted in the urine.
39. Bilirubin is a normal breakdown product of _____.
41. One major source of brain damage after prolonged hypoglycemia is _____ _____ (2 words).
43. Acronym for common causes of metabolic acidosis.
44. A high serum bicarbonate level indicates a metabolic _____.
45. Glucose move into cells by either _____ transport or cotransport.
46. Rapid changes in the serum sodium level should be corrected _____.

Down

1. Bicarbonate represents metabolic _____.
2. Glucagon stimulates glycogenolysis, inhibits glycogenesis, and stimulates _____.
2. Ethanol causes hypoglycemia by diverting resources from the process of _____.
2. Cortisol increases hepatic _____.
5. The effects of glucagon are _____ to those of insulin.
8. In hepatocellular damage, liver _____ are elevated greater than two times normal.
9. Conjugated bilirubin that does not enter the bowel leaves the body in the _____.
11. ACE blockers increase the likelihood of hypoglycemia in diabetics by decreasing the production of _____.
13. Prolonged hypoglycemia is _____.
17. The resting membrane potential occurs as a result of potassium movement with movement of _____.
19. Insulin has _____ effects while counterregulatory hormones have catabolic actions.
23. The blood sugar level at which a given patient becomes symptomatic from hypoglycemia is _____.
25. Thiamine deficiency leads to formation of inadequate brain _____.
26. Patients with total _____ jaundice have absolutely no urobilinogen in their urine.
28. Ketones dissociate in serum, resulting in free _____ ions.
29. The presence of visible clinical jaundice means that the patient's _____ level is elevated.
32. Insulin does not act through second _____.
33. Red blood cells die every 120 days via the normal process of _____.
36. The _____ a person's diabetic control, the greater the risk of hypoglycemic spells.
40. Facilitates intracellular transport of ingested nutrients.
42. Bicarbonate causes the oxyhemoglobin desaturation curve to shift to the _____.

Path Chap 3 -- Cardiovascular

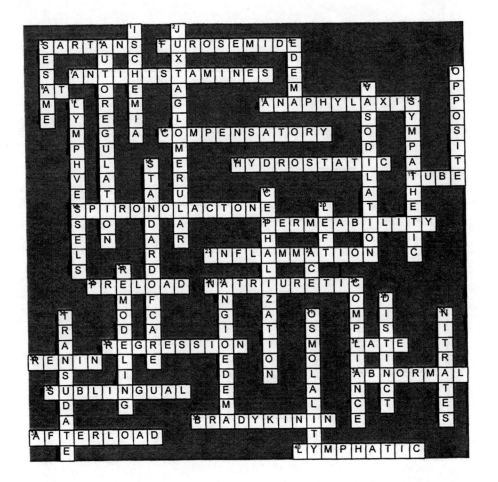

Across

3. Specific blockers of AT-1 receptors.
5. Only common drug for pulmonary edema that increases pulmonary lymphatic efferent flow.
7. Risky therapy, by themselves, for acute and progressive urticaria.
9. General type of receptors bound by angiotensin-II.
12. Any type I IgE-mediated immediate hypersensitivity reaction, regardless of the severity of the symptoms.
14. Cardiac dilation on the chest x-ray in CHF initially reflects a normal _____ mechanism.
16. _____ pressure refers to the "water pressure" either in the tubule or the surrounding tissue.
17. The Starling equation is a mathematical relationship that expresses the net direction of fluid flow into or out of a biologic _____.
19. Specific aldosterone blocker.
21. Pulmonary edema results from leaky vessels (abnormal _____), low oncotic pressure, or increased hydrostatic pressure.
22. Underlying lesion in atherosclerosis, acute and chronic.
25. The amount of blood the heart must pump.
26. Production of _____ proteins by the atria prevents fluid and sodium overload.
33. Stimulation of AT-2 receptors by angiotensin-II leads to _____ of left ventricular hypertrophy.
34. Occurrence of the _____ phase of an anaphylactic reaction depends directly upon the presence of the early phase.
35. Catalyzes the conversion of angiotensinogen to angiotensin-I.
36. You must appreciate the normal to understand the _____.
37. Potentially life-saving route of epinephrine administration in anaphylaxis.
38. Reason for cough in patients on ACE blockers.
39. The workload against which the heart must pump blood.
40. As CHF progresses, the _____ load increases.

Down

1. The underlying lesion in acute pulmonary edema is myocardial _____.
2. Receptors in the macula densa region of _____ apparatus of the kidney monitor intravascular volume and serum sodium concentration.
3. Type of oil contained in Susphrine.
4. Elevated blood pressure is a normal response to loss of cerebral _____.
6. Production of excess fluid in the interstitium or body cavities.
8. The response of the pulmonary circulation to hypoxia is _____ to that of the peripheral vessels.
10. Nitric oxide produces _____.
11. _____ _____ (2 words) are able to dilate and increase their fluid carrying capacity up to fifty times normal.
13. TNF is thought to be released due to _____ stimulation.
15. Beta-blockers are considered a _____ _____ _____ (3 words) in many patients with chronic CHF.
18. _____ of flow on the chest x-ray in CHF is a result of hypoxic vasoconstriction.
20. Side of the lymphatic circulation on which the majority of lymph fluid drains.
23. _____ (abbrev) catalyzes the conversion of AT-I to angiotensin-II.
24. An enlarged cardiac silhouette in late CHF is due to ventricular _____.
27. Life-threatening side effect of ACE blockers.
28. The most common form of hydrostatic pulmonary edema is due to acute loss of left ventricular _____.
29. ARDS is a _____ clinical entity with specific diagnostic criteria.
30. Edema fluid produced by noninflammatory mechanisms is called a _____.
31. By altering the _____ of the renal medulla, fluid is either drawn back into the body from the collecting tubules or allowed to leave as urine.
32. Sildenafil (Viagra) has a potentially life-threatening interaction with _____.

Path Chap 4 -- Respiratory

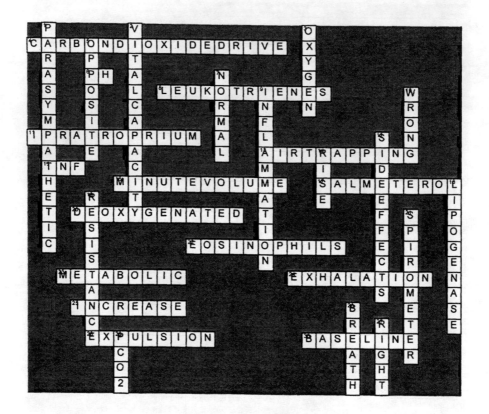

Across

Across

4. Primary normal breathing stimulus.
6. Sum of all potentially competing and compensatory respiratory and metabolic acid-base processes.
8. _____ are produced from arachidonic acid, as are prostaglandins, but via a different pathway.
11. Blocks bronchoconstriction induced by cGMP.
13. During attacks, asthma patients suffer bronchospasm with variable degrees of _____ _____ (2 words).
15. Potential mediator during acute exacerbation of COPD.
16. Total amount of new air moved into the respiratory passages each minute.
17. Inhaled beta-sympathomimetic agents indicated only for chronic therapy.
20. Cyanosis appears when the amount of _____ hemoglobin is > 5 gm per 100 ml of blood.

22. Increase in sputum 2-3 days prior to an acute exacerbation.
23. Hyperventilation is a normal respiratory compensatory mechanism for _____ acidosis.
24. FEV1 is the amount of air that can be expired in one second during a forced _____.
25. Shifts of the oxyhemoglobin dissociation curve to the left _____ the affinity of hemoglobin for oxygen.
28. Peak expiratory flow is the fastest measured rate of air _____ during a maximum forced exhalation.
30. There is a big difference between _____ and normal.

Down

1. _____ (cholinergic) stimulation leads to the formation of arachidonic acid.
2. Maximum amount of air a person can expel from the lungs after a maximum inspiration followed by maximum expiration.

3. The best treatment for a hypoxic patient.
5. The pH and the pCO2 move in _____ directions.
7. In restrictive disease, flow rates are usually _____, but the lungs are unable to expand fully.
9. Underlying chronic state in obstructive lung disease.
10. Apparent "anxiety hyperventilators" have something _____ until proven otherwise.
12. Lower risk with inhaled steroids, but still present.
14. Despite advances, the death rate from asthma continues to _____.
18. Enzyme that produces leukotrienes from arachidonic acid.
19. Persons with near fatal asthma appear to have blunted perception of increased airflow _____.

19. Obstructive lung disease is characterized by increased _____ to air flow and high lung volumes.
21. Device that measures respiratory excursions and air movement.
26. Tidal volume is the volume of air inspired or expired with each normal _____.
27. Oxygen delivery to the tissues increases when the oxyhemoglobin dissociation curve shifts to the _____.
29. Respiratory acid level in the blood.

Path Chap 5 -- Neuro

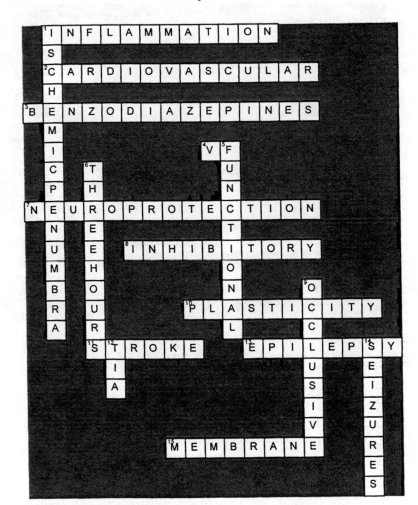

Across

1. Underlying lesion in cerebrovascular disease.
2. Neurophysiology is very similar to that of the _____ system.
3. Stop seizures by causing release of GABA.
4. The pathophysiology of a seizure in the brain is nearly identical to that of _____ (abbrev) of the heart.
7. Why we still need early identification of stroke victims.

8. GABA is an _____ neurotransmitter.
10. Reason patients with seizures become refractory to benzodiazepines.
11. Cerebral ischemic syndrome resulting from disruption of the cerebral circulation.
13. Seizures recurring spontaneously over a span of years.
15. Both lidocaine and phenytoin have _____-stabilizing actions.

Down

1. The "peri-stroke" zone.

5. Neuronal plasticity is the ability of a cell to alter its _____ properties "on the fly."
6. Usual upper limit "window of opportunity" for thrombolytic therapy in stroke.
9. The majority of vascular strokes are _____ in nature.
12. "Unstable angina of the brain" (abbrev).
14. sudden, paroxysmal episodes caused by excessive electrical discharge of cerebral neurons.

Path Chap 6 -- Shock

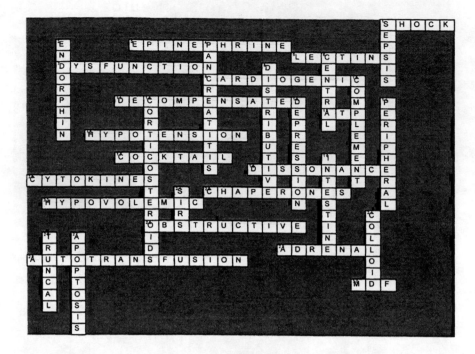

Across

1. Syndrome of inadequate delivery and use of oxygen at the cellular level.
3. The body's initial response to hypovolemia results in the release of norepinephrine and _____.
5. General term for proteins that bind carbohydrates with high affinity and specificity.
7. WBC _____ is common in the SIRS.
9. Type of shock when the cardiac pump cannot adequately circulate the available volume.
11. Phase of shock where cells switch to anaerobic metabolism.
15. Decreased production of _____ (abbrev) leads to intracellular energy failure.
16. _____ is not necessary to diagnose shock.
17. Many times, a catecholamine _____ is preferable to a single agent.
19. Immunologic _____ occurs because the patient has inappropriate and unbalanced normal regulatory systems.
20. Endogenously produced proteins of small molecular weight with multiple biological effects.
22. Molecular _____ prevent misfolding and aggregations of proteins.
23. Type of shock where the intravascular compartment is inadequately filled for proper tissue perfusion.
25. Type of shock where physical obstruction to blood flow in the heart or great vessels is present.
28. A significant number of patients with shock have acquired _____ insufficiency.
29. Capillary hydrostatic pressure decreases in early shock, allowing fluid from the interstitium to flow into the vessels.
30. General term (abbrev) for compounds produced in shock that ultimately result in cardiogenic shock and death.

Down

1. The systemic response to infection.
2. In shock, TRH acts by an antagonism of the _____ system.
4. Acute _____ is the "classic" example of a noninfectious process that leads to identical hemodynamic features of septic shock.
6. Form of shock when the heart and great vessels are unable to pump sufficient blood to maintain tissue oxygen needs.
8. Type of shock due to a major defect in arterial resistance, venous capacitance, or both with loss of vascular tone.
10. Activation leads to formation of the membrane attack complex.
12. High-dose _____ should not be used for treatment of septic shock.
13. Profound myocardial _____ has been described in the end stages of most forms of shock.
14. Type of shock that occurs at the level of the peripheral vascular bed.
18. The _____ is thought to be one of the first organs to respond to shock.
21. Acute illness characterized by generalized activation of the endothelium (abbrev).
24. Two to four times the volume of crystalloid must be infused compared with _____.
26. Unless the patient has penetrating truncal trauma, "standard" fluid therapy is still considered appropriate.
27. Neutrophil _____ is altered in the SIRS.

Path Chap 7 -- Renal

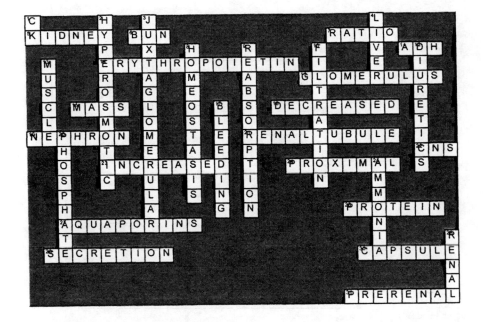

Across

5. Any rise in blood creatinine levels is a sensitive indicator of _____ malfunction.
6. A small amount of urea remains in the blood and is measured as the _____ (abbrev) level.
7. A BUN to Cr _____ of greater than 10:1 suggests prerenal azotemia.
11. The permeability to water of collecting tubules is controlled by _____ (abbrev).
14. Stimulates RBC production in the bone marrow.
15. Complex of capillaries in which fluid is filtered from the blood.
16. Urine creatinine levels can be used to estimate muscle _____.
18. Starvation leads to _____ BUN levels in the serum.
19. Structural and functional unit of the kidney.
21. Long tube in which fluid is converted into urine.
22. Ammonia is highly toxic to the _____ (abbrev).
23. Increased GI protein loads leads to _____ BUN levels in the serum.
24. The _____ tubule is normally impermeable to waste products.
26. BUN levels reflect _____ metabolism.
27. The great water permeability of the thin descending loop is due to the presence of water channels known as _____.
29. Net movement of water and solutes into the tubules.
30. Bowman's _____ is a membrane around the glomerulus.
31. "Good beans, bad water supply."

Down

1. Creatine is reversibly phosphorylated to creatine phosphate (phosphocreatine) by the enzyme _____ (abbrev).
2. Tubular fluid becomes _____ as it moves toward the medulla.
3. The first part of the distal tubule forms the _____ apparatus.
4. The majority of ammonia is converted to urea in the _____.
8. All normal renal functions serve to maintain _____.
9. Return of water and solutes from the tubules back into the blood.
10. Filtering of fluid from the glomerular capillaries into the renal tubules.
12. _____ block various membrane transporters and enzymes, leading to increased loss of electrolyte and water.
13. Creatinine levels reflect _____ metabolism.
17. An elevated BUN in the face of a normal creatinine level suggests GI _____.
20. Phosphocreatine serves as a store of high-energy _____ in muscle.
25. Accumulates during liver failure.
28. "Bad beans, good water supply."

Path Chap 8 -- Summary

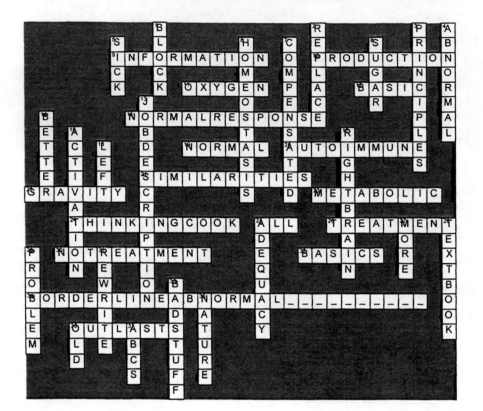

INDEX AND ABBREVIATION CROSS-REFERENCE

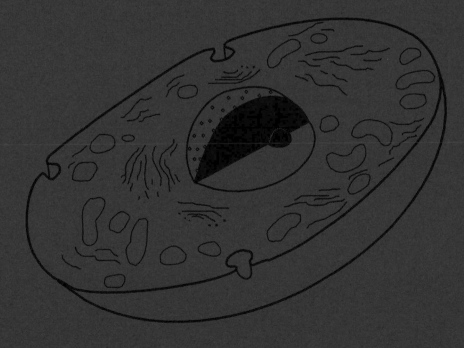

INDEX AND ABBREVIATION CROSS-REFERENCE

2

Four fixes, 1-1, 1-2, 1-55, 1-71, 1-72
Free fatty acids, 1-29, 1-30, 1-40, 2-33, 2-34
Free radicals, 1-2, 1-43, 1-47, 2-23, 4-5, 5-14, 5-17, 6-26, 6-52, 6-56, 8-7
Furosemide, 3-2, 3-37, 3-41, 7-8, 7-9

G

G6PD (glucose-6-phosphate dehydrogenase), 1-47
Gamma aminobutyric acid (GABA), 5-6, 5-7, 5-8
Gastric tonometry, 6-20
Gastrointestinal, 1-74, 6-15, 6-21, 6-45, 6-50, 7-13, 7-14, 7-15, 7-16
Gating, 1-16
GCS (Glasgow coma scale), 1-67
GDP, 1-19, 1-20, 1-23, 1-24
Gene, 1-11, 1-49, 2-10
Generalized seizure, 5-3, 8-2
Genetic code, 1-11, 1-13
GFR (glomerular filtration rate), 3-43, 3-51, 6-22, 7-7, 7-17, 7-18
GI (gastrointestinal), 1-30, 1-61, 1-62, 1-74, 2-6, 6-13, 7-10, 7-13, 7-14, 7-19
Glasgow coma scale, 1-66, 1-67
Globin, 7-14
Glomerular filtration rate (GFR), 2-35, 3-43, 3-51, 3-63, 6-22, 7-7, 7-17, 7-19
Glomerulus, 7-5, 7-6
Glucagon, 2-2, 2-5, 2-6, 2-11, 2-18, 2-29, 2-32, 2-33, 2-35, 3-55, 8-3, 8-8, 8-9
Glucocorticoids, 2-13, 6-48, 6-49
Gluconeogenesis, 2-9, 2-11, 2-13, 2-16, 2-28, 2-29, 2-35
Glucose 6-phosphate dehydrogenase (G6PD), 1-47
Glucose clamp, 2-19
Glucose transport vesicles, 2-8
Glucosuria, 2-36, 2-40
Glutamate oxaloacetate transaminase (GOT, AST), 1-38
Glutamate pyruvate transaminase (GPT, ALT), 1-37
Glutamate, 1-36, 1-38, 5-8, 6-19, 7-11
Glyburide, 2-28
Glycine, 5-19
Glycogen, 1-26, 1-34, 1-36, 2-5, 2-7, 2-9, 2-11, 2-12, 2-16, 2-33
Glycogenesis, 1-26
Glycogenolysis, 1-26, 2-9, 2-11, 2-13, 2-16, 2-29, 2-35
Glycolysis, 1-27, 1-32, 2-9, 2-11, 2-24, 2-39
Glycosylated hemoglobin, 2-39

Glycosylation, 2-39
GOT (glutamate oxaloacetate transaminase), 1-38, 1-65, 2-31, 3-29
G-protein, 1-2, 1-19, 1-20, 1-22, 1-24, 1-53, 2-12, 2-13, 3-51, 3-54
GPT (glutamate pyruvate transaminase), 1-37, 1-19, 1-20, 1-23, 1-24, 3-51
Guanine, 1-12
Guanosine diphosphate, 1-19

H

H_2-blockers, 3-2
Haldane effect, 2-37
Hb (hemoglobin), 2-39
Hct (hematocrit), 7-15
HDLs (high-density lipoproteins), 1-31
Head trauma, 3-63, 6-15
Hematocrit, 1-74, 3-40, 6-40, 6-64, 8-16
Hemodynamic instability, 6-41
Hemoglobin, 1-74, 2-37, 2-39, 3-40, 4-1, 6-13, 6-59, 7-14, 8-16
Hemolysis, 1-47
Hepatic failure, 6-53, 7-15, 7-16
Herbals, 1-60
HES (hydroxyethyl startch), 6-41
Hg (hemoglobin), 1-66, 2-38, 3-6, 3-10, 3-11, 4-15, 4-19, 6-9, 6-64
HHNC (hyperosmolar hyperglycemic nonketotic coma), 2-40, 2-41
High-density lipoproteins, 1-31
Hippocampus, 5-6, 5-7
Histamine, 1-50, 1-54, 3-41, 4-12, 6-14, 6-27, 8-10
Homeostasis, 1-1, 1-4, 1-6, 1-42, 1-43, 2-1, 2-5, 3-51, 3-52, 4-15, 6-32, 6-33, 7-3,
        8-1, 8-6, 8-7
Houston, 6-41, 6-42
Hydrocortisone, 6-49, 6-51
Hydrophilic, 1-29
Hydrostatic pressure, 3-5, 3-7, 3-9, 3-13, 3-16, 3-28, 3-29, 3-35, 3-37, 6-13
Hydrostatic pulmonary edema, 3-13
Hydroxyethyl starch (HES), 6-41
Hyperglycemia, 2-11, 2-23, 2-32, 2-41, 6-36
Hyperkalemia, 2-37
Hyperosmolar hyperglycemic nonketotic coma (HHNC), 2-40, 2-41
Hypertensive emergencies, 3-1, 3-3, 3-61
Hypertonic saline, 6-39, 6-41

Hyperventilation, 2-32, 4-1, 4-3, 8-15

Hypochlorite free radical, 1-45

Hypochlorous acid, 1-45, 1-46

Hypoglycemia, 1-46, 1-71, 1-72, 2-1, 2-2, 2-6, 2-7, 2-14, 2-17, 2-19, 2-31, 2-37, 3-55, 4-12, 8-4, 8-7, 8-8, 8-11, 8-14

Hypo-oncotic (permeability) pulmonary edema, 3-1, 3-11

Hypotension, 1-60, 2-18, 3-40, 3-41, 3-50, 3-51, 6-2, 6-5, 6-6, 6-18, 6-20, 6-27, 6-36, 6-39, 6-43, 6-45, 6-47, 6-57, 6-58, 6-62, 6-65

Hypothalamic-pituitary-thyroid axis, 6-56

Hypothermia, 1-68, 2-1, 2-32

Hypovolemia, 1-66, 1-71, 1-72, 2-36, 2-41, 3-41, 3-43, 3-51, 6-13, 6-62, 7-14, 7-16, 7-18, 8-13

Hypovolemic shock, 6-5, 6-6, 6-8, 6-12, 6-13, 6-16, 6-18, 6-21, 6-58, 6-62

Hypoxia, 1-48, 1-49, 1-71, 1-72, 1-74, 3-17, 3-26, 3-28, 4-15, 4-17, 6-34, 8-14, 8-17

Hypoxic drive, 4-15

Hypoxic injury, 1-49

Hypoxic vasoconstriction, 3-24, 3-26, 3-29

I

ICAMs (intracellular adhesion adhesion molecules), 6-30, 6-31, 6-54

ICF (intracellular fluid), 1-14, 1-15

IgE, 4-10, 8-10, 8-11

IM (intramuscular), 3-2, 8-11

Immunologic dissonance, 6-63

Immunosuppression, 6-32

Infection, 1-53, 1-61, 2-21, 2-32, 2-41, 3-2, 3-12, 3-34, 3-56, 3-58, 3-59, 4-13, 6-12, 6-15, 6-18, 6-20, 6-21, 6-27, 6-31, 6-32, 6-48, 6-50, 6-55, 6-63, 8-12

Inflammation, 1-1, 1-5, 1-21, 1-47, 1-48, 1-50, 1-53, 1-61, 1-63, 3-2, 3-6, 3-45, 3-56, 3-59, 4-1, 4-5, 4-8, 4-11, 4-14, 5-10, 5-11, 5-16, 5-17, 6-8, 6-15, 6-16, 6-26, 6-28, 6-30, 6-61, 6-63

Initial assessment, 1-65

Initiation, 1-44, 1-53, 6-22

INR (international normalized ratio), 3-60

Insulin receptor, 2-7

Insulin, 1-26, 2-2, 2-5, 2-11, 2-14, 2-17, 2-19, 2-22, 2-25, 2-27, 2-30, 2-37, 2-40, 2-41, 3-58, 6-15, 6-36, 8-2, 8-3, 8-9, 8-11, 8-13, 8-14

Integrins, 6-30, 6-31

Oxyhemoglobin dissociation curve, 2-37, 2-38, 4-3, 8-18

P/Q

Pancreas, 2-11, 2-17, 7-9, 8-9
Pancreatitis, 3-12, 6-28, 6-29, 6-31
Parasympathetic blockade, 4-9
Parasympathetic, 4-9, 6-5, 6-6, 8-10
Parasympatholytic agents, 4-1
Partial thromboplastin time, 6-15
PAWP (pulmonary artery wedge pressure), 3-16
Peak expiratory flow, 4-12, 4-13
PEF, *see:* peak expiratory flow
Pentoxifylline, 6-43, 6-44, 6-52, 6-54, 6-61, 6-65
Peripheral edema, 3-5, 3-50, 3-52, 6-40
Peripheral nervous system, 2-16
Peripheral shock, 6-10, 6-62
Peritonitis, 6-8, 6-26, 6-27, 6-53
Permeability, 1-43, 1-50, 1-53, 3-1, 3-5, 3-7, 3-9, 3-13, 6-14, 6-18, 6-19, 6-29,
            6-55, 7-6, 7-8
Peroxynitrite, 6-26
pH, 1-33, 2-34, 2-38, 2-39, 4-15, 4-19, 6-20, 6-57, 8-15, 8-17
Phosphocreatine, 7-9, 7-10
Phosphodiesterase inhibition, 2-18, 4-10
Phosphodiesterase, 2-18, 3-39, 4-10, 4-11, 6-52
Phospholipase C, 1-21, 1-24, 3-44
Phosphorylases, 1-21, 1-24, 1-26, 1-29, 1-31, 1-32, 1-40, 1-42
Phosphorylation, 2-7
Pi (high energy phosphate), 1-20, 1-22, 1-23
Pituitary gland, 6-58
Plasmin, 1-51
Platelet activating factor, 1-54, 6-22, 6-26, 6-27
Platelet aggregation, 1-52, 1-53, 3-60, 6-52
Platelets, 1-50, 1-54, 3-59, 3-60, 6-32, 6-52
Pleural effusion, 3-1, 3-31, 3-33, 8-3
Pleural space, 3-31, 3-33, 8-3
PMNs, *see:* polymorphonuclear cells
PNS (peripheral nervous system), 2-16
Polymorphonuclear cells, 6-30
Polypeptides, 1-35, 1-36

R

Septic shock, 6-12, 6-13, 6-15, 6-16, 6-18, 6-20, 6-24, 6-26, 6-27, 6-30, 6-38, 6-43, 6-50, 6-52, 6-56, 6-59, 6-60

Serevent®, 4-5

Serotonin, 1-50, 1-54, 6-14

Serum osmolality, 2-40, 2-41

Severe sepsis, 6-21, 6-48, 6-54

Severe shock, 6-5

Shock, 2-38, 3-12, 3-40, 6-1, 6-10, 6-12, 6-13, 6-15, 6-16, 6-18, 6-24, 6-26, 6-30, 6-32, 6-36, 6-38, 6-39, 6-61, 6-60, 6-62, 6-64, 7-16, 7-17, 8-7, 8-18

Shortness of breath, 4-1, 4-3, 6-35, 8-17

Signal amplification, 2-13

Sildenafil, 3-39, 3-40

Singulair®, 4-8

SIRS, *see:* systemic inflammatory response syndrome

Smoking, 4-15

Snowballs, 3-28

Sodium, 1-14, 1-15, 1-63, 1-74, 2-3, 2-8, 2-18, 2-39, 2-42, 3-40, 3-42, 3-43, 3-46, 3-49, 3-52, 6-13, 6-48, 7-3, 7-4, 7-6, 7-8

Somogyi phenomenon, 2-2, 2-20, 2-22

Sorbitol dehydrogenase, 2-39, 2-40

Sorbitol, 2-39, 2-40

Spironolactone, 3-2, 3-49, 3-53, 3-55, 8-3

Splanchnic blood flow, 6-18

Sputum eosinophil count, 4-13

SQ (subcutaneous), 3-2

Starling equation, 3-4, 3-5, 3-7, 3-10, 3-12

Starling mechanism, 3-17, 3-18, 3-21

Starling's Law, 3-1, 3-4, 3-6, 3-9, 3-17, 3-19

Starvation, 1-33, 2-34, 3-5, 7-13, 7-15, 7-19

Statins, 3-59, 5-20

Status epilepticus, 5-6, 5-7, 5-8, 5-9

Stroke, 1-46, 1-49, 1-70, 2-25, 2-41, 3-59, 3-61, 3-63, 5-1, 5-2, 5-5, 5-8, 5-10, 5-11, 5-12, 5-13, 5-14, 5-15, 5-16, 5-17, 5-18, 5-19, 5-20, 5-21, 5-22, 6-57, 8-4, 8-6, 8-7

Substance P, 1-53

Sugar, 1-26, 1-72, 2-5, 2-7, 2-11, 2-17, 2-20, 2-26, 2-29, 2-33, 2-37, 2-39, 2-40, 8-4, 8-5, 8-14

Superantigens, 6-12, 6-21, 6-53

Superoxide free radical, 1-45

SVR, *see:* systemic vascular resistance

Transient ischemic attack, 5-1, 5-11, 5-20, 5-22
Translation, 1-11, 1-13, 2-10, 2-34, 6-24
Trauma, 1-57, 2-25, 3-12, 3-63, 6-5, 6-6, 6-8, 6-10, 6-15, 6-16, 6-20, 6-22, 6-30, 6-35, 6-41, 6-42, 6-44, 6-55, 6-59, 6-63
Treat and release, 2-30
Trendelenburg position, 6-35
TRH, *see:* thyroid-releasing hormone
Triamterene, 7-9
Triglycerides, 1-29, 1-34, 1-40, 1-62, 2-5, 2-9, 2-10, 2-33
tRNA, *see:* transfer RNA
Troponin, 1-21
Trypsin, 1-35
Tubular reabsorption, 7-4, 7-5, 7-19
Tubular secretion, 7-5, 7-19
Tumor necrosis factor (TNF), 1-53, 1-54, 3-21, 4-14, 6-15, 6-19, 6-21, 6-23, 6-27, 6-28, 6-32, 6-52, 6-54, 6-61, 6-63, 8-9, 8-12
Tyrosine kinase, 2-7

U

UA (urinalysis), 2-3, 2-32
UGIB, *see:* upper gastrointestinal bleeding
Undermedication, 4-11
Unstable coronary ischemic syndromes, 3-15
Upper gastrointestinal bleeding, 7-14, 7-15, 8-16
Up-regulation, 1-49
Uracil, 1-12
Urea cycle, 1-37, 1-38, 7-12
Urea, 1-37, 1-38, 7-1, 7-4, 7-7, 7-16, 7-18
Urinary excretion, 3-51, 7-5
Urine formation, 7-1, 7-4
Urobilinogen, 2-3
Urticaria, 3-2

V

Valsartan, 3-44
Vasodilation, 1-50, 1-52, 3-27, 3-39, 3-41, 3-45, 3-46, 3-48, 3-51, 3-63, 6-8, 6-18, 6-27, 6-29, 6-32, 6-45
Ventilation, 3-1, 3-24, 3-26, 3-37, 3-38, 4-16, 6-14, 8-18
Ventricular fibrillation, 6-9, 8-2